Analysis of Variance and Covariance: How to Choose and Construct Models for the Life Sciences

Analysis of variance (ANOVA) is a core technique for analysing data in the life sciences. This reference book bridges the gap between statistical theory and practical data analysis by presenting a comprehensive set of tables for all standard models of analysis of variance and covariance with up to three treatment factors. The book will serve as a tool to help post-graduates and professionals define their hypotheses, design appropriate experiments, translate them into a statistical model, validate the output from statistics packages and verify results. The systematic layout makes it easy for readers to identify which types of model best fit the themes they are investigating, and to evaluate the strengths and weaknesses of alternative experimental designs. In addition, a concise introduction to the principles of analysis of variance and covariance is provided, alongside worked examples illustrating issues and decisions faced by analysts.

PATRICK DONCASTER is a Reader in Ecology in the School of Biological Sciences at the University of Southampton.

ANDREW DAVEY is an Environmental Scientist at the UK Water Research centre (WRc).

Analysis of Variance and Covariance

How to Choose and Construct Models
for the Life Sciences

C. PATRICK DONCASTER and ANDREW J. H. DAVEY

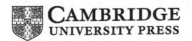

CAMBRIDGE
UNIVERSITY PRESS

CAMBRIDGE
UNIVERSITY PRESS

University Printing House, Cambridge CB2 8BS, United Kingdom

One Liberty Plaza, 20th Floor, New York, NY 10006, USA

477 Williamstown Road, Port Melbourne, VIC 3207, Australia

4843/24, 2nd Floor, Ansari Road, Daryaganj, Delhi - 110002, India

79 Anson Road, #06-04/06, Singapore 079906

Cambridge University Press is part of the University of Cambridge.

It furthers the University's mission by disseminating knowledge in the pursuit of education, learning and research at the highest international levels of excellence.

www.cambridge.org
Information on this title: www.cambridge.org/9780521684477

First published 2007

A catalogue record for this publication is available from the British Library

ISBN 978-0-521-86562-3 Hardback
ISBN 978-0-521-68447-7 Paperback

Contents

Preface

Hypothesis testing in the life sciences often involves comparing samples of observations, and analysis of variance is a core technique for analysing such information. Parametric analysis of variance, abbreviated as 'ANOVA', encompasses a generic methodology for identifying sources of variation in continuous data, from the simplest test of trend in a single sample, or difference between two samples, to complex tests of multiple interacting effects. Whilst simple one-factor models may suffice for closely controlled experiments, the inherent complexities of the natural world mean that rigorous tests of causality often require more sophisticated multi-factor models. In many cases, the same hypothesis can be tested using several different experimental designs, and alternative designs must be evaluated to select a robust and efficient model. Textbooks on statistics are available to explain the principles of ANOVA and statistics packages will compute the analyses. The purpose of this book is to bridge between the texts and the packages by presenting a comprehensive selection of ANOVA models, emphasising the strengths and weaknesses of each and allowing readers to compare between alternatives.

Our motivation for writing the book comes from a desire for a more systematic comparison than is available in textbooks, and a more considered framework for constructing tests than is possible with generic software. The obvious utility of computer packages for automating otherwise cumbersome analyses has a downside in their uncritical production of results. Packages adopt default options until instructed otherwise, which will not suit all types of data. Numerous problems can arise from incautious use of any statistics package, be it of the simplest or the most sophisticated type. In this book we will anticipate all of the following common issues:

- Wrong model or insufficient terms requested for the desired hypothesis (page 2 onwards);
- Wrong error terms calculated by default or wrongly requested (page 2 onwards);
- Data unsuitable for analysis of variance (page 14);
- Unwise pooling of error terms by default or design (page 38);
- Default analysis of effects that have no logical test (e.g., several designs in Chapter 7);
- In unbalanced designs, inappropriate default adjustment to variance estimates (page 237);
- In mixed models, undesired default use of an unrestricted model (page 242);
- Inappropriate application of analysis of variance (page 250).

Armed with precise knowledge of the structure of a desired analysis, the user can evaluate outputs from a statistics package and correct inconsistencies or finish the analysis by hand. The main chapters of this book are designed to provide the relevant information in a clearly accessible format. They are preceded by an introduction to analysis of variance that provides the context of experimental design, and followed by further topics that treat issues arising out of design choices.

Scope and approach

Whilst there is no computational limit to the complexity of ANOVA models, in practice, designs with more than three treatment factors are complicated to analyse and difficult to interpret. We therefore describe all common models with up to three treatment factors for seven principal classes of ANOVA design:

1. One-factor – replicate measures at each level of a single explanatory factor;
2. Nested – one factor nested in one or more other factors;
3. Factorial – fully replicated measures on two or more crossed factors;
4. Randomised blocks – repeated measures on spatial or temporal groups of sampling units;
5. Split plot – treatments applied at multiple spatial or temporal scales;
6. Repeated measures – subjects repeatedly measured or tested over time;
7. Unreplicated factorial – a single measure per combination of two or more factors.

For each class of ANOVA, we describe its particular applications, highlight its strengths and weaknesses, and draw comparisons with other classes. We then present a series of models covering all reasonable combinations of fixed and random factors. For each model we provide the following information:

- The model equation and its associated test hypothesis;
- A table illustrating the allocation of factor levels to sampling units;
- Illustrative examples of applications;
- Any special assumptions and guidance on analysis and interpretation;
- Full analysis of variance tables.

A systematic approach, with consistent layout and notation, makes it easy for readers to evaluate alternative models and to identify which type of model best fits the themes they are investigating.

Examples bring statistics to life as they show how particular models can be applied to answer real-life questions. Throughout the book we develop a series of examples to illustrate the similarities and differences between different ANOVA models. More detailed worked examples are also given to illustrate how the choice of model follows logically from the design of the experiment and determines the inferences that can be drawn from the results.

A multitude of statistics packages are available on the market and it is beyond the scope of this book to describe the analysis of ANOVA models in each. Rather, we encourage readers to become familiar with the approach taken by their favourite package, and to interpret its outputs with the help of the tables in the book and the sample datasets on our website.

How to use this book

The book is a reference tool to help experimental and field biologists define their hypotheses, design an appropriate experiment or mensurative study, translate it into a statistical model, analyse the data and validate the resulting output. As such, it is intended to be a companion throughout the scientific process. At the planning stage, the documented tables allow users to make informed choices about the design of experiments or fieldwork, with particular regard to the need for replication and the different scales of replication across space or over time. Different designs are directly comparable, facilitating the task of balancing costs of replication against benefits of predictive power and generality. At the analysis stage, the book shows how to construct ANOVA models with the correct *F*-ratios for testing the hypotheses, gives options for *post hoc* pooling of error terms, and highlights the assumptions underlying the predictions. Finally, by appreciating the methods used by computer packages to perform ANOVAs, users can check that their input model is appropriately structured and correctly formatted for the desired hypothesis, can verify that the output has tested the intended hypothesis with the correct error degrees of freedom, and can draw appropriate conclusions from the results.

Who should use this book?

The book is aimed at researchers of post-graduate level and above who are planning experiments or fieldwork in the life sciences and preparing to ask questions of their data. We assume that readers are familiar with the basic concepts of statistics covered by introductory textbooks (e.g., Dytham 2003; Ruxton and Colegrave 2003; McKillup 2006, amongst many). Numerous very readable texts already exist to explain the theory and mechanics underpinning analysis of variance (e.g., Kirk 1994; Underwood 1997; Crawley 2002; Grafen and Hails 2002; Quinn and Keough 2002), and we recommend that readers consult such texts in addition to this book. We expect the users of this book to analyse their data with a statistics package suitable for analysis of variance, and we assume that they will employ its tutorial and help routines sufficiently to understand its input commands and output tables.

Companion website

The book is supported by a website at www.soton.ac.uk/~cpd/anovas, which provides additional tools to help readers analyse and interpret the ANOVA models presented here. The website includes:

- *Analyses of example datasets.* The analyses illustrate how the raw data translate into tested hypotheses for each of the ANOVA models in this book. Datasets can be freely downloaded to verify the output from the reader's own statistics package.
- *Model selection and comparison tools.* A dichotomous key to the main classes of ANOVA model is provided to help readers select the right kind of ANOVA design for their needs, and a hyperlinked summary of all the ANOVA models in the book is presented to facilitate the comparison of alternative models.

Acknowledgements

We owe a great debt of thanks to the numerous people who gave us their time to discuss statistical concepts, make suggestions for improving structure and content, and correct our errors. Although we have not succeeded in following all of their recommendations, those that we have implemented have improved the book beyond recognition. We are especially grateful to Henrique Cabral, Stefano Cannicci, Tasman Crowe, Alan Grafen, Jeremy Greenwood, Laura Guichón, Stephen Hawkins, Jan Geert Hiddink, Mark Huxham, Fernando Milesi, Jonathan Newman, Susanne Plesner Jensen, Will Resetarits, Graeme Ruxton, Martin Skov, Richard Thompson, the undergraduates and postgraduates in biology and environmental sciences at Southampton University. Finally, AD would like to thank Kirsty Davey for her unfailing support during the writing of this book.

While researching this book, we have been inspired and guided by a number of standard-setting accounts of statistical methods, notably in books by Robert Sokal and F. James Rohlf, Tony Underwood, Gerry Quinn and Michael Keough, Alan Grafen and Rosie Hails, and Michael Crawley. We thank these authors, along with all those referenced in the book, for the tuition that we have gained from their works.

Introduction to analysis of variance

What is analysis of variance?

Analysis of variance, often abbreviated to ANOVA, is a powerful statistic and a core technique for testing causality in biological data. Researchers use ANOVA to explain variation in the magnitude of a response variable of interest. For example, an investigator might be interested in the sources of variation in patients' blood cholesterol level, measured in mg/dL. Factors that are hypothesised to contribute to variation in the response may be categorical or continuous. A categorical factor has levels – the categories – that are each applied to a different group of sampling units. For example, sampling units of hospital patients may be classified as male or female, representing two levels of the factor 'Gender'. By contrast, a continuous factor has a continuous scale of values and is therefore a covariate of the response. For example, age of patients may be quantified by the covariate 'Age'. ANOVA determines the influence of these effects on the response by testing whether the response differs among levels of the factor, or displays a trend across values of the covariate. Thus, blood cholesterol level of patients may be deemed to differ among male and female patients, or to increase or decrease with age of the patient.

A factor of interest can be experimental, with sampling units that are manipulated to impose contrasting treatments. For example, patients may be given a cholesterol-lowering drug or a placebo, which represent two levels of the factor 'Drug'. Alternatively, the factor can be mensurative, with sampling units that are grouped according to some pre-existing difference. For example, patients may be classified as vegetarians or non-vegetarians, which represent two levels of the factor 'Diet'.

Biologists use ANOVA for two main purposes: prediction and explanation. In predictive studies, ANOVA functions as an exploratory tool to find the best fitting set of response predictors. From a full model of all possible sources of variation in the response, procedures of model simplification allow the investigator to discard unimportant factors and so develop a model with maximum predictive power. This application of ANOVA is just one of many forms of exploratory analyses now available in standard statistics packages. ANOVA really comes into its own when it is used for hypothesis testing. In this case, the primary goal is to explain variation in a response by distinguishing a hypothesised effect, or combination of effects, from a null hypothesis of no effect. Any such test of hypothesised effects on a response has an analytical structure that is fixed by the design of data collection. Although this book provides some guidance on model simplification, its principal focus is on the hypothesis-testing applications of ANOVA in studies that have been designed to explain sources of variation in a response. More exploratory studies concerned with parameter estimation may be better suited to maximum likelihood techniques of generalised linear modelling (GLIM) and Bayesian inference, which lie beyond the scope of the book.

The great strength of ANOVA lies in its capacity to distinguish effects on a response from amongst many different sources of variation compared simultaneously, or in certain cases through time. It can identify interacting factors, and it can measure the scale of variation within a hierarchy of effects. This versatility makes it a potentially powerful tool for answering questions about causality. Of course tools can be dangerous if mishandled, and ANOVA is no exception. Researchers will not go astray provided they adhere to the principle of designing parsimonious models for hypothesis testing. A parsimonious design is one that samples the minimum number of factors necessary to answer the question of interest, and records sufficient observations to estimate all potential sources of variance amongst those chosen few factors. As you use this book, you will become aware that the most appropriate models for answering questions of interest often include nuisance variables. They need measuring too, even if only to factor them out from the effects of interest. One of the biggest challenges of experimental design, and best rewards when you get it right, is to identify and fairly represent all sources of variation in the data. True to the playful nature of scientific enquiry, this calls for building a model.

How to read and write statistical models

A statistical model describes the structure of an analysis of variance. ANOVA is a very versatile technique that can have many different structures, and each is described by a different model. Here we introduce the concept of a statistical model, and some of the terminology used to describe model components. The meanings of terms will be further developed in later sections, and all of the most important terms are defined in a Glossary on page 271.

Analysis of variance estimates the effect of a categorical factor by testing for a difference between its category means in some continuous response variable of interest. For example, it might be used to test the response of crop yield to high and low sowing density. Data on yield will provide useful evidence of an effect of density if each level of density is sampled with a representative group of independent measures, and the variation in yield between samples can be attributed solely to sowing density. The test can then calibrate the between-sample variation against the residual and unmeasured within-sample variation. A relatively high between-sample variation provides evidence of the samples belonging to different populations, and therefore of the factor explaining or predicting variation in the response. The analysis has then tested a statistical model:

$$Y = A + \varepsilon$$

We read this *one-factor* model as: 'Variation in the *response* variable [Y] is explained by [=] variation between levels of a *factor* [A] in addition to [+] *residual* variation [ε]'. This is the *test hypothesis*, H_1, which is evaluated against a mutually exclusive *null hypothesis*, H_0: $Y = \varepsilon$.

The evidence for an *effect* of factor A on variation in Y is determined by testing H_0 with a *statistic*, which is a random variable described by a probability distribution. Analysis of variance uses the F statistic to compute the probability P of an effect at least as big as that observed arising by chance from a true null hypothesis. The null hypothesis is rejected and the factor deemed to have a significant effect if P is less than some predetermined threshold α, often set at 0.05. This is known as the *Type I error rate* for the test, and $\alpha = 0.05$ means that we sanction 5% of such tests yielding false positive reports as a result of rejecting a true null hypothesis. The analysis has a complementary probability β of accepting a false null hypothesis, known as the *Type II error rate*. The value of β gives the rate of false negative reports, and a lower rate signifies a test with more power to distinguish true effects. We will expand on these important issues in later sections (e.g., pages 13 and 248); for the purposes of model building, it suffices to think of the factor A as having a significant effect if $P < 0.05$.

Analysis of variance can also estimate the effect of a continuous factor. This is done by testing for a trend in the response across values of the covariate factor. The analysis is now referred to as *regression*. For example, one might wish to test the response of crop yield to sowing density measured on a continuous scale of seeds/m^2. A single sample of independent measurements of yield over a range of sowing densities allows the effect of sowing density to be tested with a statistical model having the same structure as the one for the categorical factor:

$$Y = A + \varepsilon$$

We read this *simple linear regression* model as: 'Variation in the response variable [Y] is explained by [=] variation in a *covariate* [A] in addition to [+] residual variation [ε]'. The process of distinguishing between the test hypothesis and a null hypothesis of no effect is exactly the same for the covariate as for the categorical factor. The null hypothesis is rejected and the covariate deemed to cause a significant linear trend if $P < \alpha$.

Users of statistics employ a variety of terminologies to describe the same thing. One-factor designs may be referred to as *one-way* designs. The response may be referred to as the *data* or *dependent* variable; each hypothesised effect may be referred to as a *factor*, *predictor* or *treatment*, or *independent* or *explanatory* variable; categories of a factor may be referred to as *levels*, *samples* or *treatments*; and the observations or measures within a sample as *data points*, *variates* or *scores*. Each observation is made on a different *sampling unit* which may take the form of an individual *subject* or *plot* of land, or be one of several repeated measures on the same subject or block of land. The residual variation may be referred to as the *unexplained* or *error* variation. The precise meanings of these terms will become apparent with use of different models, for some of which residual and error variation are the same thing and others not, and so on. A summary of the standard notation for this book can be found on page 44, and further clarification of important distinctions is provided by the Glossary on page 271.

The full versatility of ANOVA becomes apparent when we wish to expand the model to accommodate two or more factors, either categorical or continuous or both. For example, an irrigation treatment may be applied to a sample of five maize fields and compared to a control sample of five non-irrigated fields. Yield is measured from a sample of three randomly distributed plots within each field. Thus, in addition to differences between plots that are the result of the irrigation treatments, plots may differ between fields within the same treatment (due to uncontrolled variables). This design has an Irrigation factor A with two levels: treatment and control, and a Field factor B with five levels per level of A. Factor B is *nested* in A, because each field belongs to only one level of A. This *two-factor nested* model is written as:

$$Y = A + B'(A) + \varepsilon$$

The model equation is read as: 'Variation in growth rate [Y] is explained by [=] variation between treatment and control fields [A], and [+] variation between fields nested within each treatment level [B'(A)], in addition to [+] residual variation between plots within each field [ε]'. This model has two test hypotheses: one for each factor. At the cost of greater design complexity, we are now able to test the region-wide applicability of irrigation, given by the A effect, even in the presence of natural variation between fields, given by the B'(A) effect.

The site factor B' is conventionally written as B-prime in order to identify it as a *random* factor, meaning that each treatment level is assigned to a random sample of fields. Factor A is without prime, thereby identifying it as a *fixed* factor, with levels that are fixed by the investigator – in this example, as the two levels of treatment and control. We will return again to fixed and random factors in a later section (page 16), because the distinction between them underpins the logic of ANOVA. A nested model such as the one above may be presented in the abbreviated form: '$Y = B'(A) + \varepsilon$', which implies testing for the main effect A as well as B'(A). Likewise, the abbreviated description: $Y = C'(B'(A)) + \varepsilon$ implies testing for A and B'(A) as well as C'(B'(A)).

As an alternative or a supplement to nesting, we use designs with *crossed* factors when we wish to test independent but simultaneous sources of variation that may have additive or multiplicative effects. For example, seedlings may be treated simultaneously with different levels of both a watering regime (A) and a sowing density (B). This is a *factorial* model if each level of each factor is tested in combination with each level of the other. It is written as:

$$Y = A + B + B*A + \varepsilon$$

The model equation is read as: 'Variation in growth rate [Y] is explained by [=] variation in watering [A], and independently [+] by variation in sowing density [B], and also [+] by an inter-dependent effect [B*A], in addition to [+] residual within-sample variation [ε]'. This model has three test hypotheses: one for each factor and one for the interaction between them. We are now able to test whether A and B act on the response as independent *main effects* A and B additively, or whether the effect of each factor on Y depends on the other factor in an *interaction* B*A. An interaction means that the effects of A are not the same at all levels of B, and conversely the effects of B differ according to the level of A. This factorial model can be written in abbreviated form: '$Y = B|A + \varepsilon$', where the vertical separator abbreviates for 'all main effects and interactions of the factors'. Likewise, the description of a three-factor model as: $Y = C|B|A + \varepsilon$ abbreviates for all three main effects and all three two-way interactions and the three-way interaction:

$$Y = A + B + B*A + C + C*A + C*B + C*B*A + \varepsilon$$

For any ANOVA with more than one factor, the terms in the model must be entered in a logical order of main effects preceding their nested effects and interactions, and lower-order interactions preceding higher-order interactions. This logical ordering permits the analysis to account for independent components in hierarchical sequence.

This book will describe all the combinations of one, two and three factors, whether nested in each other or crossed with each other. For example, the above cross-factored and nested models may be combined to give either model 3.3 on page 98: $Y = C|B(A) + \varepsilon$, which is also described with an example on page 51, or model 3.4 on page 109: $Y = C(B|A) + \varepsilon$. Throughout, we emphasise the need to identify the correct statistical model at the stage of designing data collection. It is possible, and indeed all too easy, to collect whatever data you can wherever you can get it, and then to let a statistical package find the model for you at the analysis stage. If you operate in this way, then you will have no need for this book, but the analyses will certainly lead you to draw unconvincing or wrong inferences. Effective science, whether experimental or mensurative, depends on you thinking about the statistical model when designing your study.

What is an ANOVA model?

Any statistical test of pattern requires a model against which to test the null hypothesis of no pattern. Models for ANOVA take the form: Response $=$ Factor(s) $+ \varepsilon$, where the response refers to the data that require explaining, the factor or factors are the putative explanatory variables contributing to the observed pattern of variation in the response, and ε is the residual variation in the response left unexplained by the factor(s). For each of the ANOVA designs that we describe in Chapters 1 to 7, we express its underlying model in three ways to highlight different features of its structure. For example, the two-factor nested model introduced above is described by its:

- Full model, packed up into a single expression: $Y = B'(A) + \varepsilon$;
- Hierarchical nesting of sampling units in factors: $S'(B'(A))$;
- Testable terms for analysis, unpacked from the full model: $A + B(A)$.

A statistics package will require you to specify the ANOVA model desired for a given dataset. You will need to declare which column contains the response variable Y, which column(s) contain the explanatory variable(s) to be tested, any nesting or cross factoring of multiple factors (these are the 'testable terms' above), whether any of the factors are random (further detailed on page 16) and whether any are covariates of the response (page 29). On page 259, we describe a typical dataset structure and associate it with various models.

In the event that the analysis indicates a real effect, this outcome can be described succinctly (detailed on page 260) and illustrated with a graph. Figure 1(a) shows a typical illustration of differences between group means for a model $Y = A + \varepsilon$, with three levels of A. The significance of the pattern is evident in the large differences between the three means relative to the residual variation around the means. A non-significant effect of factor A would result from larger sample variances, or sample means all taking similar values.

General principles of ANOVA

Analysis of variance tests an effect of interest on a response variable of interest by analysing how much of the total variation in the response can be explained by the effect. Differences among sampling units may arise from one or more measured factors making up the effect(s) of interest, but it will certainly also arise from other sources of unmeasured variation. Estimating the significance of a hypothesised effect on the response requires taking measurements from more than one sampling unit in each level of a categorical factor, or across several values of a covariate. The sampling units must each provide independent information from a random sample of the factor level or covariate value, in order to quantify the underlying unmeasured variation. This random variation can then be used to calibrate the variation explained by the factor of interest.

For example, we can use ANOVA to test whether gender contributes significantly to explaining variation in birth weights of babies. To assess the effect of gender as a factor in the birth-weight response, it makes sense to weigh one sample of male babies and another of female babies, with each baby picked at random from within the population of interest (perhaps a geographical region or an ethnic group). These babies serve as the replicate sampling units in each of the two levels (male and female) of the factor gender. The babies must be chosen at random from the defined population to avoid introducing any bias that might reinforce a preconceived notion, for example by selecting heavier males and lighter females. They should also contribute independent information to the analysis, so twins should be avoided where the weight of one provides information about the weight of the other. The ANOVA on these samples of independent and random replicates will indicate a significant effect of gender if the average difference in weight between the male and female samples is large compared to the variation in weight within each sample.

ANOVA works on the simple and logical principle of partitioning variation in a continuous response Y into explained and unexplained components, and evaluating the effect of a particular factor as the ratio between the two components. The method of partitioning explained from unexplained variation differs slightly depending on whether the ANOVA is used to compare the response among levels of a categorical factor or to analyse a relationship between the response and a covariate. We will treat these two methods in turn.

Analysis of variance on a categorical factor tests for a difference in average response among factor levels. The total variation in the response is given by the sum of all observations, measured as their squared deviations from the response grand mean $\bar{\bar{y}}$. This quantity is called the total sum of squares, SS_{total} (Figure 1). The use of squared deviations then allows this total variation to be partitioned into two sources. The variation explained by the factor is given by the sum of squared deviations of each group mean $\bar{y}_i$ from the grand mean $\bar{\bar{y}}$, weighted by the n values per group (where subscript i refers to the i-th level of the factor). This quantity is called the explained sum of squares, $SS_{explained}$. The residual variation left unexplained by the model is given by the sum of squared deviations of each data point y_{ij} from its own group mean $\bar{y}_i$ (where subscript ij refers to the jth observation in the i-th factor level). This quantity $SS_{residual}$ is variously referred to as the residual, error, or unexplained sum of squares.

Each sum of squares (SS) has a certain number of degrees of freedom (d.f.) associated with it. These are the number of independent pieces of

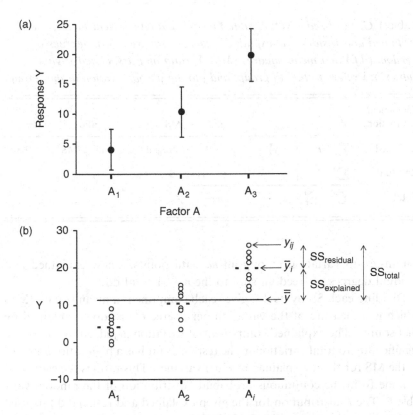

Figure 1 Dataset of three samples (a) summarised as group means and standard deviations, and (b) showing the $j = 8$ observations in each of the $i = 3$ groups. Total variation in the dataset, measured by the sum of squared deviations of each observation (y_{ij}) from the grand mean ($\bar{\bar{y}}$), is partitioned into an explained component that measures variation among the group means ($\bar{y}_i$), and an unexplained or residual component that measures variation among the data points within each group. The deviations indicated for the mean of group i and its j-th data point are summed across all data to obtain the model sums of squares.

information required to measure the component of variation, subtracted from the total number of pieces contributing to that variation. The total variation always has degrees of freedom that equal one less than the total number of data points, because it uses just the grand mean to calculate variation among all the data points. A one-factor model with n observations in each of a groups has $a - 1$ d.f. for the explained component of variation, because we require one grand mean to measure between-group variation among the a means; it has $na - a = (n - 1)a$ d.f. for the residual component, because we require a group means to measure

Table 1 *Generalised ANOVA table for testing a categorical factor, showing explained and residual (unexplained) sums of squares (SS), degrees of freedom (d.f.) and mean squares (MS), F-ratio and associated P-value. Subscript i refers to the ith group, and j to the jth observation in that group.*

Component of variation	SS	d.f.	MS	F-ratio	P
Explained	$\sum_{i=1}^{a} n \cdot (\bar{y}_i - \bar{\bar{y}})^2$	$a-1$	$SS_{expl}/d.f._{expl}$	MS_{expl}/MS_{res}	$< 0.05?$
Residual	$\sum_{i=1}^{a} \sum_{j=1}^{n} (y_{ij} - \bar{y}_i)^2$	$(n-1)a$	$SS_{res}/d.f._{res}$		
Total	$\sum_{i=1}^{a} \sum_{j=1}^{n} (y_{ij} - \bar{\bar{y}})^2$	$na-1$			

within-group variation among all *na* data points. These explained and residual degrees of freedom sum to the $na - 1$ total d.f.

Dividing each SS by its d.f. gives each component a mean square (MS) which is a measure of the variation per degree of freedom explained by that source. The explained component of variation is judged to contribute significantly to total variation in the response if it has a high ratio of its MS to the MS for the unexplained residual variance. This ratio is the estimated *F*-value from the continuous probability distribution of the random variable *F*. The *F* distribution for the given explained and residual d.f. is used to determine the probability *P* of obtaining at least as large a value of the observed ratio of sample variances, given a true ratio between variances equal to unity. Researchers in the life sciences often consider a probability of $\alpha = 0.05$ to be an acceptably safe threshold for rejecting the null hypothesis of insignificant explained variation. An effect is then considered significant if its *F*-value has an associated $P < 0.05$ (Table 1), indicating a less than 5% probability of making a mistake by rejecting a true null hypothesis of no effect (the Type I error rate). This is reported by writing $F_{a-1,(n-1)a} = \#.\#\#$, $P < 0.05$, where the subscript '$a - 1$, $(n - 1)a$' are the numbers of test and error d.f. respectively. Every *F*-value must always be reported with these two sets of d.f. (further detailed on page 260) because they provide information about the amount of replication, and therefore the power of the test to detect patterns.

The validity of the ANOVA test depends on three assumptions about the residual variance: that the random variation around sample means has the same magnitude at all levels of the factor, that the residuals contributing to this variation are free to vary independently of each other, and that the residual variation approximates to a normal distribution. These important requirements are explained on page 14.

Analysis of covariance tests for a linear trend in a continuous response Y with a factor X that varies on a continuous scale. The continuous factor X is said to be a 'covariate' of Y. The analysis is commonly referred to as 'regression analysis' unless one or more categorical factors are included in the model with the continuous factor(s). This book will describe analyses of covariance with and without categorical factors, and for the sake of consistency we will refer to them all as analyses of covariance, abbreviated 'ANCOVA'.

In the simplest case there is only one sample, comprising coordinates x, y of the covariate and response. The analysis estimates a line of best fit through the data that intersects the sample mean coordinate ($\bar{x}$, $\bar{y}$). This 'linear regression' is defined by a mathematical equation: $\hat{y} = a + b \cdot x$, where the parameter a is the 'intercept' value of $\hat{y}$ at $x = 0$ and the parameter b is the 'gradient' of $\hat{y}$ with x. We will ignore the mechanics of calculating the parameter values, other than to note that a standard analysis of variance uses the method of 'ordinary least squares' which minimises the sum of squared deviations of each response y_j from the regression line. This sum comprises the residual sum of squares, $SS_{residual}$, and it partitions out the variation left unexplained by the linear model (Figure 2). The corresponding explained sum of squares, $SS_{explained}$, is the

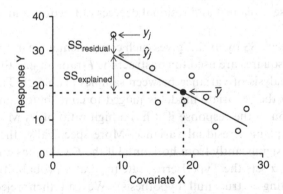

Figure 2 A sample of $n = 10$ observations on a covariate and response, with regression line fitted by analysis of covariance. Total variation, measured by the sum of squared deviations of each observation from the sample mean, is partitioned into an explained component that measures deviations of the line from horizontal, and an unexplained or residual component that measures the deviation of each data point from the line. The deviations indicated for one data point are summed across all points to obtain the model sums of squares.

sum of squared deviations of the n linear estimates $\hat{y}$ (each given by $a + b \cdot x_j$) from the sample mean response $\bar{y}$. This sum partitions out the component of variation in the data due to the slope of the regression line from horizontal. The explained and residual SS together add up to the total sum of squares, SS_{total}, given by the sum of squared deviations of the response y_j from the mean response $\bar{y}$. The proportion of explained variation: $SS_{explained}/SS_{total}$ is known as the 'coefficient of determination', and its square-root is the correlation coefficient, r, which is given a sign corresponding to a positive covariance of y with x or a negative covariance.

As with the analysis of variance between samples, each sum of squares (SS) has a certain number of degrees of freedom (d.f.) associated with it. Again, these are the number of independent pieces of information required to measure the component of variation, subtracted from the total number of pieces contributing to that variation. As before, the total variation always has degrees of freedom that equal one less than the total number of data points $(n - 1)$, because it uses just the grand mean to calculate variation among all the data points. For the analysis of covariance on a sample of n coordinates, the explained component of variation has one d.f. because it uses the grand mean to measure variation from a line defined by two parameters (so $2 - 1 = 1$). The residual component of variation has $n - 2$ d.f. because we require the two parameters that define the line in order to measure the variation of the n responses from it. These explained and residual degrees of freedom sum to the $n - 1$ total d.f.

Dividing each SS by its d.f. gives each component a mean square (MS). These mean squares are used to construct the F-ratio in just the same way as for the analysis of variance between samples (Table 2). The variation explained by the covariate model is judged to contribute significantly to total variation in the response if it has a high ratio of its MS to the MS for the unexplained residual variance. More specifically, the regression slope differs significantly from horizontal if the F-value has an associated $P < \alpha$, where α sets the Type I error rate (e.g., at a probability of 0.05 of falsely rejecting a true null hypothesis). We can then reject the null hypothesis of no change in Y with X in favour of the model hypothesis of a linear trend in Y with X. This is reported by writing $F_{1,n-2} = \#.\#\#$, $P < 0.05$, where the subscript '1, $n - 2$' refer to the d.f. of the test and error d.f. respectively.

The validity of the ANOVA test depends on three assumptions about the residual variance: that the random variation around fitted values has

Table 2 *Generalised ANOVA table for testing a covariate, showing explained and residual (unexplained) sums of squares (SS), degrees of freedom (d.f.) and mean squares (MS),* F*-ratio and associated* P*-value. Subscript* j *refers to the* jth *response in a sample of size* n.

Component of variation	SS	d.f.	MS	F-ratio	P
Explained	$\sum_{j=1}^{n}(\hat{y}_j - \bar{y})^2$	1	$SS_{expl}/d.f._{expl}$	MS_{expl}/MS_{res}	$< 0.05?$
Residual	$\sum_{j=1}^{n}(y_j - \hat{y}_j)^2$	$n-2$	$SS_{res}/d.f._{res}$		
Total	$\sum_{j=1}^{n}(y_j - \bar{y})^2$	$n-1$			

the same magnitude across the range of the covariate, that the residuals contributing to this variation are free to vary independently of each other, and that the residual variation approximates to a normal distribution.

ANOVA as a tool for hypothesis testing

An explanatory hypothesis is a proposal that something interesting is going on. The hypothesis will be testable if it can be compared to a null hypothesis of nothing interesting. In analysis of variance, the 'something' of interest takes the form of a difference in the response between levels of a categorical factor or a trend in the response across values of a covariate. The null hypothesis is that the data contain no such patterns. Analysis of variance subjects a dataset to one or more test hypotheses, described by a model. The approach is always to decide whether or not to reject the null hypothesis of no pattern in favour of the test hypothesis of a proposed pattern, with some acceptably small probability of making a wrong decision.

For example, a test of the model $Y = B|A + \varepsilon$ may reject or accept the null hypothesis H_0: no effect of A on the response. Likewise, it rejects or accepts the null hypotheses of no B effect and of no interaction effect. A decision to reject each H_0 is taken with some predetermined probability α of making a Type I error by rejecting a true null hypothesis. If $\alpha = 0.05$, for example, an effect of A with $P < 0.05$ is judged significant. Factor A is then deemed to influence the response. Conversely, a decision to accept H_0 is taken with a probability β of making a Type II error by accepting a false null hypothesis. Regardless of the size of β – which depends very much on sample sizes – an effect with $P \geq \alpha$ is deemed to have a non-significant influence on the response. In this case we have only an absence of evidence, rather than positive evidence of no effect. In general β exceeds α, with the consequence that absence of evidence is less certain than evidence of an effect. These issues are discussed more fully in the sections later in the book on statistical power (page 248) and evaluating alternative designs for data collection (page 250).

A hypothesis can be of no value in explaining data unless it has a falsifiable H_0. Consider a test for the effect of blood-sucking mites on fledgling survival in swifts. ANOVA will test the H_0: no difference in survival between nests with and without mites. Only if the evidence leads us to reject H_0 with small probability of error do we accept H_1: mites affect survival. The persuasive evidence is in the form of a difference that has been calibrated against unmeasured random variation. Seeking confirmation of H_1 directly would not permit this rigorous evaluation of the alternative, because H_1 is not falsifiable – there are innumerable ways to not see a real effect.

In this book we focus on the explanatory applications of ANOVA, using models to test evidence for the existence of hypothesised effects on the response. ANOVA can also be used in a predictive capacity, to identify parsimonious models and estimate parameter values, in which case its merits should be judged in comparison to alternative approaches of statistical inference by likelihood testing. For their explanatory applications, ANOVA models are generally structured according to the design of data collection, and magnitudes of effect take secondary importance to statistical significance. The validity of any inferences about significance then depends crucially on the assumptions underpinning the model and the test statistic.

Assumptions of ANOVA

Four assumptions underlie all analysis of variance (ANOVA) using the F statistic. These are:

(1) Random sampling from the source population;
(2) Independent measures within each sample, yielding uncorrelated response residuals;
(3) Homogeneous variances across all the sampled populations;
(4) Normal distribution of the response residuals around the model.

Two further assumptions apply to analysis of covariance (ANCOVA):

(5) Repeatable covariate values that are fixed by the investigator;
(6) Linear relation of the response to the covariate.

The first two assumptions are *design considerations*. Proper interpretation of any statistical test requires that it be based on comparisons between representative and unbiased samples, and that the measures within a sample are free to vary independently of each other. For example, a comparison of immature warthog body weights between younger females and older males has an inherent bias that falsely inflates the contrast; the design should compare like with like, or compare each level of sex with each level of age. Similarly, the presence of siblings amongst subjects introduces an inherent co-dependence within samples that falsely reduces their error variation; the design should remove siblings, or randomly disperse them amongst treatment allocations, or include 'family group' as an extra factor representing random variation from family to family. The assumption of independence drives many of the most challenging issues in constructing appropriate ANOVA models. Sub-sampling from the data, grouping observations, and repeated measures on sampling units can all lead to loss of independence unless recognised and accounted for in the analysis.

The third and fourth assumptions are features of the *parametisation of ANOVA*. The analysis uses a single error mean square to represent the residual variation around each of the sample means, which is therefore assumed to be symmetrical about the mean and to take a magnitude that does not depend on the size of the mean. The calculated F-ratio of test to error MS is tested against an F distribution which assumes that the two mean squares come from normally distributed populations. This may be far from realistic for residuals with distributions skewed from normal, or variances that increase (or decrease) with the mean, which are therefore not homogeneous.

The assumption of normality can be tested statistically using a Shapiro–Wilks test, or checked graphically using a normal probability plot. ANOVA results are generally more sensitive to the assumption of homogeneous variances. This is best checked in the first instance by plotting the residuals at each level of the fitted effect(s) to find out whether they have a similar spread at all levels. Formal statistical tests of the null hypothesis that the variances are equal across all groups (for example, Cochran's test or the F_{max} test) may be useful for simple ANOVA designs, but are sensitive to non-normality.

In the event of violation of these parametisation assumptions, it is often possible to approximate the normal distribution and homogeneous variances by applying a systematic transformation to the data. General textbooks of statistics provide recommendations on, for example, using the square root of counts, or applying an 'arcsine-root' transformation to proportions (e.g., Sokal and Rohlf 1995). However, many types of data have inherently non-normal distributions and heterogeneous variances. For example, a response measuring the frequency of occurrence of an event has positive integer values with random variation that increases with the mean. These attributes are described by the Poisson distribution, which approximates the normal distribution only at large frequencies. A response measuring proportions (or percentages) is strictly bounded between zero and one (or 100), giving a random variation that increases with distance from either boundary to peak at a proportion of 0.5. These attributes are described by a binomial distribution. A more parsimonious alternative to transformation is to use a GLIM which allows the investigator to declare error structures other than normal, including Poisson and binomial (e.g., Crawley 2002).

The fifth and sixth assumptions are features of the *parametisation of ANCOVA*, in which one or more factors vary on a continuous scale and thus are covariates of the response rather than categorical factors. These are assumed to be fixed factors (detailed in the next section) with values that are measured without variance and so could be repeated in another study. The analysis uses just two parameters to represent the response Y to a covariate X: the Y intercept at $X = 0$ and the slope of Y with X. It therefore assumes a constant slope across all values of X, giving a linear relation of Y to X. For a covariate with a curvilinear relation to the response, transformations may be applied to Y or X, or both, to linearise the relation, which will often simultaneously rectify problems of heterogeneity of variances. These are discussed in the section on uses of covariates on page 29.

An additional assumption is introduced by having unreplicated repeated measurements on individual sampling units, blocks or subjects. This is the assumption of '*homogeneity of covariances*' which applies to the randomised-block, split-plot and repeated-measures designs described in Chapters 4 to 6. The assumption is detailed in those chapters, on page 118 for randomised blocks and page 183 for repeated measures.

How to distinguish between fixed and random factors

A categorical factor can take one of two forms: fixed or random. Distinguishing between these alternatives is one of the first hurdles to understanding analysis of variance, and getting it wrong can lead to invalid conclusions. Here we describe how to identify and interpret fixed and random factors. The consequences for analysis will be detailed with model descriptions in Chapters 1 to 7.

A *fixed factor* has precisely defined levels, and inferences about its effect apply only to those levels. For example, in a test of the impact of irrigation on maize yield, Irrigation will be a fixed factor if its levels have been selected for specific comparison. Irrigation schedules of daily, weekly and monthly application might be randomly assigned to replicate plots. The null hypothesis is that there are no differences in the means of the response among levels of the factor. If the test rejects H_0, *post hoc* tests (page 245) may be used to investigate precisely how the levels differ from each other. A subsequent experiment must therefore use the same levels to re-test the same hypothesis.

In contrast, a *random factor* describes a randomly and independently drawn set of levels that represent variation in a clearly defined wider population. The precise identity and mean of each level holds no value in itself, and a subsequent analysis could draw a different set at random from the population to re-test the same hypothesis. Indeed it is assumed that the levels chosen for analysis come from a large enough population to be deemed infinite. For example, Genotype would be a random factor if a random selection of all maize genotypes were tested on the levels of irrigation in the previous experiment. The null hypothesis is that there is zero variance in the response among the genotypes. A subsequent study could therefore select at random a different set of genotypes to re-test the same hypothesis. The basic sampling unit in any study, in this case the plot, is a random variable by definition. Any other nested factors are almost always random too, in order to provide the residual variation against which to calibrate the higher-level effects. These nested factors will be assumed to have a normal distribution of sample means, and homogeneous variances. We will expand on the applications of nesting on page 21 and in Chapter 2. Random factors can also function to group together multiple sources of nuisance variation. For example, the above experiment could be run on a regional scale by repeating it across a number of replicate farms. The random factor Farm is not an experimental treatment; rather, its levels sample unmeasured spatial variation in soil characteristics, microclimate, historical land use etc. Random factors of this sort are called 'blocks', and we expand on their function on page 25 and in Chapter 4.

A factor is usually fixed if its levels are assigned randomly to sampling units. For example, Irrigation treatments are applied randomly to experimental plots in order to measure their influence on growth. Interpretation of such factors is straightforward since the manipulative nature of the experiment means the factor measures just one source of variation. Interpretation of a fixed factor is less straightforward when its levels cannot be assigned randomly to sampling units. Male–female subjects, north–south aspects, or upstream–downstream plots are all pre-assigned to their levels. Consequently, the variation due to sex, aspect or location is always confounded with unmeasured covariates of these factors, and this must be acknowledged when interpreting significant effects. Mensurative (non-experimental) studies have non-random assignment of factor levels by definition. For example, in a study comparing the tolerance to ultraviolet radiation of Caucasians and Afro-Caribbeans, Ethnicity cannot be randomly assigned to subjects with the result that it cannot be isolated and tested as a cause of tolerance. With adequate replication, however, any significant difference in tolerance among the two groups can be attributed to the factor Ethnicity as defined by all the unmeasured correlates intrinsically associated with each group, such as melanin concentration, diet, exposure to sunshine and so on.

Particular care must be taken with the distinction between fixed and random factors when factor levels cannot be randomly assigned to sampling units because they represent different locations or times. For example, a Location factor may have levels of elevation up a shore, or of blocks of land across a field; a Time factor may have levels of days, or of seasons. These factors always group together multiple sources of variation, and for this reason they must be treated as random unless each of their levels are adequately replicated. Consider the specific example of a field test in which the settlement of barnacle larvae onto inter-tidal rocks is measured at three shore elevations: upper, middle and lower. Elevation is a spatial factor that represents variation due not only to height up the shore, but also to all the correlates of height, such as immersion time, wind exposure, predation pressure and surface topography. Any effect of elevation on settlement can be attributed to the multi-dimensional natural gradient made up of these variables, provided that their variation with elevation is a consistent feature of rocky shores in general. It is the investigator's knowledge of this proviso that defines whether elevation must be random or whether it can be fixed.

If barnacle settlement is measured in replicate quadrats at each of three elevations on a single shore, then any effect of elevation will be completely confounded with random spatial variation. In other words, a settlement gradient with elevation may be due to variables that have no intrinsic association with elevation. For example, low barnacle settlement on the upper shore could be due to a band of granite there, which might equally occur at other elevations on other shores. Elevation can be fixed if one is specifically interested in testing for differences among those particular locations on that particular shore, but this sort of hypothesis is rarely useful because the confounding of elevation with random, within-shore spatial variation makes it impossible to determine the underlying cause of any significant effect. With data from only a single shore, it therefore makes sense to treat elevation as a random blocking factor.

Elevation can be fixed by distributing the quadrats at each of the three elevations across two or more randomly selected shores within the region of interest. The replication of shores removes the confounding of variation due to elevation with random spatial variation. The analysis is therefore able to partition out the combined effect of elevation and all variables that consistently co-vary with elevation across shores, from the effect of all other sources of spatial variation that are not related to elevation. A significant effect of elevation means that barnacle settlement varies in response to elevation plus all that co-varies with elevation in the region, such as immersion time and predation pressure. Without an experimental assignment of treatments to quadrats, however, it is not possible to identify which of the covariates causes variation in barnacle settlement.

Some *spatial factors* are less clearly defined than elevation and must always be random because they cannot be replicated in space. For example, consider an experiment to compare the growth of a crop under three fixed Irrigation treatments. To take account of suspected spatial variation in soil conditions, a field is divided into three blocks of land and each irrigation treatment is assigned randomly to four plots in each block. Because the blocks are arranged arbitrarily, rather than in relation to some known biological or physical feature or gradient, the natural variation that they encompass cannot be defined; it simply encompasses all random sources of spatial variation. It is therefore not possible to replicate the exact levels of that factor in other fields, and Block must be treated as a random factor.

The same logic applies to *temporal factors*. If the condition of blackbirds is measured in each of four Seasons in a single year, then unless one specifically wishes to test for differences among seasons in that particular year, Season will be random because any effect of time of year is completely confounded by short-term temporal variation. For example, low condition of birds in summer could be due to natural environmental changes that occur every summer, or due to an unusually wet spring. However, if condition is measured in each of four seasons in each of two or more years, then Season will be fixed because any consistent effect can be partitioned out and tested, over and above random within-year variation. The only caveat is that the cause of any significant Season effect cannot be identified from amongst the multiple sources of temporal variation grouped together by Season, including variations in temperature, weather, competitor abundance and so on.

Similarly, if an experiment measures the concentration span of students over the course of three, arbitrarily-selected weekdays, then Weekday will be a random factor because it encompasses all possible sources of temporal variation from day to day. Even when the investigator is specifically interested in the Monday, Wednesday and Friday, if all data are obtained from a single week, then Weekday must again be random because any systematic variation in concentration span over the course of the week is completely confounded by random temporal variation from day to day. However, if the concentration span of students is measured on the Monday, Wednesday and Friday of two or more weeks, then Weekday can be treated as fixed. This is because the replicated levels of Weekday over time now permit partitioning of variation in concentration span due to these particular days, which might represent numerous intrinsically linked variables such as prior alcohol consumption and prior sleep, from random day to day variation such as that caused by the weather. Although we still do not know the ultimate cause of any significant differences in concentration span between different days of the week, Weekday is now an interpretable effect because it has been demonstrated from replicate trials.

In summary, a categorical factor is generally fixed if it is randomly assigned to sampling units. It can be fixed even if it groups together multiple unmeasured sources of variation, provided that its levels are independently replicated in time or space. Interpretation of such grouping factors does not permit conclusions about causality, but useful descriptive information can be forthcoming with which to guide the design of future experimental manipulations. Random categorical factors group together all unreplicated spatial or temporal variation, which inherently confounds their interpretation. Although this is not a problem for main effects, it can create difficulties when interpreting interactions between fixed and random factors (further detailed in Chapters 3 and 4).

ANOVA models are classified according to the type of factors they contain, over and above the random sampling unit(s). A model that contains only fixed factors is called a 'model I ANOVA', whereas a model that contains only random factors is called a 'model II ANOVA'. Models containing both fixed and random factors are known as 'mixed models'. Covariates are always fixed, so ANCOVA models may be either 'model I' or 'mixed'. The nature of the test hypothesis will determine what is the appropriate assignment of fixed and random factors, and this must be correctly judged because it crucially influences the nature of any inferences. Fixed effects are allowed by the model to influence only the mean of the response Y; they yield inferences about the specific levels of the factor, but the results cannot be generalised to other possible levels. Random effects are allowed to influence only the variance in Y; they yield inferences only about the population from which the levels were drawn (see discussions in Beck 1997; Newman *et al.* 1997). These differences result from fixed and random factors differing in the components of variation that they estimate, which in turn affect which denominator is used to calculate a valid F-ratio (detailed in the section below on constructing F-ratios).

Nested and crossed factors, and the concept of replication

One factor is *nested* in another when its levels are grouped within each level of the nesting factor. All replicated analyses of variance have some element of nesting; even a one-factor ANOVA has sampling units (S′) nested in each level of the treatment factor (A). For example, an experiment to test the effect of irrigation on crop yield might use a randomly chosen set of 16 fields, each allocated to either a watering or a control treatment. Field is then a random factor S′ nested in Irrigation factor A because no field receives both watering treatments and thus the identity of the fields is different in each treatment group (Figure 3). In terms of a statistical model, we represent this feature of the design as S′(A). The effect of irrigation on crop yield can be tested with a straightforward one-way ANOVA by requesting a model in the form Y = A which will test the treatment effect with 1 and 14 d.f. Note that it is not necessary to specify S′ in the model request because it is the lowest level of nesting, which accounts for the residual variation.

Although nesting is involved in all ANOVA models with any form of replication, the so-called 'nested' models will have at least two scales of nesting. As an example, suppose that the two irrigation treatments have

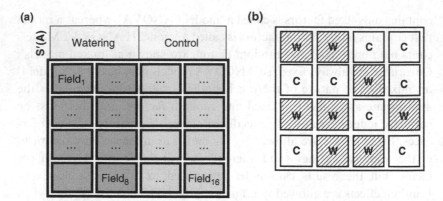

Figure 3 (a) Allocation table illustrating samples of eight fields receiving either watering or control treatments. Fields are nested in the factor Irrigation because each field is measured at only one level of the factor. (b) Experimental layout showing one possible spatial arrangement of fields randomly assigned to treatment levels of watering (W, hatched) or control (C, clear).

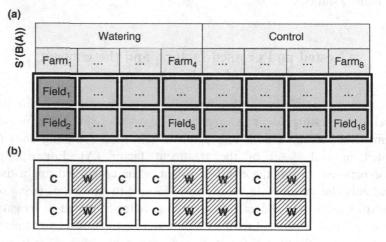

Figure 4 (a) Allocation table illustrating samples of two fields on each of eight farms receiving either watering or control treatments. Fields are nested in the factor Farm, and Farms are nested in the factor Irrigation. (b) Experimental layout showing one possible spatial arrangement of farms (columns) randomly assigned to treatment levels of watering (W, hatched) or control (C, clear).

been allocated randomly to eight whole farms, and that crop yield has been measured in two fields on each farm (Figure 4).

This design contains two levels of nesting: Fields S' are nested in Farms B', and Farms are nested in levels of Irrigation (A), all of which is denoted S'(B'(A)). The analysis of crop yield will now require a model requested in the form $Y = A + B(A)$ where B is declared as a random factor. The Irrigation effect A is tested against the random farm effect, and therefore has one and six d.f. (where previously we had one and 14 d.f.). Its reduced d.f. means that we have lost power to detect a treatment effect, but this cost has been traded against the benefit of sampling from across a wider region in order to obtain a more robust prediction. The analysis also has the possibility of *post hoc* pooling in the event that the farms within each treatment category differ little from each other, which will reinstate the 14 error d.f. (detailed on page 38).

Nested factors are an unavoidable feature of any studies in which treatments are applied across one organisational scale and responses are measured at a finer scale. For example, consider a study aiming to test whether the length of parasitic fungal hyphae depends on the genotype of a host plant. The hyphae grow in colonies on leaves of the plant, and the investigators have measured the hyphal length of ten colonies on each of two leaves from each of two plants from each of five genotypes, giving a total of 40 observations for each of the five genotypes. At the analysis stage, the investigators ignore differences between leaves and plants, which hold no inherent interest, and test for a genotype effect with the one-factor ANOVA: Length = Genotype + ε. They obtain a significant effect with four and 195 d.f. Such an analysis is flawed, because the one-factor model has ignored the reality that the 200 data points are not truly independent, but include replicate colonies from the same leaf and from the same plant. In fact, the design has two nested factors: Plant B' nested in Genotype and Leaf C' nested in Plant, in addition to the Colony sampling unit S' nested in Leaf nested in Plant, and the Genotype factor A of interest. The hierarchical structure of the design should be recognised by requesting a model in the form $Y = A + B(A) + C(B\ A)$ where B and C are declared as random factors, and the undeclared residual error $\varepsilon = S'(C'(B'(A)))$. The genotype effect of interest is now correctly tested with five error d.f. (instead of 195) because the only independent replicate information for testing an effect of genotype is the average hyphal length per plant. Had the study been planned with the correct analysis in mind, the distribution of sampling effort could have been targeted to give a more powerful test. A better design would have measured fewer colonies per leaf, because replication at this lowest organisational level is informative only about the variation among leaves, and instead would have measured more plants of each genotype, because it is the replication at this highest organisational level that determines the error d.f. for the genotype effect of interest.

In contrast to nesting, two factors are *crossed* when every level of one factor is measured in combination with every level of the other factor. The resulting design is termed 'factorial'. The simplest factorial design has sampling units nested in each combination of levels of two factors. For example, a test of crop yield uses a randomly chosen set of 16 fields, each allocated to either a watering or a control irrigation treatment and to either a high or a low sowing density (Figure 5). The two crossed factors are Irrigation (A) and Density (B), each with two levels. The study can test their simultaneous effects by allocating four fields to the watering-high combination, four to watering-low, four to control-high and four to control-low. In terms of a statistical model, we say that a random Field factor S' is nested in Treatment factors A and B, and we write this feature of the design as $S'(B|A)$. A two-factor ANOVA requested in the form $Y = B|A$ or $Y = A + B + B*A$ will test the independent and combined influences of irrigation and density on crop yield. The effect of irrigation may depend on sowing density (the $B*A$ interaction), for example if better yields come from dry–high and wet–low fields (Figure 5c). Alternatively, one or both of irrigation and density may influence crop yield independently of the other, for example if better yields generally come from high sowing densities regardless of watering regime. In this design, the three possible sources of explained variation, $A + B + B*A$, are all tested with one and 12 d.f. reflecting the two levels of each factor and the total of 16 fields grouped into four samples. Note that the tests of main effects A and B are not equivalent to two separate one-way ANOVAs, each of which would have one and 14 d.f., because the factorial design measures the effect of each factor whilst holding the other factor constant.

All of the designs considered thus far have been *fully replicated* because they take several independent and randomly selected measurements of the response at each level of each factor, or at each combination of levels of crossed factors. In terms of the statistical model, we can measure the residual variation from replicate sampling units S' nested in the factors A, B, C, etc., which is written: $S'(C\ B\ A)$, where the factors inside the parentheses may be variously nested or crossed with each other. Although full replication can be expensive to realise, its great advantage is that it allows testing of all sources of variation in the model. In the absence of full replication, a nested model will lose one or more levels of nesting, and a cross-factored model will lose the ability to test for all interactions. In the next section, we consider the strengths and weaknesses of a number of designs that usually lack full replication.

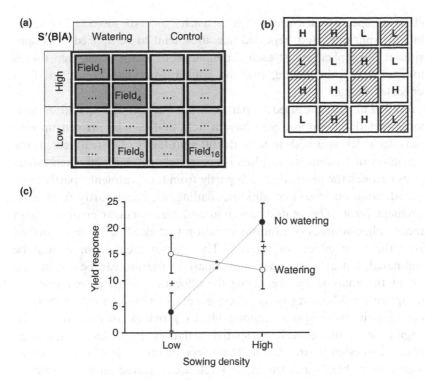

Figure 5 (a) Allocation table, and (b) experimental layout of irrigation (watering or control: hatched or clear) and sowing density (high or low: H or L) randomly assigned to four samples of four fields. Irrigation and Density are fully cross factored because measurements are taken at every combination of factor levels, in this case from four replicate fields nested in each of the four treatment combinations. (c) Example results, showing sample means and standard deviation for each of the four treatment combinations. There is a marked interaction of irrigation with sowing density: watering improves yield at low density but not at high density. The interaction exposes an effect of watering that is not apparent either in the irrigation main effect, which has negligible magnitude after pooling across sowing densities (comparing means of means given by '*'), or in the density main effect which shows a noticeable overall increase in yield after pooling irrigation levels (comparing means of means given by '+'). See also Figure 10 on page 78, showing the full range of possible outcomes from designs of this type.

Uses of blocking, split plots and repeated measures

Blocking and repeated measures are two methods used to partition out unwanted sources of random variation among sampling units in an ANOVA. Blocked designs (detailed in Chapter 4), and their associated split-plot variants (Chapter 5), and repeated-measures designs (Chapter 6), all have repeated measures taken on each block or subject. The terms 'block', 'split plot' and 'repeated measures' tend to be applied to designs without full replication at each combination of factor levels, and that is how we apply them here, drawing comparisons with equivalent fully replicated designs.

Blocked designs are used to partition out background spatial or temporal variation. Suppose you have a field that can be divided up into plots, to which you wish to allocate different levels of a treatment. If the allocation of treatments to plots is completely randomised, then differences between the plots will result partly from the treatments, partly from spatial variation in soil conditions, shading, etc., and partly from measurement error. The spatial variation and measurement error are both uncontrolled sources of random variation that need to be distinguished from the fixed effects of interest. The measurement error cannot be eliminated, but at least some of the spatial variation can be partitioned out of the analysis by organising the allocation of treatment levels to groups of neighbouring plots. These groups of plots are called 'blocks'. Variation in the response among blocks provides an estimate of the magnitude of the underlying spatial variation. In a fully randomised block, the design is stratified so that every treatment level is represented once in every block, and treatment levels are allocated randomly to plots within each block. Blocks usually group sampling units in space, but any random factor that cannot be randomly assigned to sampling units can be regarded as a block. For example, Family is a block that groups siblings; Parent plant is a block that groups seedlings (e.g., Newman *et al.* 1997; Resetarits and Bernardo 1998).

As an example, consider a two-factor experiment designed to test the response of crop yield to irrigation (factor A with two levels: watering and control) and sowing density (factor B with two levels: high and low). A total of sixteen plots of land are available for the experiment. A naturally homogeneous landscape, with little natural variation between plots, will suit a completely randomised design in which each of the four combinations of treatment levels is allocated randomly to four plots (Figure 6a). A natural variation amongst plots that is more marked, however, will give large residual MS and an experiment with low power to detect treatment effects. Moreover, any pattern to the natural variation, such as a gradient in soil moisture, may bias the predictions of the completely randomised model.

A randomised-block design partitions out this unwanted background variation by grouping plots into four groups of four in such a way that

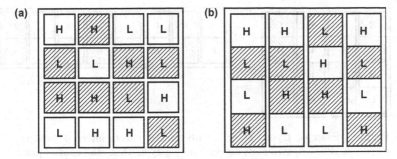

Figure 6 Example layouts of plots to test effects on crop yield of irrigation, with watered plots designated by grey hatching and control plots unhatched, and of sowing density, with high density designated by H and low density by L. (a) Completely randomised design for a homogeneous landscape with 16 plots (the squares), and treatment combinations randomly assigned to replicate plots. (b) Randomised-block design for partitioning out a left–right environmental gradient, with four plots (separated by single lines) in each of four blocks (double lines), and treatment combinations randomly assigned to plots within each block.

the plots within each block are as homogeneous as possible. Each of the four combinations of treatment levels is then represented once in each block, with treatment levels randomly allocated to plots within each block (Figure 6b). The blocks are modelled in the analysis as a random factor with four levels. The variation in the response from block to block is then partitioned out of the residual MS to provide a more powerful test for the main treatment effects. It is essential to include the blocking factor in the analysis because plots are not truly independent of each other, since they belong to a particular block, and are randomly assigned to treatment levels per block. To omit the block will result in falsely inflated error degrees of freedom, and consequently an increased likelihood of falsely rejecting a true null hypothesis (termed 'pseudoreplication' by Hurlbert 1984). Note that blocking can only serve its purpose if the investigator has some knowledge of the pattern of landscape hetero-geneity. The visible habitat structure may not suffice to describe relevant landscape heterogeneity, in which case a set of pre-measures of the response taken across the experimental area can inform the placement of blocks.

Split-plot designs are an extension of randomised-block designs in which treatments are applied at different spatial or temporal scales. For instance, logistical considerations may favour irrigating a larger unit of area than the unit for sowing density. This is likely to be the case if the

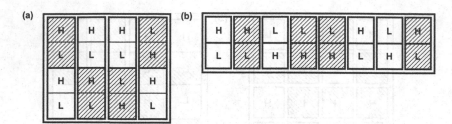

Figure 7 Example layout of split plots to test effects on crop yield of irrigation, with irrigated plots designated by grey hatching and control plots unhatched, and of sowing density, with high density designated by H and low density by L. (a) Split-plot design I, with two sub-plots (demarked by thin line) within each of two plots (thick line) within each of four blocks (double lines), showing irrigation applied to one plot randomly selected in each block and sowing density applied to one sub-plot randomly selected in each plot. (b) Split-plot design II, with two plots (demarked by single line) within each of eight blocks (double lines), showing irrigation assigned at random to replicate whole blocks and sowing density applied to one plot selected at random within each block.

irrigation is provided by a piped water sprayer, whereas sowing density is manipulated by hand. Continuing the example from above, irrigation could be randomly allocated to one plot per block comprising half of its area, and sowing density is then randomly allocated to one of two sub-plots within each plot (Figure 7a). Alternatively, for an experimental area with a smaller scale of natural variation, watering may be applied to replicate whole blocks and sowing density to plots within blocks. For example, four out of eight blocks could be chosen at random to receive extra watering and one of the two plots in each block chosen at random to receive high sowing density (Figure 7b). Such designs require care with the construction of appropriate statistical models. In the first case, blocks are crossed with both watering and density treatments, whereas in the second case blocks are nested within watering and crossed with density treatment.

Repeated-measures designs partition out variation among experimental subjects by applying more than one treatment level to each subject. Treatment levels are applied to the subject in temporal or spatial sequence. The subject acts as a random blocking factor, but the sequential application of treatment levels distinguishes this design from randomised-block and split-plot designs, both of which have a random allocation of treatment levels within each block. Repeated-measures designs are otherwise directly analogous to randomised-block and split-plot designs; in the same way that observations are not fully independent when they come from the same block, so repeated measurements may be correlated when made on the same subject.

Both blocking and repeated measures can greatly increase the power of an analysis to detect treatment effects because the variation among blocks or among subjects can be measured and partitioned out. They also allow a study to be performed block-by-block rather than simultaneously testing all combinations of factors which can prove impractical for large designs. The disadvantage of these techniques is that any interaction of block or subject with the treatment factors will complicate the interpretation of the analysis, and may not be testable unless the design is fully replicated by having multiple, independent observations of each treatment level in each block or on each subject. These difficulties should be anticipated at the design stage, because tighter controls may eliminate the need for blocking or repeated measures, and a fully replicated design will greatly facilitate estimation and interpretation of interactions. The non-independence of observations within a block or on a subject also requires that the ANOVA meets an additional assumption, of homogeneity of covariances. This is explained for randomised-block designs on page 118, for split-plot models on page 143 and for repeated-measures designs on page 183.

The analysis of randomised-block, split-plot and repeated-measures designs differs from that of their equivalent fully randomised models only when the design lacks full replication. With or without full replication, however, their interpretation is less straightforward than for fully randomised models. A treatment effect cannot be fully interpreted in the presence of a significant interaction with a block or repeated-measures variable, because that random variable groups together multiple unmeasured sources of variation. This problem is treated in more detail in the descriptions of fully randomised models (Chapter 3) and blocked, split-plot and repeated-measures models (Chapters 4 to 6).

Uses of covariates

A covariate is a predictor variable that is measured on a continuous scale such as kg, km, hrs, etc., as opposed to a categorical scale, such as male/female or low/medium/high. All of the ANOVA models in this book can be adapted to include one or more covariates; the generic term for parametric models that involve a combination of factors and covariates is a general linear model (GLM).

Covariates may be of interest in their own right. For example, a study of male and female body sizes might aim to test whether sex differences depend on age. Alternatively, covariates may serve to partition out an unwanted source of variation in order to increase power to detect treatment effects, in a similar fashion to blocking. For example, a study of sex differences in body size might include age as a covariate if samples of males and females cannot have individuals all of the same age.

Covariates of inherent interest are included as predictors in the model in the same way as a categorical factor, with all interactions. For example, a design with a single covariate X and a single factor A is tested with the model:

$$Y = X + A + A*X + \varepsilon$$

In effect, the model fits a separate linear regression between the covariate and the response at each level of A. The main effect X tests for a non-zero slope of the response across the range of the covariate after pooling across all levels of A, the main effect A tests for differences among the *a* means of factor A after pooling across all X, and the A*X interaction tests whether all levels of A have the same regression slope. Figure 8 shows an example. Note that analysis of main effects and interaction does not require replicate subjects for each level of factor A at each value of covariate X, nor the same values of X to be sampled within each level of A. However, the *n* subjects within each level of A must sample a minimum of three values of X to allow testing of the assumption of linearity.

The structure of the analysis of variance table is the same as that for a factorial design with two categorical factors A and B, except for the degrees of freedom. A linear covariate always has one d.f., because it comprises two pieces of information: the regression slope and its intercept, and one piece is required to measure its variation: the mean value of the response (so $2 - 1 = 1$ d.f.). The d.f. for the categorical factor A are $a - 1$, just as in a conventional ANOVA, whilst the d.f. for A*X interaction are the product of the d.f. for the component terms: $(a - 1) \times 1 = a - 1$. The residual variation will then have $(n - 2)a$ d.f., because unexplained variation is measured by deviations of the *n* replicates from their sample regression line which is fixed by the two parameters of slope and intercept. Thus a covariate X measured on five replicates in each of three levels of a treatment A will allow testing of the main effects and the interaction against $(5 - 2) \times 3 = 9$ residual d.f.

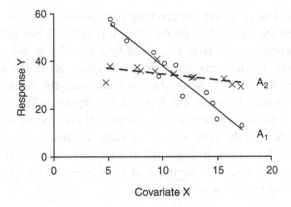

Figure 8 Relationship of the response to a covariate X (e.g., age in years) measured on subjects nested in two levels of treatment A (e.g., sex: males and females). For these data, analysis of covariance indicates a significant main effect of X but a non-significant main effect of A. The non-significance reflects the similar mean responses of A_1 and A_2 when data for each sample are pooled across all covariate values (i.e., ignoring the covariate values). The analysis produces a significant A*X interaction, which reflects the different slopes of Y with X at each level of A. This interaction indicates that factor A does indeed influence the response, with a switch in relative effect across the range of X. See also Figure 10 on page 78, showing the full range of possible outcomes from designs of this type.

Covariates of no inherent interest are included to partition out unwanted variation in designs that are conventionally termed analysis of covariance ('ANCOVA', though all models containing continuous factors are in fact analyses of covariance). An ANCOVA partitions out the effect of the covariate by adjusting the data for the regression relationship between the response and the covariate. For a design with two crossed factors A and B, the model is:

$$Y = X + A + B + B*A + \varepsilon$$

The continuous variable is conventionally entered as the first term in the model, in order to partition out the unwanted covariation before testing the factors of interest. Although this will only make a difference to the results of non-orthogonal designs, ANCOVA is likely to be non-orthogonal when it is unbalanced by having levels of the covariate that are not set by the study design but measured separately on each randomly selected subject or sampling unit. The imbalance is caused by not having exactly repeated values of the covariate at each combination of levels of the categorical factors, and the resulting loss of orthogonality affects the calculation of SS. This is discussed further on page 237, but will not be an issue if the nuisance covariate is entered first into the model.

Because this model tests only the main effect X, it fits a common regression relationship between the covariate and the response for all groups or samples. It makes the implicit assumption of no interactions between the covariate and any of the categorical factors, meaning that all category levels have the same slope of Y with X. This assumption should be tested, which requires fitting a full model that includes all covariate-by-factor interactions. For the two-factor example above, the covariate interactions are tested using the model:

$$Y = X + A + B + A*X + B*X + B*A + B*A*X + \varepsilon$$

Any non-significant interaction terms can be omitted and the model refitted with the interaction SS pooled into the residual SS. Any significant interaction terms should be retained in the model, and interpreted by plotting out the within-factor regression slopes. A significant interaction indicates that the magnitude of treatment effects depends on position along the covariate scale. Although significant interactions can complicate interpretation of the analysis, they are often of considerable biological interest and tend to be easier to interpret than interactions with blocks, because the nature of the variation is more clearly defined.

An ANCOVA should always be used to partition out unwanted variation in a continuous variable rather than any kind of 'residuals analysis' involving the creation of a new data set made up of regression residuals. Analysing residuals is fundamentally flawed because factors used to explain residual variation may interact with the covariate (García-Berthou 2001), or be correlated with it (Darlington and Smulders 2001) leading to biased parameter estimates (Freckleton 2002).

All GLMs assume *linear responses to the covariate*, which can be checked visually by plotting the raw data. Some relationships are intrinsically non-linear, such as those comparing variables with different dimensions (volume or weight to length or area, etc.). These are likely also to violate the assumptions of a normal distribution and homogeneous variance of response residuals along the regression slope. Transforming the response and/or the predictor can often correct all of these problems, but remember always to plot the data again after any transformation to check that it has had the desired effect.

The value of a covariate analysis depends on its underlying linear model having some biological meaning. When considering transformations, it is therefore sensible to think about the process that you hypothesise is driving the observed pattern, and then find a way to present it in linear form. For example, a Volume response will have a cubic relation to a Length covariate if length is representative of the dimensions that make up the volume. The hypothesis that Volume $\propto$ Length^3 will be tested by a linear regression of log(Volume) against log(Length) with a predicted regression coefficient $b = 3$ defining the slope. Alternatively, one might accept the existence of a cubic relation $V = a \cdot L^3$, and cube the length measures in order to test only the value of the parameter a – for example, whether it differs significantly from zero or between different treatments. One or other transformation should be applied even if the distribution of raw data is not obviously non-linear, unless you intend to test the biologically more complex hypothesis that the volume–length relation is represented by a constant of proportionality. Note that transformations can change the structure of the model from an interpretive point of view. Logging the response, for instance, alters the data points from being additive to being multiplicative.

Other relationships may require more subtle transformations based on an underlying mechanistic model to ensure interpretable predictions. This is well illustrated by an example of predator responses to prey density. Predators generally respond to increased prey density with an increased ingestion rate, but for many species their responsiveness diminishes as prey density increases. The positive relationship between ingestion rate and prey density consequently takes a decelerating (concave) form, known as a saturation response (Figure 9a). Such data are clearly not suitable for analysis using the model Rate = Density + ε without suitable transformation. In this case we have no biological justification for log-transforming prey density, even though it may well straighten out the relationship. Instead, linearity is achieved more rationally by taking the inverse of both the response and the covariate (Figure 9b). A simple model of the underlying mechanism demonstrates why this is a biologically meaningful transformation. We partition the time interval between consecutive ingestions into a search time that is inversely proportional to prey density D, and a constant handling time a required to manipulate and ingest each item. The linear regression of Interval on the y-axis against $1/D$ on the x-axis then yields a prediction: Interval = $b/D + a$, with slope b and intercept a. Since the inverse of the interval is the rate of ingestion, we have Rate = $D/(b + aD)$, which is the concave predictor to

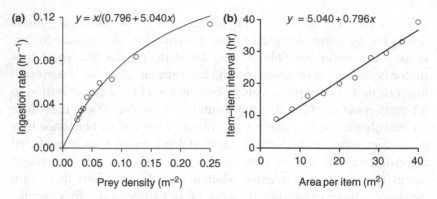

Figure 9 (a) Saturation response of predator ingestion rate to prey density, D. (b) Inverse transformations of both axes yield a relationship suitable for linear regression if the predator has search time inversely proportional to prey density (here with a predicted constant of proportionality $b = 0.796$) and constant handling time (here taking a predicted value of $a = 5.040$ hrs). The curved line in (a), with its equation above the graph, is derived from the linear regression line in (b), with its equation above the graph.

fit through the data on rate against density. Note that a sampling effort designed to give an approximately equal spread of prey densities will yield values of search time that are skewed towards the origin, which is not ideal for estimating the linear regression. This problem can be avoided by weighting sampling effort towards lower prey densities (as in Figure 9), but it requires thinking through the analysis before collecting the data.

Wave functions from circular relationships can also be linearised, for example if the wave is symmetrical and gives a straight-line response to sine(X). Many other curvilinear relationships with peaks and troughs cannot be transformed to a linear relationship in principle. These will not suit linear models unless they can be represented by a polynomial of the form $Y = X|X + \varepsilon$, or $Y = A|X|X + \varepsilon$, etc. Non-linear models lie beyond the scope of this book, but they can be tested with specialist statistics packages (e.g., see Crawley 2002; Motulsky and Christopoulos 2004).

Some kinds of data may require a comparison of models from alternative transformations in order to explore underlying processes. For example, perhaps the density of a population appears to show a linear increase over time despite an expectation of exponential growth. It is then useful to compare the fit of the linear model: Density = Time + ε to the fit of the linearised exponential model: ln(Density) = Time + ε. The better fitting model is the one with the higher proportion of explained variation, given by the coefficient of determination: $r^2 = SS_{explained}/SS_{total}$. In general, however, a study with a focus on model comparison and parameter estimation may be better suited to the likelihood approaches of GLIM or Bayesian inference.

Models with covariate and categorical factors are *unbalanced* if the covariate takes different values for one treatment level than for another. Type II SS should then be used to take account of any resulting correlation between covariates and factors (detailed on page 240). In extreme cases, where the covariate takes lower values for one treatment level than for another, the adjustment to the SS in an ANCOVA involves extrapolation of the regression line beyond the range of the covariate values in one or more groups. Interpretation of the results therefore requires appropriate caveats about the assumptions made by this extrapolation. ANCOVA is very sensitive to the assumption of homogeneity of variances if the design is further unbalanced by having different numbers of observations in each treatment level, for example if a factor Sex has different sample sizes for male and female body weights measured against the covariate Age.

Covariates are generally analysed as *fixed factors*, meaning that the values are set by the design and measured without error (just like a fixed categorical factor). This may not be the reality, particularly where a covariate takes the role of a randomly sampled nuisance factor, in which case regression slopes may be underestimated (e.g., Quinn and Keough 2002).

How *F*-ratios are constructed

The model designs shown in this book all adhere to a standard protocol for constructing each *F*-ratio with an error MS that comprises all relevant components of random variation (Schultz 1955). We give it here, because it yields the correct *F*-ratios for any balanced ANOVA model with categorical factors, including designs with more than three factors. It adapts readily to include covariates, as we will describe. For protocols that show the weightings on each independent component of variation, see for example Winer *et al.* (1991); Kirk (1994); Underwood (1997).

To find the correct error mean square for each *F*-ratio, make up a table with as many rows as sources of variation. Table 3 below shows a completed example for the cross-factored fully replicated model $Y = C|B'(A) + \varepsilon$. These are the steps to filling out the four columns in turn:

Column I: Source of variation. List all of the sources, one per line, in their hierarchical order from main effects and their nested effects through their constituent interactions to the highest-order interactions and nested components within them.

Column II: Degrees of freedom. For each source of variation, calculate its degrees of freedom by multiplying together the number of levels for any factors within parentheses, and the number of levels minus one for any factors outside parentheses. For example, a source of variation given by the interaction of two factors: B*A, with b and a levels respectively, has $(b-1)(a-1)$ degrees of freedom; a source of residual variation given by n subjects nested in three factors: S'(C'(B*A)), with c, b and a levels respectively, has $(n-1)cba$ degrees of freedom. The column sum is the number of degrees of freedom for the total variation, which equals one minus the product of n with all factor levels. For example, all models with three factors have $ncba - 1$ total degrees of freedom, regardless of nesting or factoring, or repeated measures.

Column III: Components of variation estimated in the population. For each source of variation in turn, list all of the components of variation estimated in the population by the mean square for this source. These are identified from amongst the sources of variation in lower rows. Start with the bottom row and work upwards towards the current row, adding each source only if (*i*) it contains all of the factor(s) in the current row source, and (*ii*) any other factors outside parentheses are random, or if no parentheses, any other factors are random. Finally add in the source for the current row.

Column IV: F-ratio. For each source of variation, identify its F-ratio from a numerator comprising the mean square of the row source, and a denominator comprising the mean square of the error variation. Identify the source of error variation from whichever row beneath the test row contains all of the same components of variation in the population (in Column III), except for the test component. This error variation is always the source that contains all of the factors in the test component plus one and only one random factor (Keppel and Wickens 1973). No exact test exists if there is more than one such source.

Some models present complications beyond the remit of this protocol. Type II and mixed models allow pooling of error terms under appropriate conditions, detailed in the next section. Other models have sources of variation with no exact error MS, which can be analysed with quasi F-ratios described below on page 40. Mixed models can use an alternative set of rules for constructing the error MS of random factors, detailed in the section on unrestricted models on page 242. We signal these complications as they arise in Chapters 1 to 7, in footnotes to the ANOVA tables.

If a factor is a linear *covariate*, then it will always have one d.f., because the linear regression is defined by two pieces of information: its intercept and slope, and one piece of information is required to sum its deviations from horizontal: the grand mean. The residual error for each regression is calculated with $n - 2$ d.f. because it sums the squared deviations of n observations from their regression defined by an intercept and slope. Table 3 demonstrates how the ANOVA table is influenced by factor C being a categorical factor or a covariate in the model $C|B'(A) + \varepsilon$.

Table 3 *ANOVA tables for the fully replicated, cross-factored with nesting model* $Y = C|B'(A) + \varepsilon$ *(model 3.3 on page 98). (a) All factors are categorical; (b) factor C is a covariate of the response. Differences between the two tables are indicated by shading. Worked example 3 on page 51 shows a specific application with specified numbers of factor levels and sample sizes.*

Mean square	d.f.	Components of variation estimated in population	F-ratio
(a) I	II	III	IV
1 A	$a-1$	$S'(C*B'(A)) + B'(A) + A$	**1/2**
2 B'(A)	$(b-1)a$	$S'(C*B'(A)) + B'(A)$	**2/6**
3 C	$c-1$	$S'(C*B'(A)) + C*B'(A) + C$	**3/5**
4 C*A	$(c-1)(a-1)$	$S'(C*B'(A)) + C*B'(A) + C*A$	**4/5**
5 C*B'(A)	$(c-1)(b-1)a$	$S'(C*B'(A)) + C*B'(A)$	**5/6**
6 S'(C*B'(A))	$(n-1)cba$	$S'(C*B'(A))$	–
Total variation	$ncba - 1$		
(b) I	II	III	IV
1 A	$a-1$	$S'(C*B'(A)) + B'(A) + A$	**1/2**
2 B'(A)	$(b-1)a$	$S'(C*B'(A)) + B'(A)$	**2/6**
3 C	1	$S'(C*B'(A)) + C*B'(A) + C$	**3/5**
4 C*A	$(a-1)$	$S'(C*B'(A)) + C*B'(A) + C*A$	**4/5**
5 C*B'(A)	$(b-1)a$	$S'(C*B'(A)) + C*B'(A)$	**5/6**
6 S'(C*B'(A))	$(n-2)ba$	$S'(C*B'(A))$	–
Total variation	$nba - 1$		

Use of *post hoc* pooling

The power of an F test is the ability to detect a specified difference between two or more population means, or a linear trend across values of a covariate, with a specified level of confidence. *Post hoc* pooling is a technique applied to models with ramdom factors to improve their power to detect treatment effects by increasing the denominator degrees of freedom.

How does pooling work?

Planned *post hoc* pooling involves eliminating non-significant components of variation from the ANOVA model and then pooling mean square terms that estimate identical components of variation. When pooling down – the most common and useful form of pooling – the pooled error MS for a term is calculated by taking a weighted average of the original denominator MS and the error MS of this non-significant term, which is equivalent to summing the sums of squares (SS) of the original terms and dividing by the sum of their degrees of freedom:

$$MS_{pooled} = \frac{(df_1 \cdot MS_1) + (df_2 \cdot MS_2)}{df_1 + df_2} = \frac{SS_1 + SS_2}{df_1 + df_2}$$

The pooled MS has degrees of freedom equal to $df_1 + df_2$. The F-ratio is then recalculated and tested as normal. The precise criteria for choosing which error terms can be pooled with which are detailed in footnotes to the ANOVA tables in this book (following Underwood 1997).

Although pooling is designed to improve power, statisticians do not agree either about its desirability in principle, or about the criteria for identifying non-significant components of variation for elimination. Pooling can substantially increase the statistical power of a test to detect difference among treatments. Pooling can also increase the power of subsequent multiple comparison tests and may therefore be desirable even if the original analysis is already powerful enough to detect differences among treatments. On the other hand, *post hoc* pooling results in the investigator seeking differences between treatments with a design that has been modified in response to the results from the original design for which the data were collected. Moreover, power is not always improved by pooling, and falsely pooling a term when its effect is not zero (the result of a Type II error) can inflate the Type I error rate for subsequent tests (Underwood 1997; Janky 2000).

Given that pooling is a mixed blessing, when should it be used? In an ideal world you would avoid compromising the integrity of your design by ensuring sufficient replication to detect differences with the a priori analysis, including all terms in the model. This should be the aim for any experimental manipulation, but it may not be always achievable in the presence of unmanipulated components such as blocks, or in mensurative studies. Be wary of designs that rely on pooling to provide an exact denominator to test a main effect or, more generally, that rely on pooling to provide a reasonable number of denominator degrees of freedom to test a main effect. Weigh the benefits of including random factors to test across greater spatial scales against the costs of needing replicate samples from across these scales, and the risk of failing to test a main effect powerfully if the criteria for pooling are not met (see below). We recommend pooling only when logistical considerations severely limit the replication possible for an essential random block. For example, when it is not possible to find, or impractical to sample, many replicate locations nested in each level of a main effect, then *post hoc* pooling may be necessary to provide a powerful test of the main effect. These considerations are discussed in worked example 3, on page 51.

Statistical power is likely to be increased only by '*pooling down*' (*sensu* Hines 1996), which involves pooling the original denominator with an MS that estimates fewer components of variation (i.e., one located lower down in the ANOVA table). If the design accommodates *post hoc* pooling in principle, appropriate terms and criteria should be identified in advance to avoid the temptation to keep eliminating terms until the null hypothesis is rejected. Terms and criteria for *post hoc* pooling are identified in the footnotes to tables in this book. Components of variation should be eliminated only if there is a reasonable likelihood of detecting the variation that is present among units. A common rule of thumb, which we adopt, is to control the Type II error rate by pooling only if $P > 0.25$, having set $\alpha = 0.25$ (Underwood 1997; Janky 2000). A more conservative set of rules for deciding when to pool is given in Sokal and Rohlf (1995).

The alternative method: '*pooling up*', involves pooling the original denominator with an MS that has more components of variation (i.e., one located higher up in the ANOVA table). This generally produces a higher MS which more than offsets any benefit associated with increasing the denominator degrees of freedom. More fundamentally, finding a non-significant interaction is not a good justification on its own for dropping the interaction from the analysis (in effect, pooling up the original error term with the interaction). This is because the failure to detect a significant interaction from the samples does not necessarily mean that there is no interaction in the population. If it is there, and you are making a Type II error in not finding it, then removing the interaction biases the error MS and consequently the validity of the treatment F-ratios.

Likewise, it is not advisable to drop higher-order interactions a priori, without testing significance. Doing so has two main shortcomings. Firstly, assuming a lack of interaction between factors changes the test hypothesis (see discussion in Newman *et al.* 1997). In effect, undeclared terms are pooled up untested into the error MS, which compromises the integrity of the analysis and can render meaningless any attempt to interpret causality from the main effects. Secondly, if factors do interact, their pooling into the error term can reduce the power of the analysis to detect main effects (Hines 1996). Keep test questions simple in order always to estimate all potential sources of variation.

The need to report all potential sources of variation applies particularly to models that are designed to test experimental hypotheses, and especially to those that include blocking factors. It may be less relevant to mensurative studies aiming to isolate the factors that most influence a response and to identify the most parsimonious explanatory model. In this case, the ANOVA functions as a tool for *model simplification* and prediction rather than for hypothesis testing. Complex, often unbalanced, models may be simplified by testing higher-order interactions first, followed by lower-order interactions and main effects. Each term is tested by comparing a full model to a reduced model without that term. Non-significant terms are dropped from the model and their variation pooled into the residual (Grafen and Hails 2002; Crawley 2002). Since the removal of a main effect necessitates also removing any of its higher-order interactions, this approach upholds the fundamental principle of ANOVA that terms be tested in hierarchical order (known as the principle of marginality).

Use of quasi F-ratios

For some mixed and random models there is no exact F-ratio denominator for certain tests. In such cases it may be possible to add and subtract mean squares to construct an error mean square with the appropriate estimated components of variation. This error mean square is then used to obtain a quasi F-ratio. The corresponding error d.f. are also estimated from these additions and subtractions of k mean squares, using the following formula (e.g., Kirk 1994):

$$df = integer \left[\frac{(MS_1 \pm \cdots \pm MS_k)^2}{MS_1^2/df_1 + \cdots + (MS_k^2/df_k)} \right]$$

Examples of quasi F-ratios are given in ANOVA tables wherever they apply in Chapters 3 to 7. Quasi F-ratios produce only crude approximations to valid tests, and *post hoc* pooling can often provide a more favourable alternative (Underwood 1997). We will identify these alternatives where they arise in ANOVA tables in Chapters 3 to 7.

Introduction to model structures

In the following Chapters 1 to 7, we will describe all common models with up to three treatment factors for seven principal classes of ANOVA design:

(1) One-factor – replicate measures at each level of a single explanatory factor;
(2) Nested – one factor nested in one or more other factors;
(3) Factorial – fully replicated measures on two or more crossed factors;
(4) Randomised blocks – repeated measures on spatial or temporal groups of sampling units;
(5) Split plot – treatments applied at multiple spatial or temporal scales;
(6) Repeated measures – subjects repeatedly measured or tested in temporal or spatial sequence;
(7) Unreplicated factorial – a single measure per combination of two or more factors.

For each model we provide the following information:

- The model equation;
- The test hypothesis;
- A table illustrating the allocation of factor levels to sampling units;
- Illustrative examples;
- Any special assumptions;
- Guidance on analysis and interpretation;
- Full analysis of variance tables showing all sources of variation, their associated degrees of freedom, components of variation estimated in the population, and appropriate error mean squares for the F-ratio denominator;
- Options for pooling error mean square terms.

As an introduction to Chapters 1 to 7, we first describe the notation used, explain the layout of the allocation tables, present some worked examples and provide advice on identifying the appropriate statistical model.

Notation

Chapters 1 to 3 describe fully randomised and replicated designs. This means that each combination of levels of categorical factors (A, B, C) is assigned randomly to n sampling units (S′), which are assumed to be selected randomly and independently from the population of interest. The sampling unit is therefore the subject or plot from which a single data point is taken. These replicate observations provide a measurable residual error, which is denoted by ε in the model description and by S′(C B A) in the ANOVA table. The ANOVA tables in Chapters 1 to 3 are appropriate also to fully replicated versions of blocked designs in Chapters 4 to 6, and this will be signalled where relevant.

Chapters 4 to 7 describe designs without full replication. This means that each combination of levels of categorical factors is tested on just a single independent sampling unit, leaving no measurable residual error (residual d.f. $= 0$). In addition, the designs in Chapters 4 to 6 are not fully randomised: those in Chapters 4 and 5 involve one or more blocking factors that group sampling units together spatially or temporally, whilst those in Chapter 6 involve repeated measurements taken sequentially from the same subject. These blocking factors/subjects are denoted by S′ because they represent the only true form of replication in the model, and the sampling units nested hierarchically within them are termed plots (P′), sub-plots (Q′) and sub-sub-plots (R′).

The full notation used in Chapters 1 to 7 is listed in Table 4. For meanings of 'd.f.', 'SS', 'MS', '*F*', and '*P*' in the ANOVA tables, see the general principles of ANOVA on page 7. The Glossary on page 271 provides further summary definitions of these and other terms.

Allocation tables

For each model in Chapters 1 to 7, an allocation table shows the allocation of treatment levels amongst replicate sampling units, illustrated with two or more levels of each factor. We have used a consistent number of factor levels and replicates across all allocation tables in order to facilitate comparison

Table 4 *Notation used in Chapters 1 to 7.*

Symbol	Meaning
Y	Continuous response variable.
A, B, C	Fixed factor (e.g., Treatment A of watering regime).
A', B', C'	Random factor (e.g., Treatment B' of crop genotype).
a, b, c	Number of sample levels of factor A, B, C (e.g., factor A may have $a = 2$ levels, corresponding to 'low' and 'high').
S', P', Q', R'	Random factor representing randomly selected subjects/blocks (S'), plots (P'), sub-plots (Q'), or sub-sub-plots (R'), to which treatments are applied.
S_i, P_i, Q_i, R_i,	Independent and randomly chosen subject/block, plot, sub-plot or sub-sub-plot which provides a replicate observation of the response.
n	The size of each sample, given by the number of measures of the response in each combination of factor levels (including any repeated measures), or by the number of measures across all values of a covariate.
N	Total number of measures of the response across all factor levels.
$B'(A)$	Hierarchical nesting of one factor in another (here, B' is nested in A).
B*A	Interaction between factors in their effects on the response (here, interaction of B with A).
ε	Residual variation left unexplained by the model, taking the form $S'(\ldots)$, $P'(\ldots)$, $Q'(\ldots)$ or $R'(\ldots)$.
$Y = C\|B\|A + \varepsilon$	Full model (here, variation in Y around the grand mean partitions amongst the three main effects A, B, C plus the three two-way interactions B*A, C*A, C*B plus the one three-way interaction C*B*A, plus the unexplained residual (error) variation $\varepsilon = S'(C*B*A)$ around each sample mean. This would not be a full model if only main effects were tested, or only main effects and two-way interactions).

across models, but these should not be taken to indicate adequate replication for testing effects. The amount of replication required for a given error d.f. can be judged from inspection of the ANOVA tables. The example allocation tables below apply to fully replicated models. Models with blocking factors or repeated measures have allocation tables with at least one extra level of nesting. These will be explained as they arise in Chapters 4 to 6.

The allocation for the factorial model below shows $n = 4$ subjects (S) in each of $a = 2$ levels of factor A, cross factored with $b = 2$ levels of factor B, as identified by column and row headers.

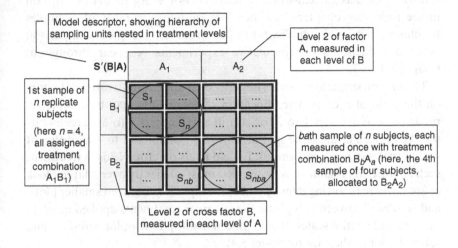

The allocation for the factorial-with-nesting model below shows $n = 2$ subjects (S) in each of $b = 2$ levels of factor B nested in each of $a = 2$ levels of factor A, and cross factored with $c = 2$ levels of factor C, as identified by column and row headers.

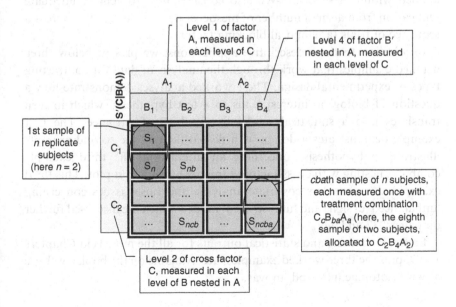

Examples

Examples are a valuable tool for understanding how to apply abstract statistical models to real-world situations. For every model description in the following chapters, we therefore outline a number of examples to illustrate possible applications. In order to facilitate comparison between models, two manipulative experiments reappear throughout Chapters 1 to 7.

The first experiment hypothesises effects of up to three treatment factors on the yield of a crop. The allocation of treatments may be completely randomised (Chapters 1 to 3) or stratified (Chapters 4 to 6). Treatments may be applied at the same spatial scale (e.g., Chapters 1 to 4) or different spatial scales (Chapters 5 and 6). In field trials on crop yields, a treatment such as watering regime may be applied most efficiently over a large block of area, whereas sowing density can be manipulated between smaller plots, and fertiliser between sub-plots. We consider treatments applied at up to three nested spatial scales: block, plot and sub-plot (or plot, sub-plot and sub-sub-plot in the case of model 5.4).

The second experiment describes the effects of up to three treatment factors on the growth of plants within laboratory mesocosms (controlled-environment rooms). We consider treatment levels of temperature applied between mesocosms, and treatment levels of light and fertiliser that can be applied within mesocosms. We also consider how to achieve adequate replication from a small number of mesocosms, by re-using them across a sequence of trials (a temporal blocking factor).

In addition to these descriptive applications, we present below three detailed examples that work through the analysis of data for contrasting types of experimental design. These worked analyses demonstrate how a question of biological interest leads to a test hypothesis, which in turn translates into a statistical model for analysis of variance. The first example demonstrates a design with nested factors; the second example illustrates a hypothesis concerning an interaction; the third example combines nesting with cross-factored treatments in a split plot. This third example also considers covariate analysis, and raises issues concerning 'unbalanced' designs and 'unrestricted' models which are discussed further on pages 237 and 242.

Example datasets and statistical outputs for all the models in Chapters 1 to 7, plus the three worked examples, are available on the book's website at www.soton.ac.uk/~cpd/anovas.

Worked example 1: Nested analysis of variance

Farm chickens are susceptible to many sources of stress even with free-range access to an outdoor pen. Any form of suffering is clearly undesirable from a welfare point of view, and it can also reduce the quantity and quality of eggs and meat for the farmer. One approach to reducing stress is to add complexity to the animals' environment of a type that might have been faced by their wild ancestors, and to which they may have evolved behavioural and physiological adaptations. The experiment below tests whether the wellbeing of free-range hens improves with a challenge to their foraging skills in the form of a less predictable availability of food. The response variable is the concentration of the hormone cortisol, which can be sampled from blood or saliva and is a good indicator of an individual's state of stress.

Test hypothesis

Does higher uncertainty in the location of food reduces physiological stress? The hypothesis was tested experimentally by measuring cortisol levels in hens subjected to predictable and unpredictable distributions of their food. Food predictability was manipulated in communal outdoor pens by distributing the same volume of grain either evenly or in small and randomly sited patches over the ground. Pens were randomly assigned to treatment levels and hens were randomly assigned to pens. Although the design has a single treatment factor it does not suit one-way ANOVA because responses were measured per individual, whereas the treatment levels of food predictability were applied to pens. This mismatch between the scale of treatment application and the scale of measurement means that pen must be declared as a second factor in the model. Each pen received just one food treatment, so the random factor Pen was nested in treatment factor Food. Each hen was present in just one pen, so the random factor Hen was nested in Pen. This gives model 2.1 (page 68):

Model

$$\text{Cortisol} = \text{Pen}'(\text{Food}) + \varepsilon$$

Factors	Levels	Values
A. Food	2	'Even' and 'Patchy'
B. Pen(Food)	4	'1', '2', '3', '4' in Even, '5', '6', '7', '8' in Patchy

Allocation table

The table shows Cortisol concentration (μg/dl) in samples of $n = 3$ replicate hens (S') in each of $b = 4$ Pens (B') at each of $a = 2$ levels of Food treatment (A).

S'(B(A))	Even				Patchy			
	1	2	3	4	5	6	7	8
	15.5	18.7	12.0	12.4	16.1	7.5	5.2	8.8
	16.2	15.0	15.0	10.4	7.3	7.2	9.4	10.3
	15.0	20.8	13.2	9.5	10.5	10.8	5.5	9.9

The data were arranged in three columns: Food, Pen and Cortisol concentration. Although the experiment used a total of eight pens, these were coded as numbers 1 to 4 repeated in each level of Food, as demanded by some software packages to reflect the balanced design.

Food	Pen	Cortisol
1	1	15.5
1	1	16.2
1	1	15.0
1	2	18.7
...	...	...
...	...	...
2	4	9.9

A balanced ANOVA was computed, requesting analysis of Y against the terms: $A + B(A)$, with B declared random.

ANOVA table

Food is a fixed factor, Pen is a random factor:

Source of variation	d.f.	Mean square	F-ratio	F	P
1 Food	1	177.127	**1/2**	8.64	0.026
2 Pen'(Food)	6	20.498	**2/3**	3.78	0.016
3 Hen'(Pen'(Food))	16	5.424			
Total variation	23				

The analysis shows that the mean cortisol concentration differed among pens within each treatment level ($F_{6,16} = 3.78$, $P = 0.016$). Over and above the variation at this scale, however, cortisol concentration was influenced by food predictability ($F_{1,6} = 8.64$, $P = 0.026$). Mean cortisol concentration was lower on average in pens with a patchy distribution of food than in pens with an even distribution of food. Note that the error d.f. for the treatment effect depend on the number of replicate pens per treatment level (*F*-ratio: **1/2**) and not on the number of replicate hens per pen. Thus the power of the test could have been improved with more replicate pens, but not directly with more replicate hens.

The experiment suggests an impact of food predictability on welfare, which now requires further exploration. The patchily distributed food caused the hens to spend longer foraging and to interact more with each other, and either time or interaction could have been primary causes of the observed differences. The timing of sampling, the number of hens per pen, and the previous history of the hens may all influence the result. These could be investigated further with tests for changes in cortisol concentration associated with swapping from one regime to the other (see repeated-measures models in Chapter 6). Although stress tends to raise cortisol levels, a history of trauma can cause unusually low levels. It would thus be sensible to test for long-term benefits of food predictability with complementary measures of welfare such as weight gain or egg production.

Worked example 2: Cross-factored analysis of variance

Bullheads (*Cottus gobio*) and stone loach (*Barbatula barbatula*) are sympatric stream fish that prey on benthic macro-invertebrates such as Chironomid larvae. Although ecologically similar to each other, they have contrasting foraging strategies. Bullheads are sit-and-wait ambush predators, whereas stone loach actively search for prey. Predation can be important in limiting the abundance of prey species. Moreover, predators may facilitate each other's prey capture if behavioural responses of prey to one predator make them more vulnerable to attack from the other.

Test hypothesis

The test hypothesis is that bullheads and stone loach both reduce the density of Chironomid larvae, and their combined effect is greater than the summed effects of the two species in isolation.

The hypothesis was tested experimentally by stocking five bullheads, five stone loach, or five bullheads plus five stone loach into enclosures in a stream. A fish exclosure treatment was used as a control. Each of the four treatments was replicated five times. Fish were held in the cages for 21 days. At the end of the experiment, the gravel substrate in the base of each enclosure was sampled to estimate densities of Chironomid larvae remaining. Prey density was expressed as individuals/m^2 and log-transformed to normalise residuals. The data were analysed by two-factor ANOVA, with presence and absence of bullheads and presence and absence of stone loach as fixed factors (model 3.1(*i*) on page 82). This design is orthogonal since each predator is held with and without the other. Because the enclosures contain different densities of fish, the influence of consumer density confounds the influence of species presence or absence. However, the effect of all individuals consuming Chironomids equally will show up in the analysis of variance as equally strong main effects for each species. The interesting test in this analysis is the interaction between species, with a significant interaction indicating that one species hinders or facilitates the other's access to the food resource.

Model

Density = Bullhead | Stone loach + ε

Factors	Levels	Values
A. Bullhead	2	'Absent' and 'Present'
B. Stone loach	2	'Absent' and 'Present'

Allocation table

The table shows Chironomid density ($\log_{10}$(individuals/m^2)) in samples of $n = 5$ replicate cages in each of $ba = 4$ combinations of levels of Stone loach*Bullhead.

		Bullhead									
S'(B|A)		Absent					Present				
Stone loach	Absent	3.89	3.94	4.19	3.99	4.04	3.94	4.01	4.21	4.10	4.02
	Present	3.48	3.81	4.08	3.63	3.64	3.60	3.94	3.86	3.96	3.62

The analysis was computed by requesting the model $Y = B|A$, after arranging the data in three columns: Bullhead, Stone loach and Chironomid density:

Bullhead	Stone loach	Density
Absent	Absent	3.89
Absent	Absent	3.94
Absent	Absent	4.19
Absent	Absent	3.99
...	...	...
...	...	...
Present	Present	3.62

ANOVA table

Bullhead and Stone loach are both fixed factors:

Source of variation	d.f.	Mean square	*F*-ratio	*F*	*P*
1 Bullhead	1	0.01624	**1/4**	0.61	0.446
2 Stone loach	1	0.36721	**2/4**	13.79	0.002
3 Stone loach*Bullhead	1	0.00061	**3/4**	0.02	0.882
4 Cage′(Stone loach*Bullhead)	16	0.02663			
Total variation	19				

The analysis shows no interaction between the fish species in their impacts on Chironomid larvae in the cage enclosures ($F_{1,16} = 0.02$, $P = 0.882$). This non-significant result was obtained despite high power to detect a real effect, given by the 16 error d.f. (see page 248 for further discussion of statistical power). The density of larvae was reduced in the presence of stone loach ($F_{1,16} = 13.79$, $P = 0.002$), by an amount that was unaffected by the addition of bullheads, which had no discernable impact on larval abundance ($F_{1,16} = 0.61$, $P = 0.446$). The full analysis described in Davey (2003) included water velocity as a covariate to control for variation in physical conditions between enclosures.

Worked example 3: Split-plot, pooling and covariate analysis

The inter-tidal barnacle *Semibalanus balanoides* is a small crustacean abundant on European rocky shores. With an entirely sessile adult stage and internal cross-fertilisation, adults can reproduce only if they live within a penis-reach of neighbours. Although they are hermaphrodite and have penises up to ten times their body length, this mode of reproduction is likely to cause larvae to aggregate close to adult conspecifics when they settle out from pelagic waters onto inter-tidal rocks. Larvae may be less strongly influenced by the presence of adults on shores that have a generally high level of recruitment, however, because of the greater chance of other larval settlers recruiting close by.

Test hypothesis

The test hypothesis is that adult clusters influence larval settlement, with an effect of cluster size that depends on background levels of recruitment.

The hypothesis was tested experimentally by measuring the densities of barnacles settling onto replicate patches of inter-tidal rock face during the spring settlement season. Each patch had been scraped clean of barnacles, except for a central cluster left untouched, which comprised either two, eight or 32 adults. To test for an influence of background levels of recruitment, patches were prepared on replicate shores of high and low recruitment. Analysis called for an ANOVA that cross factored the treatment with shores nested in recruitment type, which is split-plot model 5.6(i) on page 167. Because the design is fully replicated, however, it can be analysed using the equivalent completely randomised design (model 3.3(i) on page 98). We will show the analysis first with treatment as a fixed factor and then with treatment as a covariate.

With a limited budget for the experiment, it was decided to sample just two independent replicate shores within each level of recruitment. The Recruitment effect has an F-ratio denominator given by the MS for Shore$'$(Recruitment), and the low replication means it is tested with only two error d.f.; in other words, with little power to detect a difference. This is apparent from inspection of the table for model 3.3(i) on page 101, where factor A (= Recruitment) has an F-ratio denominator given by the MS for B$'$(A) (= Shore$'$(Recruitment)), with $(b-1)a$ error d.f. (= $(2-1)\times2$). Preliminary observations had suggested, however, that the two high recruitment shores were similarly high, and the two low were similarly low, which could then permit pooling error terms (see footnote a to the ANOVA table for model 3.3(i) on page 101). With three replicate patches per sample and three samples per shore, this apparent similarity between shores could be tested with 24 error d.f. giving a high power to avoid falsely accepting the null hypothesis of no difference between shores. The Treatment effect has an *F*-ratio denominator given by the MS for Treatment*Shore'(Recruitment), and having three treatment levels means it will be tested with only four error d.f., unless there is no variation between shores in the treatment effect. Doing the analysis will illustrate this weakness, and point to design improvements.

Model

$$\text{Density} = \text{Treatment} \mid \text{Shore}'(\text{Recruitment}) + \varepsilon$$

Samples of three replicate Patches (S') are nested in each level of the Treatment (C) on each shore (B'), which is nested in background Recruitment (A).

Factors	Levels	Values
A. Recruitment	2	'High' and 'Low' background recruitment of barnacles
B. Shore(Recruitment)	2	'Cowes' and 'Seaview' in High, 'Totland' and 'Ventnor' in Low
C. Treatment	3	'2', '8' and '32' adult barnacles in remnant cluster

Allocation table

The table shows larval settlement density (square-root(cm^{-2})) in samples of $n = 3$ replicate Patches in each of $c = 3$ levels of Treatment C for each of $b = 2$ levels of Shore B nested in each of $a = 2$ levels of Recruitment A.

S'(C|B(A))	High recruitment						Low recruitment					
	Cowes			Seaview			Totland			Ventnor		
Treatment 2	0.386	0.397	0.432	0.279	0.411	0.260	0.190	0.177	0.300	0.304	0.302	0.278
Treatment 8	0.484	0.482	0.514	0.625	0.531	0.478	0.268	0.261	0.396	0.402	0.351	0.254
Treatment 32	0.484	0.520	0.569	0.738	0.570	0.620	0.384	0.319	0.334	0.244	0.401	0.324

The data were arranged in four columns: Recruitment, Shore, Treatment and the numeric Density:

Recruitment	Shore	Treatment	Density
High	Cowes	2	0.386
High	Cowes	2	0.397
High	Cowes	2	0.432
High	Cowes	8	0.484
...	...	...	...
...	...	...	...
Low	Ventnor	32	0.324

Mean squares were computed in a statistics package by requesting analysis of terms: $C|A + C|B(A)$, with Shore (B) declared a random factor. In the table below, the F-ratios were calculated using the 'restricted model', which follows the protocol for constructing F-ratios described on page 35. The issue of restricted and unrestricted models is discussed on page 242.

ANOVA table

Recruitment and Treatment are fixed factors, Shore is a random block:

Source of variation	d.f.	Mean square	F-ratio	F	P
1 Recruitment	1	0.3008 52	**1/pooled(2 + 6)**[a]	79.60	<0.001
2 Shore'(Recruitment)	2	0.0031 36	**2/6**[b]	0.82	0.453
3 Treatment	2	0.0720 71	**3/5**[c]	7.18	0.047
4 Treatment*Recruitment	2	0.0166 22	**4/5**[c]	1.66	0.299
5 Treatment*Shore' (Recruitment)	4	0.0100 32	**5/6**	2.62	0.060
6 Patch'(Treatment* Shore'(Recruitment))	24	0.0038 33	–		
Total variation	35				

[a] The MS Shore'(Recruitment) gives a Recruitment effect $F_{1,2} = 95.93$, $P = 0.010$. Because Shore'(Recruitment) has $P > 0.25$, however, we assume negligible variance between nested shores, and make a more powerful test from the pooled error MS:[SS{Shore'(Recruitment)} + SS{Patch'(Treatment*Shore' (Recruitment))}]/[2 + 24] with 26 d.f. See page 38.

[b] Many packages default to an unrestricted model of random effects, which uses Treatment*Shore'(Recruitment) as the error MS, giving a Shore'(Recruitment) effect $F_{2,4} = 0.31$, $P = 0.748$. See page 242.

[c] Treatment*Shore'(Recruitment) has $P < 0.25$, ruling out *post hoc* pooling for Treatment or Treatment*Recruitment.

The analysis indicates that the response density of settling barnacles depended on the background level of recruitment ($F_{1,26} = 79.60$, $P < 0.001$) irrespective of shore ($F_{2,24} = 0.82$, $P > 0.05$), and it depended on the treatment of remnant cluster size ($F_{2,4} = 7.18$, $P < 0.05$) also irrespective of shore ($F_{4,24} = 2.62$, $P > 0.05$). Settlement density increased with cluster size irrespective of background recruitment ($F_{2,4} = 1.66$, $P > 0.05$).

Note that the design allowed only four error d.f. for testing the treatment effect and its interaction with recruitment. This meant that a significant effect could be detected only from an explained component of variation that had more than seven times the magnitude of the unexplained component (because the result: $F_{2,4} = 7.18$ gave $P = 0.047$, which lies just within the 0.05 threshold for significance). In fact, the full experiment described in Kent *et al.* (2003) had six levels of treatment, with cluster sizes of '0', '2', '4', '8', '16', '32', and the three extra levels gave ten d.f. for the error MS of Treatment*Shore'(Recruitment) in row 5. The greater range of treatment levels resulted in a much stronger treatment main effect of $F_{5,10} = 7.05$, $P = 0.005$; in other words, the six extra error d.f. helped to reduce the probability of falsely rejecting the null hypothesis by a factor of ten. Could the same improvement have been achieved by instead increasing the replication of patches to six per sample? Most likely not, since the within-sample replication does not directly influence the tests for Treatment and Treatment*Recruitment. These considerations illustrate the value of planning for analysis of variance at the design stage, in order to make the best use of available resources.

The analysis can also be done with Treatment as a covariate. We will describe the ANCOVA for the purposes of comparison, although it will be seen to provide an inferior analysis. Where previously we had three patches in each of 12 samples, we now have nine patches in each of four samples, because the three levels of Treatment now belong to one sample (instead of three), from which a regression is calculated at each level of Shore. As before, the Treatment effects in rows 3 and 4 below are tested against Treatment*Shore'(Recruitment) in row 5. In effect, the slope of the single regression for the Treatment main effect (row 3), and the variation in slopes of the two regressions for Treatment*Recruitment (row 4), are both calibrated against the variation in slopes between the shores within each level of Recruitment. This time the calibration is accomplished with only two error d.f. (compared to four with a categorical treatment), because of the reduced number of samples. The residual d.f. are correspondingly larger, at $(n-2) \times (1 \times 2 \times (2)) = 28$, with $n = 9$ responses per regression per shore and a total of four shores.

Note that some statistics packages will show 'adjusted SS' for Recruitment and Shore′(Recruitment) that differ from the 'sequential SS', even though the design is balanced and should be analysed with the sequential SS. The difference is caused by the statistics package employing a Type III adjustment, which adjusts each main effect for its interaction as well as for the other main effects. The issues of balance and adjusted SS are discussed in more detail on page 237. Some packages will use the residual term in row **6** as the default error MS for testing the main effects in rows **3** and **4**, in effect ignoring the designation of shore as a random factor for the purposes of the regressions.

ANCOVA table

Recruitment is a fixed factor, Shore is a random block, Treatment is a covariate:

Source of variation	d.f.	Mean square	*F*-ratio	*F*	*P*
1 Recruitment	1	0.3008 52	**1/pooled(2 + 6)**[a]	55.73	<0.001
2 Shore′(Recruitment)	2	0.0031 36	**2/6**	0.56	0.575
3 Treatment	1	0.0972 97	**3/5**	6.30	0.129
4 Treatment* Recruitment	1	0.0256 29	**4/5**	1.66	0.327
5 Treatment* Shore′(Recruitment)	2	0.0154 46	**5/6**[b]	2.78	0.079
6 Patch′(Treatment* Shore′(Recruitment))	28	0.0055 60	–		
Total variation	35				

[a] Pooling as in the previous table.

[b] Treatment*Shore′(Recruitment) has $P < 0.25$, ruling out *post hoc* pooling for Treatment or Treatment*Recruitment.

With only two error d.f. for testing the treatment main effect, this now appears as a non-significant covariate. These reduced error d.f. mean that the ANCOVA has lost power to distinguish the treatment effects of interest, and this time there are no gains in error d.f. to be had from testing more levels of Treatment. In addition, graphing the response against Treatment at each shore reveals a decelerating rise in settlement density with cluster size, at least on some shores. There is thus little biological information to be gained even from an ANCOVA that treats Shore as a fixed factor for the purposes of the regressions (the default option in many packages), and consequently deploys the 28 residual d.f. for measuring the regression errors. For this particular experimental design, a much more powerful and informative test was obtained from the ANOVA with Treatment as a categorical factor. The categories of Treatment moreover allow further *post hoc* testing (see page 245) to show that Density is most sensitive to smaller cluster sizes.

In general, designating a factor as a covariate may decrease its error d.f., and hence reduce the power of the analysis to distinguish effects of interest, if the model includes random cross factors (as here). Conversely, designating a factor as a covariate may increase its error d.f. if the factor would otherwise be treated as a random block or if any other cross factors are fixed, and always assuming that the covariation describes a linear response. These differences will be signalled as they arise in Chapters 1 to 3 of the model structures.

Key to types of statistical models

Use the key below to identify the appropriate chapter of model structures on the following pages, then peruse the illustrations of alternative designs to find one that matches your data structure.

(1) Can you randomly sample from a population with independent observations? *Yes* → 2; *No* → the data may not suit statistical analysis of any sort (see design considerations on page 15).
(2) Are you interested either in differences between sample averages or in relationships between covariates? *Yes* → 3; *No* → the data may not suit ANOVA or ANCOVA.
(3) Does one or more of your explanatory factors vary on a continuous scale (e.g., distance, temperature etc.) as opposed to a categorical scale (e.g., taxon, sex etc.)? *Yes* → consider treating the continuous factor as a covariate and using ANCOVA designs in Chapters 1 to 3; this will be the only option if each sampling unit takes a unique value of the factor; *No* → 4.
(4) Can all factor levels be randomly assigned to sampling units without stratifying any crossed factors and without taking repeated measures on plots or subjects? *Yes* → 5; *No* → 9.
(5) Are all combinations of factor levels fully replicated? *Yes* → 6; *No* → use an unreplicated design (Chapter 7).

Fully randomised and fully replicated designs

(6) Do your samples represent the levels of more than one explanatory factor? *Yes* → 7; *No* → use a one-factor design (Chapter 1).

(7) Is each level of one factor present in each level of another? *Yes* → 8; *No* → use a nested design with each level of one factor present in only one level of another (Chapter 2).

(8) Use a fully replicated factorial design (Chapter 3), taking account of any nesting within the cross factors (models 3.3 to 3.4).

Stratified random designs

(9) Are sampling units grouped spatially or temporally and all treatment combinations randomly assigned to units within each group? *Yes* → use a randomised-block design (Chapter 4), with analysis by corresponding Chapter-3 ANOVA tables if fully replicated; *No* → 10.

(10) Are treatments applied at different spatial scales and their levels randomly assigned to blocks or to plots within blocks, etc.? *Yes* → use a split-plot design (Chapter 5), taking account of nesting among sampling units. *No* → use a repeated-measures design (Chapter 6), taking account of repeated measures on each sampling unit in a temporal or spatial sequence. Analyse with corresponding Chapter-3 ANOVA tables if fully replicated.

How to describe a given design with a statistical model

Follow these steps to work out the statistical model associated with a given design. Then go to the appropriate chapter of the book to evaluate the amount of replication needed to give sufficient error d.f. for testing the effects of interest (see also page 248 on choosing experimental designs).

(1) Define your independent and random sampling units (S′, usually subjects or plots) from which you measure the response variable (Y), and decide how many factors contribute to explaining variation in Y. This book deals with up to three factors, so let's imagine you have three, which we will label A, B and C.

(2) You will have a fully replicated design if each sample has $n > 1$ replicates each measured once. The model then has S′ nested in all of

the explanatory factors, in the form $Y = S'(C\ B\ A)$, where the factors within the parenthesis are variously crossed or nested with each other as illustrated in Chapters 1 to 3. For example, factor B is nested in A if each level of B belongs to (or is treated to) only one level of A; factor C is cross factored with B if each level of C is represented in (or treated to) each level of B. These models are conventionally described without direct reference to S', as '$Y = C|B'(A) + \varepsilon$', etc. Here, the term ε refers to the unexplained (residual) variation of the S' around their sample means: $S'(C|B'(A))$. In a statistics package, request the model without reference to ε, as '$C|A + C|B(A)$', etc. (further detailed on page 258).

(3) If the design is not fully replicated, it may have repeated measures at one or more levels, or be fully unreplicated. Your design will have repeated measures if you measure each subject or plot, or level of a blocking factor, at more than one level of a crossed factor. For example, with repeated measures on subjects over time (C), the model takes the form $Y = C|S'(B\ A)$. The subjects S' are nested in the remaining factors A and B, because each subject belongs to (or is treated to) only one level or combination of levels of these factors. We now decide whether B is nested in A, meaning that each level of B belongs to (or is treated to) one level of A, giving the full model: $Y = C|S'(B'(A))$ as described on page 214. Alternatively, B may be cross factored with A, meaning that each level of B is represented in (or treated to) each level of A, giving the full model $Y = C|S'(B|A)$ as described on page 220. The lack of full replication means that these models have no true residual variation ε. Your statistics package may fail to complete the analysis on account of this, unless you declare all terms except the highest-order term (always the last numbered row with non-zero d.f. in the ANOVA tables in this book; see also page 258). If the repeated measures are taken within spatial blocks, then you will have a randomised-block or split-plot design, which has various forms illustrated in Chapters 4 to 6.

(4) The design is fully unreplicated if you have just one data point at each combination of levels of the factors ($n = 1$). These models of the form $Y = C|B|A$ are described in Chapter 7. As with repeated measures, the lack of replication means that they have no true residual variation ε.

A suitable statistics package can calculate SS for any of the models in this book if you declare all of the numbered terms shown in the relevant ANOVA table except for the last numbered term with non-zero d.f. (which the package will use as residual variation), and any terms with zero d.f. Use the package with care when applying it to a complex model, and check its outputs by comparing them to the relevant ANOVA table in the book. If necessary, calculate the correct F-ratios by hand.

In worked example 1 on page 47, the response of cortisol concentration was measured on replicate hens S'. There were two factors: food predictability (A), with two levels: even and patchy food, and pen (B'), with four levels per level of A. Each level of B was tested at only one level of A so the design was nested (as opposed to cross-factored). The hierarchical structure of nesting is therefore $Y = S'(B(A))$, which we conventionally write as $Y = B(A) + \varepsilon$. Because of the nesting, it may need to be requested in a statistics package in a more expanded form: $A + B(A)$, declaring B random.

In worked example 2 on page 49, the response of Chironomid larval density was measured in replicate cages S'. There were two factors: bullhead (A) and stone loach (B), each with two levels: present or absent. The design was fully replicated, with samples of $n = 5$ replicate cages, each measured once. Each level of B was treated to each level of A so the design was cross factored (as opposed to nested). The hierarchical structure of nesting is therefore $Y = S'(B|A)$, which we conventionally write as $Y = B|A + \varepsilon$, and which can be requested in a statistics package as $Y = B|A$.

In worked example 3 on page 51, the response of barnacle settlement density was measured in replicate patches (S') of cleared rock face. There were three factors: background recruitment (A), shore (B') and treatment (C). The design was fully replicated, with samples of $n = 3$ replicate patches, each measured once, so it takes the form: $Y = S'(C\ B\ A)$. Within the parenthesis, each shore was present in only one level of background recruitment, giving a nested component: $B'(A)$; each level of treatment was present in each shore and level of recruitment, adding a cross-factored component: $C|B'(A)$. The hierarchical structure of nesting is therefore $Y = S'(C|B'(A))$, which we conventionally write as: $Y = C|B'(A) + \varepsilon$. Because of the nesting, it may need to be requested in a statistics package in a more expanded form: $C|A + C|B(A)$, declaring B random.

1

One-factor designs

The simplest form of analysis of variance is the one-factor ANOVA, which seeks to compare the means of a levels of a single factor A. Each sampling unit (S′) is tested or measured in just one level of factor A, so sampling units are nested within A. In manipulative experiments, in which the investigator actively creates differences among sampling units by imposing treatments, a levels of factor A are assigned randomly amongst na sampling units, giving n independent replicate measures for each level of A. For example, to investigate the effect of herbivore attack on leaf chemistry, na plants are each subjected to one of a types of mechanical defoliation. In mensurative studies, in which the investigator exploits preexisting differences among sampling units, n independent subjects are drawn randomly from each of a populations. For example, the effect of herbivore attack on leaf chemistry could be examined by comparing n randomly selected plants showing evidence of herbivore browsing with n randomly selected undamaged control plants.

The sampling unit for a given factor level is the subject or plot:

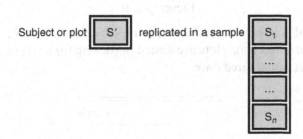

Assumptions

One-factor designs have no assumptions other than those common to all ANOVA models (page 14). Most importantly, every sampling unit or observation should be independent of all others. Repeated measurements taken from the same sampling unit are nested within that unit and should be analysed using a nested model (Chapter 2). For example, multiple leaves measured on the same plant will be correlated; treating them as independent instead of nested replicates constitutes pseudoreplication (Hurlbert 1984) and will inflate the Type I error rate.

Analysis

In the table below, we assume that samples sizes are balanced (i.e., equal n for each level of factor A). Outputs are identical for unbalanced sample sizes, except that the error d.f. $= N - a$, where $N =$ the total number of measures of the response across all factor levels. Such designs are nevertheless more sensitive to violation of the assumptions of ANOVA (page 14), particularly homogeneity of variances.

1.1 One-factor model

Model

$$Y = A + \varepsilon$$

Test hypothesis

Variation in the response Y is explained by a single factor A.

Description

Each level of A has n independent replicate subjects or plots (S'). In effect, samples of n subjects or plots are nested in (belong to) levels of factor A. Each subject is measured once.

Factors	Levels
A	a

Allocation table

The table illustrates samples of $n = 4$ replicate subjects nested in each of $a = 4$ levels of A.

S'(A)	A_1	A_2	A_3	A_4
	S_1	...	...	...
	...	...	...	...
	...	...	...	...
	S_n	...	...	S_{na}

Examples

(1) H_1: Stress in free-range hens depends upon uncertainty in the distribution of their grain, tested by measuring cortisol levels of hens housed in n replicate Pens (S') at each of a levels of food Patchiness (A). Worked example 1 on page 47 describes the experimental design in more detail. One-factor ANOVA on a response variable comprising the mean cortisol level of each cage will yield an A effect identical to that from the two-factor analysis shown in the worked example.

(2) H_1: Crop yield depends on Watering regime (A), with a regimes randomly assigned amongst na Plots (S'). The response is the yield from each plot, measured at the end of the experiment.

(3) H_1: Plant growth depends on Temperature (A), with a Temperatures randomly assigned amongst na Mesocosms (S'). The response is the mean growth of plants in each mesocosm.

(4) H_1: Breeding success of gull pairs (S') is influenced by a commercial egg Harvest (A), with three levels of impact: undisturbed control, disturbed by collectors, harvested by collectors. Planned contrasts can test for a general effect of disturbance compared to the control, and a difference in the effects of removing eggs compared to disturbance only (see page 245 for uses of contrasts). If it were possible to remove eggs without disturbance, then disturbance and harvest could have been treated as independent and fully crossed factors using model 3.1.

Comparisons

When $a = 2$, the analysis is equivalent to a Student's t test with $N - 2$ d.f. and the statistic $t = \sqrt{F}$.

Model 1.1 can be extended to include replicate measurements taken on each sampling unit (model 2.1) or a second, crossed factor applied to sampling units (model 3.1). Levels of a second, crossed factor may also be tested simultaneously in sub-plots (P′) within each plot (S′), giving split-plot model 5.6, or tested sequentially on each subject (S′), giving repeated measures model 6.3.

In testing the effect of a single treatment factor A, model 1.1 has similar objectives to randomised-block model 4.1 and repeated-measures model 6.1. Crucially it differs from both in that the assignment of the a levels of factor A to sampling units is completely randomised. Randomised-block model 4.1 accounts for sources of unwanted background variation among plots by grouping them into blocks either spatially or temporally. The random assignment of treatments to sampling units (plots within blocks) is then stratified so that every level of factor A is represented once in every block. Repeated-measures model 6.1 achieves the same goal by testing the levels of A sequentially on each subject. The order in which the treatments are assigned to sampling units (times within each subject) is randomised within each subject.

Notes

Care should be taken when testing and interpreting the effect of factors that represent different locations or times. For example, consider a study in which barnacle settlement density is measured on replicate patches of rock at three elevations (A) on a single shore. Because shore elevation is confounded by other sources of spatial variation across the shore, such as trampling intensity or predation pressure, any significant effect of A can be interpreted only as indicating differences in barnacle density with elevation on that particular shore, not as general differences among elevations on all shores. Moreover, the cause of any variation among elevations cannot be determined without further experimentation. Similarly, in a study in which the condition of blackbirds is measured in each of four seasons (A) of a year, season is confounded by other sources of temporal variation such as short-term weather events or longer-term climatic fluctuations. Any significant effect of A can be interpreted only as indicating differences in condition with season in that particular year. The null hypothesis being tested is therefore 'no difference among positions or times', rather than 'no difference among elevations or seasons'. To test the more general second hypothesis would require an experimental design in which the levels of elevation or season are replicated independently in space or time (see page 16 for details). This could be achieved by repeating the barnacle settlement study at the same three elevations on a number of replicate shores (B'), or measuring the condition of blackbirds in spring, summer, autumn and winter in a number of replicate years (B'). The design is then analysed with model 3.1 if it has replicates at each level of B'*A or otherwise by model 6.1 in a subject-by-trial design. The power to identify a main effect of elevation or season now depends on the number of replicate shores or years (b) rather than the number of replicate patches of rock at each elevation or the number of individual birds measured in each season (n).

An alternative method is to measure elevation as a covariate on a continuous scale as opposed to categorical levels, in order to seek a linear trend in barnacle settlement with elevation. Provided the elevation of each plot is measured without error, the covariate ceases to block unmeasured variation and can be treated as a fixed factor (see page 29 on uses of covariates).

ANOVA table for analysis of the term A

Model 1.1(i) *A is a fixed or random factor:*

Mean square	d.f.	Components of variation estimated in population	F-ratio
1 A	$a-1$	S′(A) + A	**1/2**
2 S′(A)	$(n-1)a$	S′(A)	–
Total variation	$na-1$		

ANCOVA table for analysis of the term A

Examples 2 and 3 above could designate A as a covariate.

The model describes a linear regression on A. Figure 2 on page 11 illustrates an example of a regression analysis with single covariate of the response. The allocation table below illustrates one sample of $n = 16$ subjects each taking one of $a = 4$ values of covariate A. Note that a full analysis is possible with or without replicate subjects for each value of A. The n subjects must sample a minimum of three values of A to allow evaluation of the assumption of a linear response.

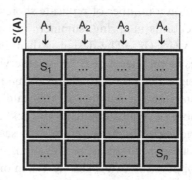

Model 1.1(*ii*) *A is a covariate of the response:*

Mean square	d.f.	Components of variation estimated in population	*F*-ratio
1 A	1	S'(A) + A	**1/2**
2 S'(A)	$n - 2$	S'(A)	–
Total variation	$n - 1$		

2

Nested designs

Nested designs extend one-factor ANOVA to consider two or more factors in a hierarchical structure. Nested factors cannot be cross factored with each other because each level of one factor exists only in one level of another (but see models 3.3 and 3.4 for cross-factored models with nesting). Nested designs allow us to quantify and compare the magnitudes of variation in the response at different spatial, temporal or organisational scales. They are used particularly for testing a factor of interest without confounding different scales of variation. For example, spatial variation in the infestation of farmed salmon with sea lice could be compared at three scales – among farms (A'), among cages within each farm (B') and among fish within each cage (S') – by sampling n fish in each of b cages on each of a farms. Similarly, seasonal variation (A) in infestation of farmed salmon by sea lice, over and above short term fluctuations in time (B'), could be measured by sampling n independent fish on b random occasions in each of a seasons.

Designs are inherently nested when treatments are applied across one organisational scale and responses are measured at a finer scale. For example the genotype of a plant may influence the mean length of its parasitic fungal hyphae. A test of this hypothesis must recognise the fact that hyphae grow in colonies (S') that are nested within leaves (C'), which in turn are nested within plants (B'), which in turn are nested in genotype (A') (discussed further on page 23). In effect, the nested design accounts for correlation among repeated measurements taken from the same plant or leaf.

Nested factors are generally random in order to ensure that higher-order factors are sampled representatively. Fixed nested factors are unusual but may be needed if levels of the nested factor are not selected at random; for example if the purpose is to control for variation between taught classes of students nested within year-group. The fixed classes must then be designated such that the random subjects nested within them also sample the higher-order factors representatively.

The sampling unit for a given combination of factor levels is the subject or plot:

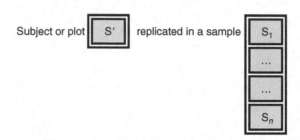

Assumptions

Nested designs have no assumptions other than those common to all ANOVA models (page 14). Note, however, that the levels of any random factors are deemed to be drawn from an infinite (or effectively infinite) population, and that if the factor is used as an error term, its samples of level means are assumed to be normally distributed with homogeneous variances between samples.

Analysis

The nested designs below all have the nested factor being measured at the same number of levels in each level of the higher-order factor. Imbalance in nested designs results in inexact F tests for all but the last term in the model. Consider using Satterthwaite's approximation (Sokal and Rohlf 1995), or deleting data points at random to reinstate balance (see page 237).

2.1 Two-factor nested model

Model

$$Y = B(A) + \varepsilon$$

Test hypothesis

Variation in the response Y is explained by treatment A and by grouping factor B nested in A.

Description

Samples of n subjects or plots (S′) are nested in levels of grouping factor B which are nested in levels of treatment A. Each subject is measured once.

Factors	Levels
A	a
B(A)	b

Allocation table

The table illustrates samples of $n = 4$ replicate subjects in each of $b = 2$ levels of B nested in each of $a = 2$ levels of A.

Examples

(1) H_1: Academic performance of students depends upon Tutorial system (A), tested by assigning each of b randomly selected Tutors (B′) of each of a Systems (A) to n randomly selected Pupils (S′).

(2) H_1: Fungal infestation of horticultural plants depends upon Fungicide (A), tested by measuring the number of fungal colonies per leaf for n Leaves (S′) randomly selected on each of b Plants (B′) subjected to one of a Fungicide treatments.

(3) H_1: Crop yield depends on Watering regime (A) with a regimes randomly assigned amongst ba Fields (B′) sampled at random across a region. Crop yield is measured in n replicate Plots (S′) in each Field. The response is the total yield from each plot measured at the end of the experiment.

(4) H_1: Plant growth depends on Temperature (A), with a Temperatures randomly assigned amongst ba Mesocosms (B′), each containing n

replicate Trays of plants (S′). The response is the mean growth of plants in each of the *nba* trays.

(5) See worked example 1 on page 47.

Comparisons

Model 2.1 is an extension of model 1.1 to include sub-sampling of each sampling unit. If there is only one observation for each level of B′, then the model reverts to model 1.1.

The design is useful when sampling units (B′) are costly or time consuming to set up, but collection of replicate observations (S′) is relatively easy. If there is little variation among levels of B′, B′(A) may be pooled into the residual error term, producing potentially substantial gains in power to test A. If *post hoc* pooling is not possible, the error d.f. for testing fixed factor A will be set by the number of levels of B′, and it is therefore a good principle of design to anticipate this eventuality by investing most effort in replication at the level of B′. Nevertheless, some replication at the lowest level of the design can usefully improve the precision of estimates for levels of B′.

Model 2.1 can be extended to include further sub-sampling (model 2.2), a third factor crossed with B′ (model 3.3) or a third factor crossed with A (model 3.4).

If B′ is a random factor that represents different locations or times then it may be regarded as a blocking factor (S′), with subjects as plots (P′) nested within blocks. Applying levels of a second treatment factor to the plots within each block then yields split-plot model 5.6.

ANOVA table for analysis of terms A + B(A)

Model 2.1(*i*) A *is fixed or random, B′ is random:*

Mean square	d.f.	Components of variation estimated in population	*F*-ratio
1 A	$a-1$	$S'(B'(A)) + B'(A) + A$	1/2[a]
2 B′(A)	$(b-1)a$	$S'(B'(A)) + B'(A)$	2/3
3 S′(B′(A))	$(n-1)ba$	$S'(B'(A))$	–
Total variation	$nba - 1$		

[a] Planned *post hoc* pooling is permissible for A if B′(A) has $P > 0.25$. Obtain the pooled error mean square from $[SS\{B'(A)\} + SS\{S'(B'(A))\}]/[a(nb-1)]$ and use $a(nb-1)$ d.f. See page 38.

ANCOVA table for analysis of terms $A + B(A)$, with A as a covariate

Factor A may be treated as a covariate, for example in measuring the diversity of arboreal arthropods in relation to woodland area A. The diversity response is measured by fumigating n trees in each of b woods of different sizes.

The model describes a linear regression on A of the mean response at each level of B. The allocation table illustrates samples of $n = 4$ replicate subjects in each of $b = 4$ samples of B each taking a unique value of covariate A. Note that a full analysis is possible with or without replicate observations (levels of B) for each value of A. The b levels of factor B must sample a minimum of three values of A to allow evaluation of the assumption of a linear response.

Model 2.1(*ii*) *A is a covariate of the response, B′ is a random factor:*

Mean square	d.f.	Components of variation estimated in population	F-ratio
1 A	1	$S'(B'(A)) + B'(A) + A$	$1/2^a$
2 B′(A)	$b - 2$	$S'(B'(A)) + B'(A)$	$2/3$
3 S′(B′(A))	$(n-1)b$	$S'(B'(A))$	–
Total variation	$nb - 1$		

[a] Planned *post hoc* pooling is permissible for A if B′(A) has $P > 0.25$. Obtain the pooled error mean square from $[SS\{B'(A)\} + SS\{S'(B'(A))\}]/[(b-2) + (n-1)b]$. See page 38.

2.2 Three-factor nested model

Model

$$Y = C(B(A)) + \varepsilon$$

Test hypothesis

Y responds to all or any of factor C' nested in factor B', or B' nested in treatment A, or A.

Description

Samples of n subjects or plots (S') are nested in levels of grouping factor C which are nested in levels of super-grouping factor B which in turn are nested in levels of treatment A. Each subject is measured once.

Factors	Levels
A	a
B(A)	b
C(B)	c

Allocation table

The table illustrates samples of $n = 4$ replicate subjects in each of $c = 2$ levels of C nested in each of $b = 2$ levels of B nested in each of $a = 2$ levels of A.

S'(C(B(A)))	A_1				A_2			
	B_1		B_2		B_3		B_4	
	C_1	C_2	C_3	C_4	C_5	C_6	C_7	C_8
S_1	...	...	...	...	...	...	...
...	...	...	...	...	...	...	...
...	...	...	...	...	...	...	...
S_n	S_{nc}	...	S_{ncb}	...	...	...	S_{ncba}

Examples

(1) H_1: Stress in laboratory mice depends upon animal husbandry practices (A), tested by measuring cortisol levels in saliva samples from n mice randomly assigned to each of c Cages (C′) maintained by b Technicians (B′) at each of $a = 2$ levels of diet Enrichment treatment: hazelnuts with shells either intact or broken.

(2) H_1: Fungal infection of horticultural plants depends upon Fungicide (A), tested by measuring the sizes of n fungal Colonies (S′) on each of c Leaves (C′) randomly selected on each of b Plants (B′) subjected to one of a Fungicide treatments.

(3) H_1: Crop yield depends on Watering regime (A), with a regimes randomly assigned amongst ba Farms (B′). Each farm contains c replicate Fields (C′), and each field contains n replicate Plots (S′). The response is the yield from each plot, measured at the end of the experiment.

(4) H_1: Plant growth depends on Temperature (A), with a temperatures randomly assigned amongst ba Mesocosms (B′). Each mesocosm contains c replicate Trays (C′), each containing n replicate plants. The response is growth of each of the $ncba$ individual Plants.

Comparisons

Model 2.2 is an extension of model 2.1 to include further sub-sampling. If there is only one observation for each level of C′, then the model reverts to model 2.1.

With C′ and B′ both random, the analysis effectively comprises a separate ANOVA at each scale in the nesting. The design is useful when sampling units (C′) are costly or time consuming to set up, but collection of replicate observations (S′) is relatively easy. If there is little variation among levels of C′, C′(B′(A)) may be pooled into the residual error term, producing potentially substantial gains in power to test A and B′(A). Likewise, if there is little variation among levels of B′, B′(A) may be pooled with C′(B′(A)), producing potentially substantial gains in power to test A. If *post hoc* pooling is not possible, the error d.f. for testing fixed factor A will be set by the number of levels of B′, and it is therefore a good principle of design to anticipate this eventuality by investing most effort in replication at the level of B′. Nevertheless, some replication at lower levels of the design can usefully improve the precision of estimates at higher levels.

If B′ and C′ are random factors that represent different locations or times then they may be regarded as blocking factors (blocks S′ and plots P′, respectively), with subjects as sub-plots (Q′) nested within plots nested within blocks. Applying levels of a second treatment factor to the plots within each block and levels of a third treatment factor to the sub-plots within each block then yields split-plot model 5.5.

ANOVA table for analysis of terms $A + B(A) + C(B\ A)$

Model 2.2(*i*) A *is fixed or random,* B′ *and* C′ *are random factors:*

Mean square	d.f.	Components of variation estimated in population	F-ratio
1 A	$a - 1$	$S'(C'(B'(A))) + C'(B'(A)) + B'(A) + A$	$1/2^a$
2 B′(A)	$(b - 1)a$	$S'(C'(B'(A))) + C'(B'(A)) + B'(A)$	$2/3^b$
3 C′(B′(A))	$(c - 1)ba$	$S'(C'(B'(A))) + C'(B'(A))$	$3/4$
4 S′(C′(B′(A)))	$(n - 1)cba$	$S'(C'(B'(A)))$	–
Total variation	$ncba - 1$		

[a] Planned *post hoc* pooling is permissible for A if B′(A) has $P > 0.25$. Obtain the pooled error mean square from $[SS\{B'(A)\} + SS\{C'(B'(A))\}]/[cb - 1)a]$. See page 38.

[b] Planned *post hoc* pooling is permissible for B′(A) if C′(B′(A)) has $P > 0.25$. Obtain the pooled error mean square from $[SS\{C'(B'(A))\} + SS\{S'(C'(B'(A)))\}]/[(nc - 1)ba]$. See page 38.

ANCOVA table for analysis of terms $A + B(A) + C(B\ A)$, with A as a covariate

Factor A may be treated as a covariate, for example in measuring the diversity of gall wasps in relation to woodland area A. The diversity response is measured by counting galls on *n* leaves from each of *c* trees in each of *b* woods of different sizes.

The model describes a linear regression on A of the mean response at each level of B. The allocation table illustrates samples of $n = 4$ replicate subjects in each of $c = 2$ samples of C in each of $b = 4$ samples of B each taking a unique value of covariate A. Note that a full analysis is possible with or without replicate observations (levels of B) for each value of A. The *b* levels of factor B must sample a minimum of three values of A to allow evaluation of the assumption of a linear response.

Model 2.2(*ii*) *A is a covariate of the response, B′ and C′ are random factors:*

Mean square	d.f.	Components of variation estimated in population	*F*-ratio
1 A	1	$S'(C'(B'(A))) + C'(B'(A)) + B'(A) + A$	**1/2**[a]
2 B′(A)	$b - 2$	$S'(C'(B'(A))) + C'(B'(A)) + B'(A)$	**2/3**[b]
3 C′(B′(A))	$(c - 1)b$	$S'(C'(B'(A))) + C'(B'(A))$	**3/4**
4 S′(C′(B′(A)))	$(n - 1)cb$	$S'(C'(B'(A)))$	–
Total variation	$ncb - 1$		

[a] Planned *post hoc* pooling is permissible for A if B′(A) has $P > 0.25$. Obtain the pooled error mean square from $[SS\{B'(A)\} + SS\{C'(B'(A))\}]/[(b - 2) + (c - 1)b]$. See page 38.

[b] Planned *post hoc* pooling is permissible for B′(A) if C′(B′(A)) has $P > 0.25$. Obtain the pooled error mean square from $[SS\{C'(B'(A))\} + SS\{S'(C'(B'(A)))\}]/[(c - 1)b + (n - 1)cb]$. See page 38.

3

Fully replicated factorial designs

Factorial models test multiple independent effects simultaneously. The models in this chapter are orthogonal designs with crossed factors, meaning that each level of each factor is tested in combination with each level of the other(s). Fully replicated orthogonal designs allow us to test whether factors influence the response additively as main effects, or whether the effect of one factor is moderated by another in an interaction. Non-orthogonal designs that cannot test interactions are best organised as a nested model. Further details of factorial designs are given on page 24.

The sampling unit for a given combination of factor levels is the subject or plot:

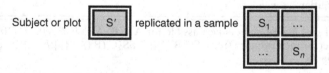

Assumptions

Fully replicated factorial designs have no assumptions other than those common to all ANOVA models (page 14). Note, however, that the levels of any random factors are deemed to be drawn from an infinite (or effectively infinite) population, and that if the factor is used as an error term, its samples of level means are assumed to be normally distributed with homogeneous variances between samples.

Analysis

Factorial designs must be analysed with respect to their hierarchy of interactions. Each interaction is entered into the model only after entering its component main effects; likewise, higher-order interactions are entered after their component lower-order interactions. The SS then account for independent components in sequence, and are aptly named 'sequential SS'. In contrast, the tabulated outputs from factorial designs should be read from the bottom upwards, in order to interpret higher-order interactions first, and lower-order interactions before main effects. This is because a significant interaction can render unnecessary further interpretation of its constituent effects. For example, in the allocation table for the two-factor model 3.1 on page 79, a response with increasing magnitude from left to right in the upper rows and from right to left in the lower rows can result in a strong interaction with apparently insignificant main effects. The interaction is all important, because each main effect is obscured by pooling across levels of the other factor. Although a main effect should not be interpreted without reference to its interactions, it may have interest in addition to them, insofar as it indicates the overall response averaged across levels of the other factor(s). Where one or more cross factors are random, significant main effects are interpretable even without reference to a significant interaction term, provided that the interaction is present in the estimated components of variation for the main effect. For example, main effect A in model 3.1(ii): $Y = B'|A + \varepsilon$ is tested against an error MS of the interaction $B'*A$, and its significance is therefore reported over and above that of the interaction. This is not the case for model 3.1(i). For both types of model, any non-significant factors should be interpreted with respect to higher-order interactions, since a significant interaction may mask real treatment effects.

The interaction plots in Figure 10 encompass the full range of possible outcomes from model 3.1: $Y = B|A + \varepsilon$, depending on which combinations of main effects and interactions are significant (shown in each equation above the graph). For each of three levels of a factor A, the lines join response means for two levels of a factor B. If factor B is a covariate, and so measured on a continuous scale on the x axis, then these lines represent linear regressions fitted to the responses at each level of A. These graphs illustrate the importance of interpreting main effects with respect to their higher-order interactions. The second row shows three alternative outcomes in which A and B both influence the response even though only one, or neither, is significant as a main effect.

With factorial designs involving several factors, the temptation to simplify models by not declaring some or all interactions should be avoided, because these terms are then pooled – untested – into the error MS (see page 40). The analysis is invalidated altogether by testing for interactions without declaring their component main effects.

Here we treat only symmetrical designs. If two factors cannot be fully crossed in principle, the existing combinations can be redefined as levels of a

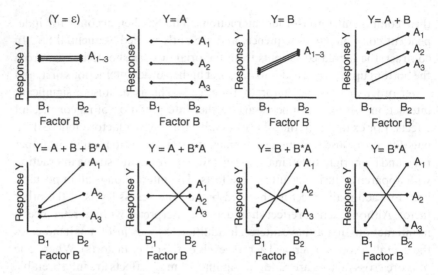

Figure 10 Alternative interaction plots for a two-factor ANOVA, showing how relationships can vary according to the influence of factors A and B additively and interactively. Statistically significant components are indicated in equations above each graph.

single factor and analysed with a priori contrasts (see page 245). Asymmetry also arises unplanned from missing data or from inherent co-dependence between factors, in which case the loss of orthogonality compromises the independence of the constituent components of variation. General linear models (GLM) accommodate this non-independence by using SS that have been adjusted for other components of the same or lower orders in the model hierarchy. When using the 'adjusted SS' of computer packages, care must be taken to ensure that the SS have not been adjusted for higher-order interactions, as to do so can invalidate the test hypotheses (see page 241).

3.1 Two-factor fully cross-factored model

Model

$$Y = B|A + \varepsilon$$

Test hypothesis

Variation in the response Y is explained by the combined effects of factor A and factor B.

Description

Samples of n subjects or plots (S') are nested in each combination of levels of B cross factored with A. Each subject is measured once.

Factors	Levels
A	a
B	b

Allocation table

The table illustrates samples of $n = 4$ replicate subjects in each of $ba = 4$ combinations of levels of B*A.

Examples

(1) H_1: Crop yield depends on a combination of Watering regime (A) and sowing Density (B) treatments, with ba combinations of levels randomly assigned amongst nba Plots (S'). The response is the yield from each plot, measured at the end of the experiment. Figure 5 on page 25 shows an example design and result.

(2) H_1: Plant growth depends on a combination of Temperature (A) and Light (B), with ba combinations of levels randomly assigned amongst nba Mesocosms (S'). The response is the mean growth of plants in each mesocosm.

(3) H_1: Condition of birds depends on Sex (A) and Species (B'), with n birds of each sex sampled for each of b randomly selected species.

(4) H_1: Seedling growth depends on fertiliser Treatment (A) and parental Genotype (B'). A total of b randomly chosen Plants (B') are grown

under identical conditions until mature, when *na* seeds are collected from each plant and sown individually into a total of *nba* Pots (S′). Each of *a* fertiliser Treatments (A) is allocated to *n* randomly selected seeds from each plant. The response is the growth of each individual seedling. Note that this design isolates the effect of parental genotype from random environmental variation arising from different locations of parent plants.

(5) A drug has been designed to treat a medical condition with a difficult diagnosis; its safety is tested by randomly assigning each of two levels of Treatment A (drug or placebo) to two samples each of *n* randomly selected volunteers, divided by Condition B (with or without the medical condition). The health response to the treatments is monitored for all individuals. A significant B*A interaction signals potential dangers of administering the drug without a definitive diagnosis, for example if it causes an improvement in health for those with the condition but provokes illness in those without the condition.

(6) See worked example 2 on page 49.

(7) See also examples to randomised-block model 4.1 on page 122 and repeated-measures model 6.1 on page 188, which are analysed with model 3.1 ANOVA tables if they are fully replicated or designate one or both factors as covariates.

Comparisons

Model 3.1 is an extension of model 1.1 to include a second crossed factor applied to subjects or plots. If there is only one observation for each of the *ba* levels of factors A and B, then the design is unreplicated and should be analysed using model 7.1.

Model 3.1 can be extended to include a third crossed factor, levels of which may be assigned randomly to subjects or plots (model 3.2), assigned randomly to replicate sampling units within each plot (model 5.9, where each plot, S′, becomes a blocking factor), or tested sequentially in random order on each subject (model 6.7). Model 3.1 can also be extended to include sub-sampling of each sampling unit (model 3.4).

In testing the combined effect of two crossed factors, model 3.1 has similar objectives to randomised-block model 4.2, split-plot models 5.1 and 5.6 and repeated-measures models 6.2 and 6.3. Crucially, however, the assignment of the *ba* levels of factors B and A to sampling units is completely randomised. Model 4.2 accounts for sources of unwanted background variation among sampling units (plots) by grouping them into blocks either spatially or temporally. The random assignment of treatments to plots within blocks is then stratified so that every combination of levels of factors A and B is represented once in every block. Split-plot models 5.1 and 5.6 achieve the same goal, but assign levels of factors A and B to sampling units at different scales. Repeated-measures models 6.2 and 6.3 account for sources of unwanted background variation among sampling units (subjects) by testing the levels of one or both factors sequentially on each subject. The order of assignment of treatments to sampling units (times within each subject) may be randomised between subjects.

If B' is a random factor that represents different locations or times then it is more properly regarded as a random blocking factor because it measures multiple sources of random spatial or temporal variation and constrains the random allocation of levels of factor A to plots. The model is then a one-factor randomised-block design (model 4.1). Full replication at each level of B'*A allows analysis by model 3.1, however, provided levels of A are randomly assigned to sampling units (plots) within each level of B'. The special assumption of homogeneity of covariances (page 118) that usually applies to randomised-block designs is then subsumed into the general assumption of homogeneity of sample variances. The principal advantage of full replication is that it allows testing of the B'*A interaction, and in the event of it being non-significant, validation of the main effect A. The B'*A interaction cannot be interpreted, however, because B' measures multiple sources of variation. The main effect of factor A may therefore be tested more efficiently with unreplicated model 4.1 which assumes a non-significant B'*A interaction for the purpose of interpreting a non-significant main effect of A.

Notes

Analysis and interpretation require care when factors are not randomly assigned to sampling units, but instead represent different locations or times, such as elevation on a shore or season of the year (see page 18 and notes to model 1.1 on page 64 for details). For example, if barnacle settlement is measured in replicate plots of different surface Rugosity (A) at three inter-tidal Elevations (B) on a single shore, then unless the objective is to test for differences among those specific locations on that particular shore, B must be regarded as a random block because any effect of elevation is completely confounded with unmeasured spatial variation across the shore. Elevation can be fixed by repeating the study at the same three elevations on two or more randomly selected shores (C′) within the region of interest. The design is then analysed with model 3.2 if it has replicate plots at each level of C′*B*A or otherwise by model 6.2 in a subject-by-trial design. The power to identify a main effect of elevation or season now depends on the number of replicate shores (c) rather than the number of replicate plots at each elevation (n).

ANOVA tables for analysis of terms B|A

Model 3.1(i) *A and B are both fixed factors:*

Mean square	d.f.	Components of variation estimated in population	F-ratio
1 A	$a-1$	$S'(B*A)+A$	1/4
2 B	$b-1$	$S'(B*A)+B$	2/4
3 B*A	$(b-1)(a-1)$	$S'(B*A)+B*A$	3/4
4 S′(B*A)	$(n-1)ba$	$S'(B*A)$	–
Total variation	$nba-1$		

Model 3.1(ii) *A is a fixed factor, B′ is a random factor (mixed model):*

Mean square	d.f.	Components of variation estimated in population	F-ratio
1 A	$a-1$	$S'(B'*A)+B'*A+A$	1/3[a]
2 B′	$b-1$	$S'(B'*A)+B'$	2/4[b]
3 B′*A	$(b-1)(a-1)$	$S'(B'*A)+B'*A$	3/4
4 S′(B′*A)	$(n-1)ba$	$S'(B'*A)$	–
Total variation	$nba-1$		

[a] Planned *post hoc* pooling is permissible for A if B′*A has $P>0.25$. Obtain the pooled error mean square from $[SS\{B'*A\}+SS\{S'(B'*A)\}]/[(b-1)(a-1)+(n-1)ba]$. See page 38.

[b] An unrestricted model tests the MS for B′ over the MS for its interaction with A (F-ratio = **2/3**). See page 242.

Model 3.1(*iii*) A' *and* B' *are both random factors:*

Mean square	d.f.	Components of variation estimated in population	F-ratio
1 A'	$a-1$	$S'(B'*A') + B'*A' + A'$	$1/3^a$
2 B'	$b-1$	$S'(B'*A') + B'*A' + B'$	$2/3^a$
3 $B'*A'$	$(b-1)(a-1)$	$S'(B'*A') + B'*A'$	$3/4$
4 $S'(B'*A')$	$(n-1)ba$	$S'(B'*A')$	–
Total variation	$nba-1$		

[a] Planned *post hoc* pooling is permissible for A' and B' if $B'*A'$ has $P > 0.25$. Obtain the pooled error mean square from $[SS\{B'*A'\} + SS\{S'(B'*A')\}]/[(b-1)(a-1) + (n-1)ba]$. See page 38.

ANCOVA tables for analysis of terms B|A, with B as a covariate

Examples 1 and 2 above could measure factor B as a covariate on a continuous scale. Figure 8 on page 31 illustrates an example of a covariate interaction.

The model describes a linear regression on B at each level of A. The allocation table illustrates $a = 2$ samples of $n = 8$ subjects, with each subject taking one of $b = 4$ values of covariate B. Note that analysis of main effects and interaction does not require replicate measures for each level of factor A at each value of covariate B, nor does it require the same values of B to be sampled within each level of A. The assumption of a linear response can only be evaluated, however, if the covariate takes more than two values. Use adjusted SS rather than sequential SS if the design is not fully orthogonal. Non-orthogonality arises from unequal replication, unequal sample sizes, or because each sampling unit takes a unique value of B (see page 237).

Model 3.1(*iv*) *A is a fixed factor, B is a covariate of the response:*

Mean square	d.f.	Components of variation estimated in population	F-ratio
1 A	$a-1$	$S'(B*A) + A$	**1/4**
2 B	1	$S'(B*A) + B$	**2/4**
3 B*A	$a-1$	$S'(B*A) + B*A$	**3/4**
4 $S'(B*A)$	$(n-2)a$	$S'(B*A)$	–
Total variation	$na-1$		

Model 3.1(*v*) *A' is a random factor, B is a covariate of the response:*

Mean square	d.f.	Components of variation estimated in population	F-ratio
1 A'	$a-1$	$S'(B*A') + A'$	**1/4**
2 B	1	$S'(B*A') + B*A' + B$	**2/3**[a]
3 B*A'	$a-1$	$S'(B*A') + B*A'$	**3/4**
4 $S'(B*A')$	$(n-2)a$	$S'(B*A')$	–
Total variation	$na-1$		

[a] Planned *post hoc* pooling is permissible for B if B*A' has $P > 0.25$. Obtain the pooled error mean square from $[SS\{B*A'\} + SS\{S'(B*A')\}]/[(a-1) + (n-2)a]$. See page 38.

Model (*v*) describes a linear regression on B at each level of A. The variation in regression slopes among levels of A provides the error term for measuring the deviation from horizontal of the average regression slope for covariate B (pooled across levels of A). Note that the default for some statistics package is to take the residual term (row **4**) as the error for the covariate main effect rather than the B*A' interaction (row **3**). Using this term requires a priori justification, because it effectively ignores the random designation of factor A. If covariate B can be redefined as a categorical factor with more than two levels, this will increase the d.f. for B*A', and therefore the error d.f. for the main effect of B, whilst decreasing the d.f. for the residual variation, which is the error term only for random effects A' and B*A'.

ANCOVA table for analysis of terms B|A, with A and B as covariates

Examples 1 and 2 above could measure factors A and B as covariates.

The model describes a plane in the dimensions of Y, A and B. The plane may tilt with Y in the A dimension (significant A effect) and/or in the B dimension (significant B effect), and/or may warp across its surface (significant B*A effect). The model can be applied to a curvilinear relationship in one-dimension by requesting the covariates as a single polynomial predictor: A|A, and taking sequential SS.

The allocation table illustrates one sample of $n = 16$ subjects each taking one of $a = 4$ values of covariate A and one of $b = 4$ values of covariate B. Note that analysis of main effects and interaction does not require replicate subjects at each combination of levels of the covariates A and B, nor does it require the same values of B to be sampled at each value of A. The assumption of linear responses can only be evaluated, however, if the covariates each take more than two values. Use adjusted SS rather than sequential SS if the design is not fully orthogonal. Non-orthogonality may arise from unequal replication or incomplete cross factoring between the covariates, or because each sampling unit takes unique values of A and B (see page 237).

Model 3.1(*vi*) *A and B are both covariates of the response:*

Mean square	d.f.	Components of variation estimated in population	F-ratio
1 A	1	$S'(B*A) + A$	1/4
2 B	1	$S'(B*A) + B$	2/4
3 B*A	1	$S'(B*A) + B*A$	3/4
4 S'(B*A)	$n - 2^2$	$S'(B*A)$	–
Total variation	$n - 1$		

3.2 Three-factor fully cross-factored model

Model

$$Y = C|B|A + \varepsilon$$

Test hypothesis

Variation in the response Y is explained by the combined effects of factors A, B and C.

Description

Samples of n subjects or plots (S') are nested in each combination of levels of C and B cross factored with A. Each subject is measured once.

Factors	Levels
A	a
B	b
C	c

Allocation table

The table illustrates samples of $n = 2$ replicate subjects in each of $cba = 8$ combinations of levels of C*B*A.

Examples

(1) H_1: Crop yield depends on a combination of Watering regime (A), sowing Density (B) and Fertiliser (C) treatments, with cba combinations

of levels randomly assigned amongst *ncba* Plots (S'). The response is the yield from each plot, measured at the end of the experiment.

(2) *Fully replicated spatial block*: H_1: Crop yield depends on a combination of sowing density (A) and Fertiliser (C) treatments, with *ca* combinations of levels randomly assigned amongst *nca* Plots (S') in each of *b* Blocks (B'). The blocks stratify a natural environmental gradient in soil moisture from top to bottom of a sloping field. The response is the yield from each plot, measured at the end of the experiment.

(3) H_1: Plant growth depends on a combination of Temperature (A), Light (B) and Fertiliser (C), with *cba* combinations of levels randomly assigned amongst *ncba* Mesocosms (S'). The response is the mean growth of plants in each mesocosm.

(4) A drug has been designed to treat a medical condition with a difficult diagnosis; its safety is tested by randomly assigning each of two levels of Treatment A (drug or placebo) to four samples each of *n* randomly selected volunteers. The four samples are divided by Condition B (with or without the medical condition) and Gender C (male or female). The health response to the treatments is monitored for all individuals. A significant C*B*A interaction signals potential dangers of administering the drug without a definitive diagnosis, for example if it improves health for females with the condition but provokes illness in males without it. Likewise, significant two-way interactions signal condition-specific and gender-specific responses to the drug.

(5) See also examples to randomised-block model 4.2 on page 129 and repeated-measures model 6.2 on page 191, which are analysed with model 3.2 ANOVA tables if they are fully replicated or designate one or more factors as covariates.

Comparisons

Model 3.2 is an extension of model 3.1 to include a third crossed factor applied to subjects or plots. If there is only one observation for each of the *cba* combinations of levels of factors A, B and C, then the design is unreplicated and should be analysed using model 7.2.

In testing the combined effect of three crossed factors, model 3.2 has similar objectives to randomised-block model 4.3, split-plot models 5.2 to 5.5, 5.7 and 5.9, and repeated-measures models 6.5 and 6.7. Crucially, however, the assignment of the *cba* levels of factors C, B and A to sampling units is completely randomised. Model 4.3 accounts for sources of unwanted background variation among plots by grouping them into blocks either spatially or temporally. The random assignment of treatments to plots within blocks is then stratified so that every combination of levels of factors A, B and C is represented once in every block. The various split-plot models achieve the same goal, but assign levels of factors A, B and C to sampling units at different scales. The repeated-measures models account for sources of unwanted background variation among subjects by testing the levels of one or more factors sequentially on each subject.

If C' is a random factor that represents different locations or times then it is more properly regarded as a random blocking factor because it measures multiple sources of random spatial or temporal variation and stratifies the random allocation of levels of factors A and B within blocks. The model is then a two-factor randomised-block design (model 4.2). Full replication at each level of $C'*B*A$ allows analysis by model 3.2, however, provided levels of A and B are randomly assigned to sampling units (plots) within each level of C'. The special assumption of homogeneity of covariances (page 118) that usually applies to randomised-block designs is then subsumed into the general assumption of homogeneity of sample variances. The principal advantage of full replication is that it allows testing of interactions with C', and in the event of their being non-significant, validation of the B|A effects. Interactions involving C' cannot be interpreted, however, because C' measures multiple sources of variation. The effect of factors A and B and their interaction B*A may therefore be tested more efficiently with unreplicated model 4.2 which assumes non-significant block-by-treatment interactions for the purpose of interpreting non-significant treatment effects.

ANOVA tables for analysis of terms C|B|A

Model 3.2(i) *A, B and C are all fixed factors:*

Mean square	d.f.	Components of variation estimated in population	F-ratio
1 A	$a-1$	$S'(C*B*A)+A$	**1/8**
2 B	$b-1$	$S'(C*B*A)+B$	**2/8**
3 B*A	$(b-1)(a-1)$	$S'(C*B*A)+B*A$	**3/8**
4 C	$c-1$	$S'(C*B*A)+C$	**4/8**
5 C*A	$(c-1)(a-1)$	$S'(C*B*A)+C*A$	**5/8**
6 C*B	$(c-1)(b-1)$	$S'(C*B*A)+C*B$	**6/8**
7 C*B*A	$(c-1)(b-1)(a-1)$	$S'(C*B*A)+C*B*A$	**7/8**
8 $S'(C*B*A)$	$(n-1)cba$	$S'(C*B*A)$	–
Total variation	$ncba-1$		

Model 3.2(ii) *A and C are fixed, B' is a random factor:*

Mean square	d.f.	Components of variation estimated in population	F-ratio
1 A	$a-1$	$S'(C*B'*A)+B'*A+A$	1/3[a]
2 B'	$b-1$	$S'(C*B'*A)+B'$	2/8[d]
3 B'*A	$(b-1)(a-1)$	$S'(C*B'*A)+B'*A$	3/8[e]
4 C	$c-1$	$S'(C*B'*A)+C*B'+C$	4/6[b]
5 C*A	$(c-1)(a-1)$	$S'(C*B'*A)+C*B'*A+C*A$	5/7[c]
6 C*B'	$(c-1)(b-1)$	$S'(C*B'*A)+C*B'$	6/8[e]
7 C*B'*A	$(c-1)(b-1)(a-1)$	$S'(C*B'*A)+C*B'*A$	7/8
8 S'(C*B'*A)	$(n-1)cba$	$S'(C*B'*A)$	–
Total variation	$ncba-1$		

[a] Planned *post hoc* pooling is permissible for A if B'*A has $P > 0.25$. Use the pooled error mean square: $[SS\{B'*A\} + SS\{S'(C*B'*A)\}]/$
$[(b-1)(a-1)+(n-1)cba]$. See page 38.

[b] Planned *post hoc* pooling is permissible for C if C*B' has $P > 0.25$. Use the pooled error mean square: $[SS\{C*B'\} + SS\{S'(C*B'*A)\}]/$
$[(c-1)(b-1)+(n-1)cba]$. See page 38.

[c] Planned *post hoc* pooling is permissible for C*A if C*B'*A has $P > 0.25$. Use the pooled error mean square: $[SS\{C*B'*A\} + SS\{S'$
$(C*B'*A)\}]/[[(c-1)(b-1)(a-1)+(n-1)cba]$. See page 38.

[d] An unrestricted model has an inexact F-ratio denominator (see page 242).

[e] An unrestricted model tests the MS for B'*A and for C*B' over the MS for the interaction term C*B'*A. See page 242.

Model 3.2(iii) A is a fixed factor, B' and C' are random factors:

Mean square	d.f.	Components of variation estimated in population	F-ratio
1 A	$a-1$	$S'(C'*B'*A)+C'*B'*A+C'*A+B'*A+A$	$1/(3+5-7)$[a]
2 B'	$b-1$	$S'(C'*B'*A)+C'*B'+B'$	$2/6$[bd]
3 B'*A	$(b-1)(a-1)$	$S'(C'*B'*A)+C'*B'*A+B'*A$	$3/7$[c]
4 C'	$c-1$	$S'(C'*B'*A)+C'*B'+C'$	$4/6$[bd]
5 C'*A	$(c-1)(a-1)$	$S'(C'*B'*A)+C'*B'*A+C'*A$	$5/7$[c]
6 C'*B'	$(c-1)(b-1)$	$S'(C'*B'*A)+C'*B'$	$6/8$[e]
7 C'*B'*A	$(c-1)(b-1)(a-1)$	$S'(C'*B'*A)+C'*B'*A$	$7/8$
8 S'(C'*B'*A)	$ncba$	$S'(C'*B'*A)$	–
Total variation	$ncba - 1$		

[a] There is no exact denominator for this test (see page 40). If B'*A and/or C'*A have $P>0.25$, however, then post hoc pooling can be used to derive an exact denominator for A. If B'*A has $P>0.25$ (but C'*A has $P<0.25$), eliminate B'*A from the mean square for A, making C'*A its error mean square. If C'*A has $P>0.25$ (but B'*A has $P<0.25$), then eliminate C'*A from the mean square for A, making B'*A its error mean square. If both B'*A and C'*A have $P>0.25$, use the pooled error mean square: $[SS\{B'*A\}+SS\{C'*A\}+SS\{C'*B'*A\}]/[(b-1)(a-1)+(c-1)(a-1)+(c-1)(b-1)(a-1)]$. See page 38.

[b] Planned post hoc pooling is permissible for B' and C' if C'*B' has $P>0.25$. Use the pooled error mean square: $[SS\{C'*B'\}+SS\{S'(C'*B'*A)\}]/[(c-1)(b-1)+(n-1)cba]$. See page 38.

[c] Planned post hoc pooling is permissible for B'*A and C'*A if C'*B'*A has $P>0.25$. Use the pooled error mean square: $[SS\{C'*B'*A\}+SS\{S'(C'*B'*A)\}]/[(c-1)(b-1)(a-1)+(n-1)cba]$. See page 38.

[d] An unrestricted model has an inexact F-ratio denominator (see page 242).

[e] An unrestricted model tests the MS for C'*B' over the MS for its interaction with A (F-ratio = **6/7**). See page 242.

90

Model 3.2(iv) A′, B′ and C′ are all random factors:

Mean square	d.f.	Components of variation estimated in population	F-ratio
1 A′	$a-1$	S′(C′*B′*A′) + C′*B′*A′ + C′*A′ + B′*A′ + A′	1/(3 + 5−7)[a]
2 B′	$b-1$	S′(C′*B′*A′) + C′*B′*A′ + C′*B′ + B′*A′ + B′	2/(3 + 6−7)[a]
3 B*A′	$(b-1)(a-1)$	S′(C′*B′*A′) + C′*B′*A′ + B′*A′	3/7[b]
4 C′	$c-1$	S′(C′*B′*A′) + C′*B′*A′ + C′*B′ + C′*A′ + C′	4/(5 + 6−7)[a]
5 C*A′	$(c-1)(a-1)$	S′(C′*B′*A′) + C′*B′*A′ + C′*A′	5/7[b]
6 C*B′	$(c-1)(b-1)$	S′(C′*B′*A′) + C′*B′*A′ + C′*B′	6/7[b]
7 C′*B′*A′	$(c-1)(b-1)(a-1)$	S′(C′*B′*A′) + C′*B′*A′	7/8
8 S′(C′*B′*A′)	$ncba$	S′(C′*B′*A′)	−
Total variation	$ncba-1$		

[a] There is no exact denominator for this test (see page 40). If higher-order interactions contributing to the mean square have $P > 0.25$, however, then they can be removed from the mean square in *post hoc* pooling to derive an exact denominator (applying the same technique as for A in model (iii) above; see page 38).

[b] Planned *post hoc* pooling is permissible for B*A′, C*A′ and C*B′ if C′*B′*A′ has $P > 0.25$. Use the pooled error mean square: [SS {C′*B′*A′} + SS{S′(C′*B′*A′)}]/[[(c−1)(b−1)(a−1) + (n−1)cba]. See page 38.

91

ANCOVA tables for analysis of terms C|B|A, with C as a covariate

Examples 1 and 3 above could measure factor C as a covariate if it is measured on a continuous scale of application rate.

The model describes a linear regression on C at each level of B|A. If a factor has more than two levels on a numerical scale, designating it as a covariate will decrease error d.f. for covariate effects, and hence reduce the power of the analysis to distinguish these effects, if the model includes random cross factors. Conversely, designating it as a covariate will increase the power of the analysis if it would otherwise be treated as a random block, or if any other cross factors are fixed, always assuming it meets the assumption of a linear response.

The allocation table illustrates $ba = 4$ samples of $n = 4$ subjects, with each subject taking one of $c = 4$ values of covariate C. Note that analysis of main effects and interactions does not require replicate measures for each combination of levels of factors A and B at each value of covariate C, nor does it require the same value of C to be sampled at each level of B|A. The assumption of a linear response can only be evaluated, however, if the covariate takes more than two values. Use adjusted SS rather than sequential SS if the design is not fully orthogonal. Non-orthogonality may arise from unequal replication or unequal sample sizes, or because each sampling unit takes a unique value of C (see page 237).

S'(C|B|A)	A_1		A_2	
	B_1	B_2	B_1	B_2
$C_1 \rightarrow$	S_1	...	...	...
$C_2 \rightarrow$	...	...	...	...
$C_3 \rightarrow$	...	...	...	...
$C_4 \rightarrow$	S_n	S_{nb}	...	S_{nba}

Model 3.2(*v*) *A and B are fixed factors, C is a covariate of the response:*

Mean square	d.f.	Components of variation estimated in population	F-ratio
1 A	$a-1$	$S'(C*B*A)+A$	**1/8**
2 B	$b-1$	$S'(C*B*A)+B$	**2/8**
3 B*A	$(b-1)(a-1)$	$S'(C*B*A)+B*A$	**3/8**
4 C	1	$S'(C*B*A)+C$	**4/8**
5 C*A	$(a-1)$	$S'(C*B*A)+C*A$	**5/8**
6 C*B	$(b-1)$	$S'(C*B*A)+C*B$	**6/8**
7 C*B*A	$(b-1)(a-1)$	$S'(C*B*A)+C*B*A$	**7/8**
8 S'(C*B*A)	$(n-2)ba$	$S'(C*B*A)$	–
Total variation	$nba-1$		

Model 3.2(*vi*) *A is a fixed factor, B' is a random factor, C is a covariate of the response:*

Mean square	d.f.	Components of variation estimated in population	F-ratio
1 A	$a-1$	$S'(C*B'*A)+B'*A+A$	**1/3**[a]
2 B'	$b-1$	$S'(C*B'*A)+B'$	**2/8**[d]
3 B'*A	$(b-1)(a-1)$	$S'(C*B'*A)+B'*A$	**3/8**
4 C	1	$S'(C*B'*A)+C*B'+C$	**4/6**[b]
5 C*A	$(a-1)$	$S'(C*B'*A)+C*B'*A+C*A$	**5/7**[c]
6 C*B'	$(b-1)$	$S'(C*B'*A)+C*B'$	**6/8**
7 C*B'*A	$(b-1)(a-1)$	$S'(C*B'*A)+C*B'*A$	**7/8**
8 S'(C*B'*A)	$(n-2)ba$	$S'(C*B'*A)$	–
Total variation	$nba-1$		

[a] Planned *post hoc* pooling is permissible for A if B'*A has $P>0.25$. Use the pooled error mean square: $[SS\{B'*A\}+SS\{S'(C*B'*A)\}]/[(b-1)(a-1)+(n-2)ba]$. See page 38.

[b] Planned *post hoc* pooling is permissible for C if C*B' has $P>0.25$. Use the pooled error mean square: $[SS\{C*B'\}+SS\{S'(C*B'*A)\}]/[(b-1)+(n-2)ba]$. See page 38.

[c] Planned *post hoc* pooling is permissible for C*A if C*B'*A has $P>0.25$. Use the pooled error mean square: $[SS\{C*B'*A\}+SS\{S'(C*B'*A)\}]/[(b-1)(a-1)+(n-2)ba]$. See page 38.

[d] An unrestricted model tests the MS for B' over the MS for B'*A (*F*-ratio = **2/3**). See page 242.

Model 3.2(*vii*) *A' and B' are random factors, C is a covariate of the response:*

Mean square	d.f.	Components of variation estimated in population	F-ratio
1 A'	$a-1$	S'(C*B'*A') + B'*A' + A'	1/3[a]
2 B'	$b-1$	S'(C*B'*A') + B'*A' + B'	2/3[a]
3 B'*A'	$(b-1)(a-1)$	S'(C*B'*A') + B'*A'	3/8
4 C	1	S'(C*B'*A') + C*B'*A' + C*B' + C*A' + C	4/(5+6−7)[b]
5 C*A'	$(a-1)$	S'(C*B'*A') + C*B'*A' + C*A'	5/7[c]
6 C*B'	$(b-1)$	S'(C*B'*A') + C*B'*A' + C*B'	6/7[c]
7 C*B'*A'	$(b-1)(a-1)$	S'(C*B'*A') + C*B'*A'	7/8
8 S'(C*B'*A')	$(n-2)ba$	S'(C*B'*A')	—
Total variation	$nba-1$		

[a] Planned *post hoc* pooling is permissible for A' and B' if B'*A' has $P > 0.25$. Use the pooled error mean square: [SS{B'*A'} + SS{S'(C*B'*A')}]/[$(b-1)(a-1) + (n-2)ba$]. See page 38.

[b] There is no exact denominator for this test (see page 40). If C*A' and/or C*B' have $P > 0.25$, however, then *post hoc* pooling can be used to derive an exact denominator for C. If C*A' has $P > 0.25$ (but C*B' has $P < 0.25$), eliminate C*A' from the mean square for C, making C*B' its error mean square. If C*B' has $P > 0.25$ (but C*A' has $P < 0.25$), then eliminate C*B' from the mean square for C, making C*A' its error mean square. If both C*B' and C*A' have $P > 0.25$, use the pooled error mean square: [SS{C*B'} + SS{C*A'} + SS{C*B'*A'}]/[$(b-1) + (a-1) + (b-1)(a-1)$]. Further pooling can be done if C*B'*A' has $P > 0.25$. See page 38.

[c] Planned *post hoc* pooling is permissible for C*A' and C*B' if C*B'*A' has $P > 0.25$. Use the pooled error mean square: [SS{C*B'*A'} + SS{S'(C*B'*A')}]/[$(b-1)(a-1) + (n-2)ba$]. See page 38.

94

ANCOVA tables for analysis of terms C|B|A, with B and C as covariates

Examples 1 and 3 above could measure factors B and C as covariates if C is measured on a continuous scale of application rate.

The model describes one plane in the dimensions of Y, B and C for each level of A. The planes may tilt with Y in the B dimension (significant B effect) and/or in the C dimension (significant C effect), and/or may warp across their surfaces (significant C*B effect), and these tilts and warps may variously differ according to the level of A (significant interactions with A). The model can be applied to a curvilinear relationship in one-dimension by treating the covariates as a single polynomial predictor and requesting analysis of terms: B|B|A with sequential SS.

The allocation table illustrates $a = 2$ samples of $n = 8$ subjects, with each subject taking one of $b = 2$ values of covariate B and one of $c = 4$ values of covariate C. Note that analysis of main effects and interactions does not require replicate measures for each level of A at each combination of values of the covariates B and C, nor does it require the same values of B and C to be sampled at each level of A. The assumption of linear responses can only be evaluated, however, if the covariates each take more than two values. Use adjusted SS rather than sequential SS if the design is not fully orthogonal. Non-orthogonality may arise from unequal replication or unequal sample sizes, or because each sampling unit takes unique values of B and C (see page 237).

$S'(C|B|A)$	A_1		A_2	
	B_1 ↓	B_2 ↓	B_1 ↓	B_2 ↓
$C_1 →$	S_1	...	...	...
$C_2 →$	...	...	...	...
$C_3 →$	...	...	...	...
$C_4 →$	...	S_n	...	S_{na}

Model 3.2(viii) *A is a fixed factor, B and C are covariates of the response:*

Mean square	d.f.	Components of variation estimated in population	F-ratio
1 A	$a-1$	$S'(C*B*A) + A$	**1/8**
2 B	1	$S'(C*B*A) + B$	**2/8**
3 B*A	$a-1$	$S'(C*B*A) + B*A$	**3/8**
4 C	1	$S'(C*B*A) + C$	**4/8**
5 C*A	$a-1$	$S'(C*B*A) + C*A$	**5/8**
6 C*B	1	$S'(C*B*A) + C*B$	**6/8**
7 C*B*A	$a-1$	$S'(C*B*A) + C*B*A$	**7/8**
8 S'(C*B*A)	$(n-2^2)a$	$S'(C*B*A)$	–
Total variation	$na-1$		

Model 3.2(ix) *A' is a random factor, B and C are covariates of the response:*

Mean square	d.f.	Components of variation estimated in population	F-ratio
1 A'	$a-1$	$S'(C*B*A') + A'$	**1/8**
2 B	1	$S'(C*B*A') + B*A' + B$	**2/3**[a]
3 B*A'	$a-1$	$S'(C*B*A') + B*A'$	**3/8**
4 C	1	$S'(C*B*A') + C*A' + C$	**4/5**[b]
5 C*A'	$a-1$	$S'(C*B*A') + C*A'$	**5/8**
6 C*B	1	$S'(C*B*A') + C*B*A' + C*B$	**6/7**[c]
7 C*B*A'	$a-1$	$S'(C*B*A') + C*B*A'$	**7/8**
8 S'(C*B*A')	$(n-2^2)a$	$S'(C*B*A')$	–
Total variation	$na-1$		

[a] Planned *post hoc* pooling is permissible for B if B*A' has $P > 0.25$. Use the pooled error mean square: $[SS\{B*A'\} + SS\{S'(C*B*A')\}]/[\ (a-1) + (n-4)a]$. See page 38.

[b] Planned *post hoc* pooling is permissible for C if C*A' has $P > 0.25$. Use the pooled error mean square: $[SS\{C*A'\} + SS\{S'(C*B*A')\}]/[1 + (n-4)a]$. See page 38.

[c] Planned *post hoc* pooling is permissible for C*B if C*B*A' has $P > 0.25$. Use the pooled error mean square: $[SS\{C*B*A'\} + SS\{S'(C*B*A')\}]/[(a-1) + (n-4)a]$. See page 38.

ANCOVA table for analysis of terms C|B|A, with A, B and C as covariates

Examples 1 and 3 above could measure factors A, B and C as covariates if C is measured on a continuous scale of application rate.

The model describes a volume in the four-dimensional space of Y, A, B and C. Sections through the volume at a given level of A may tilt with Y in the B dimension (significant B effect) and/or in the C dimension (significant C effect), and/or may warp across their surfaces (significant C*B effect), and these tilts and warps may variously differ according to the level of A (significant interactions with A). The model can be applied to a curvilinear relationship in one-dimension by treating the three covariates as a single polynomial predictor and requesting analysis of terms: A|A|A with sequential SS. Alternatively, it can be applied to a curvilinear relationship in two-dimensions by requesting two of the covariates as a single polynomial predictor: B|B|A, and taking sequential SS.

The allocation table illustrates one sample of $n = 16$ subjects each taking one of $a = 2$ values of covariate A, one of $b = 2$ values of covariate B, and one of $c = 4$ values of covariate C. Note that analysis of main effects and interactions does not require replicate subjects at every combination of values of the covariates A, B and C. The assumption of linear responses can only be evaluated, however, if the covariates each take more than two values. Use adjusted SS rather than sequential SS if the design is not fully orthogonal. Non-orthogonality may arise from unequal replication, or because each sampling unit takes unique values of A, B and C (see page 237).

S'(C|B|A)	A_1 ↓	A_1 ↓	A_2 ↓	A_2 ↓
	B_1 ↓	B_2 ↓	B_1 ↓	B_2 ↓
C_1→	S_1	...	...	...
C_2→	...	...	...	...
C_3→	...	...	...	...
C_4→	...	...	...	S_n

Model 3.2(*x*) *A, B and C are all covariates of the response:*

Mean square	d.f.	Components of variation estimated in population	F-ratio
1 A	1	$S'(C*B*A) + A$	1/8
2 B	1	$S'(C*B*A) + B$	2/8
3 B*A	1	$S'(C*B*A) + B*A$	3/8
4 C	1	$S'(C*B*A) + C$	4/8
5 C*A	1	$S'(C*B*A) + C*A$	5/8
6 C*B	1	$S'(C*B*A) + C*B$	6/8
7 C*B*A	1	$S'(C*B*A) + C*B*A$	7/8
8 S'(C*B*A)	$n - 2^3$	$S'(C*B*A)$	–
Total variation	$n - 1$		

3.3 Cross-factored with nesting model

Model

$$Y = C|B(A) + \varepsilon$$

Test hypothesis

Variation in the response Y is explained by the combined effects of treatments C and A, with levels of C measured at each level of B nested in A.

Description

Samples of *n* subjects or plots (S') are nested in each level of treatment C for each level of grouping factor B, which is nested in treatment A. Each subject is measured once.

Factors	Levels
A	*a*
B(A)	*b*
C	*c*

Allocation table

The table illustrates samples of $n = 2$ replicate subjects in each of $c = 2$ levels of C for each of $b = 2$ levels of B nested in each of $a = 2$ levels of A.

Examples

(1) H_1: Seedling growth depends upon watering regime experienced by the parent plant and fertiliser concentration. The experiment tests a levels of Watering regime (A), each allocated to b randomly chosen Plants (B'). When the plants have matured, nc seeds are collected from each of the ba plants and individually sown into a total of $ncba$ Pots (S'). Each of c concentrations of Fertiliser (C) is allocated to n pots from each of the ba plants. The response is seedling growth rate in each pot.

(2) H_1: Maternal nourishment influences subsequent dispersal distance by offspring. The experiment tests a levels of Diet quality (A), each assigned to b female Lizards (B') selected at random from the population. From each female, a random sample of n offspring of each Sex (C) is fitted with radio transmitters for monitoring subsequent dispersal.

(3) H_1: Academic performance of students depends upon tutorial system (A) and gender (C), tested by assigning each of b randomly selected Tutors (B') of each of a Systems (A) to n randomly selected Pupils (S') of each Gender (C, with two levels: male and female).

(4) See worked example 3 on page 51, which is a fully replicated split-plot analysed with model 3.3 ANOVA tables.

(5) See other examples to split-plot model 5.6 on page 168 and repeated-measures model 6.3 on page 196, which may all be analysed with model 3.3 ANOVA tables if they are fully replicated or designate one or both cross factors as covariates.

Comparisons

Model 3.3 is an extension of model 2.1 to include a third factor (C) crossed with B′. It has a similar structure to split-plot model 5.6 (where B′ corresponds with S′, and C corresponds with B) in that it tests the effect of two nested factors crossed with a third factor. It differs from model 5.6, however, in two important respects: (i) the assignment of treatments to sampling units is completely randomised, which permits full interpretation of all terms in the model; (ii) all combinations of treatment levels are fully replicated, which removes the need for a special assumption of homogeneity of covariances that would otherwise apply (page 143). In example 1, above, for instance, sowing seeds from b randomly chosen plants (B′) into individual pots (S′) isolates the variation among parent plants from all other sources of random spatial and temporal variation, which allows a significant C*B′ interaction to be interpreted unambiguously as an effect of fertiliser concentration that varies between parent plants.

If B′ is a random factor that represents different locations or times then it is more properly regarded as a random blocking factor because it measures multiple sources of random spatial or temporal variation and constrains the random allocation of levels of factor C to sampling units. The model is then a split-plot design (model 5.6). Full replication at each level of C*B′(A) nevertheless allows analysis by model 3.3, provided levels of C are randomly assigned to sampling units (plots) within each level of B′. The special assumption of homogeneity of covariances (page 143) that usually applies to split-plot designs is then subsumed into the general assumption of homogeneity of sample variances. Nonetheless, the C*B′(A) interaction cannot be interpreted because B′ measures multiple sources of variation. The main effect of factor C may therefore be tested more efficiently with unreplicated model 5.6 which assumes a non-significant C*B′(A) interaction for the purpose of interpreting a non-significant main effect of C.

Notes

Care must be taken not to inadvertently confound the effect of treatment factor B' with a random blocking factor. For instance, if the seeds from each parent plant in example 1 are all sown in the same grow-bag, then watering treatment A will be applied to whole bags (B') and fertiliser treatment C will be applied to individual seedlings within bags. The n replicates at each level of C*B'(A) allow measurement of the interaction but not its interpretation because factor B' measures both variation among parent plants and variation among grow-bags.

   Likewise, a field-based version of example 1 might allow the seeds from each plant to germinate where they fall in the vicinity of the plant. The extra realism gained by working in the field comes at the cost of reduced interpretability because B' now measures two sources of variation – random variation among parent plants and random variation among locations of parent plants – making it impossible to distinguish genetic and environmental contributions to subsequent growth.

ANOVA tables for analysis of terms C|A + C|B(A)

Model 3.3(i) A and C are fixed factors, B' is a random factor:

Mean square	d.f.	Components of variation estimated in population	F-ratio
1 A	$a-1$	$S'(C*B'(A)) + B'(A) + A$	$1/2^a$
2 B'(A)	$(b-1)a$	$S'(C*B'(A)) + B'(A)$	$2/6^c$
3 C	$c-1$	$S'(C*B'(A)) + C*B'(A) + C$	$3/5^b$
4 C*A	$(c-1)(a-1)$	$S'(C*B'(A)) + C*B'(A) + C*A$	$4/5^b$
5 C*B'(A)	$(c-1)(b-1)a$	$S'(C*B'(A)) + C*B'(A)$	5/6
6 S'(C*B'(A))	$(n-1)cba$	$S'(C*B'(A))$	–
Total variation	$ncba - 1$		

[a] Planned *post hoc* pooling is permissible for A if B'(A) has $P > 0.25$. Use the pooled error mean square: $[SS\{B'(A)\} + SS\{S'(C*B'(A))\}]/[(b-1)a + (n-1)cba]$. See page 38.

[b] Planned *post hoc* pooling is permissible for C and C*A if C*B'(A) has $P > 0.25$. Use the pooled error mean square: $[SS\{C*B'(A)\} + SS\{S'(C*B'(A))\}]/[(c-1)(b-1)a + (n-1)cba]$. See page 38.

[c] An unrestricted model tests the MS for B'(A) over the MS for its interaction with C (F-ratio = 2/5). See page 242.

Model 3.3(ii) A is a fixed factor, B' and C' are random factors:

Mean square	d.f.	Components of variation estimated in population	F-ratio
1 A	$a-1$	S'(C'∗B'(A)) + C'∗B'(A) + C'∗A + B'(A) + A	1/(2 + 4 − 5)[a]
2 B'(A)	$(b-1)a$	S'(C'∗B'(A)) + C'∗B'(A) + B'(A)	2/5[b]
3 C'	$c-1$	S'(C'∗B'(A)) + C'∗B'(A) + C'	3/5[b c]
4 C'∗A	$(c-1)(a-1)$	S'(C'∗B'(A)) + C'∗B'(A) + C'∗A	4/5[b]
5 C'∗B'(A)	$(c-1)(b-1)a$	S'(C'∗B'(A)) + C'∗B'(A)	5/6
6 S'(C'∗B'(A))	$(n-1)cba$	S'(C'∗B'(A))	–
Total variation	$ncba-1$		

[a] There is no exact denominator for this test (see page 40). If B'(A) and/or C'∗A have $P > 0.25$, however, then *post hoc* pooling can be used to derive an exact denominator for A. If B'(A) has $P > 0.25$ (but C'∗A has $P < 0.25$), then eliminate B'(A) from the mean square for A, making C'∗A its error mean square. If C'∗A has $P > 0.25$ (but B'(A) has $P < 0.25$), eliminate C'∗A from the mean square for A, making B'(A) its error mean square. If both B'(A) and C'∗A have $P > 0.25$, use the pooled error mean square: [SS{B'(A)} + SS {C'∗A} + SS{C'∗B'(A)}]/[$(b-1)a + (c-1)(a-1) + (c-1)(b-1)a$]. Further pooling can be done if C'∗B'(A) has $P > 0.25$. See page 38.

[b] Planned *post hoc* pooling is permissible for B'(A), C' and C'∗A if C'∗B'(A) has $P > 0.25$. Use the pooled error mean square: [SS{C'∗B' (A)} + SS{S'(C'∗B'(A))}]/[$(c-1)(b-1)a + (n-1)cba$]. See page 38.

[c] An unrestricted model tests the MS for C' over the MS for its interaction with A (*F*-ratio = **3/4**). See page 242.

Model 3.3(*iii*) A' and B' are random factors, C is a fixed factor:

Mean square	d.f.	Components of variation estimated in population	F-ratio
1 A'	$a-1$	$S'(C*B'(A')) + B'(A') + A'$	$1/2^{a\ d}$
2 $B'(A')$	$(b-1)a$	$S'(C*B'(A')) + B'(A')$	$2/6^{e}$
3 C	$c-1$	$S'(C*B'(A')) + C*B'(A') + C*A' + C$	$3/4^{b}$
4 $C*A'$	$(c-1)(a-1)$	$S'(C*B'(A')) + C*B'(A') + C*A'$	$4/5^{c}$
5 $C*B'(A')$	$(c-1)(b-1)a$	$S'(C*B'(A')) + C*B'(A')$	$5/6$
6 $S'(C*B'(A'))$	$(n-1)cba$	$S'(C*B'(A'))$	–
Total variation	$ncba-1$		

[a] Planned *post hoc* pooling is permissible for A' if $B'(A')$ has $P > 0.25$. Use the pooled error mean square: $[SS\{B'(A')\} + SS\{S'(C*B'(A'))\}]/[(b-1)a + (n-1)cba]$. See page 38.
[b] Planned *post hoc* pooling is permissible for C if $C*A'$ has $P > 0.25$. Use the pooled error mean square: $[SS\{C*A'\} + SS\{C*B'(A')\}]/[(c-1)(a-1) + (c-1)(b-1)a]$. See page 38.
[c] Planned *post hoc* pooling is permissible for $C*A'$ if $C*B'(A')$ has $P > 0.25$. Use the pooled error mean square: $[SS\{C*B'(A')\} + SS\{S'(C*B'(A'))\}]/[(c-1)(b-1)a + (n-1)cba]$. See page 38.
[d] An unrestricted model has an inexact F-ratio denominator (see page 242).
[e] An unrestricted model tests the MS for $B'(A')$ over the MS for its interaction with C (F-ratio $= 2/5$). See page 242.

Model 3.3(*iv*) A', B' and C' are all random factors:

Mean square	d.f.	Components of variation estimated in population	F-ratio
1 A'	$a-1$	$S'(C'*B'(A')) + C'*B'(A') + C'*A' + B'(A') + A'$	$1/(2+4-5)^{a}$
2 $B'(A')$	$(b-1)a$	$S'(C'*B'(A')) + C'*B'(A') + B'(A')$	$2/5^{b}$
3 C'	$c-1$	$S'(C'*B'(A')) + C'*B'(A') + C'*A' + C'$	$3/4^{c}$
4 $C'*A'$	$(c-1)(a-1)$	$S'(C'*B'(A')) + C'*B'(A') + C'*A'$	$4/5^{b}$
5 $C'*B'(A')$	$(c-1)(b-1)a$	$S'(C'*B'(A')) + C'*B'(A')$	$5/6$
6 $S'(C'*B'(A'))$	$(n-1)cba$	$S'(C'*B'(A'))$	–
Total variation	$ncba-1$		

[a] There is no exact denominator for this test (see page 40). If $B'(A')$ and/or $C'*A'$ have $P > 0.25$, however, then *post hoc* pooling can be used to derive an exact denominator for A'. If $B'(A')$ has $P > 0.25$ (but $C'*A'$ has $P < 0.25$), then eliminate $B'(A')$ from the mean square for A', making $C'*A'$ its error mean square. If $C'*A'$ has $P > 0.25$ (but $B'(A')$ has $P < 0.25$), eliminate $C'*A'$ from the mean square for A', making $B'(A')$ its error mean square. If both $B'(A')$ and $C'*A'$ have $P > 0.25$, use the pooled error mean square: $[SS\{B'(A')\} + SS\{C'*A'\} + SS\{C'*B'(A')\}]/[(b-1)a + (c-1)(a-1) + (c-1)(b-1)a]$. Further pooling can be done if $C'*B'(A')$ has $P > 0.25$. See page 38.
[b] Planned *post hoc* pooling is permissible for $B'(A')$ and $C'*A'$ if $C'*B'(A')$ has $P > 0.25$. Use the pooled error mean square: $[SS\{C'*B'(A')\} + SS\{S'(C'*B'(A'))\}]/[(c-1)(b-1)a + (n-1)cba]$. See page 38.
[c] Planned *post hoc* pooling is permissible for C' if $C'*A'$ has $P > 0.25$. Use the pooled error mean square: $[SS\{C'*A'\} + SS\{C'*B'(A')\}]/[(c-1)(a-1) + (c-1)(b-1)a]$. See page 38.

ANCOVA tables for analysis of terms $C|A + C|B(A)$, with C as a covariate

Example 1 above could measure factor C as a covariate on a continuous scale. If a covariate C can be redefined as a categorical factor with more than two levels, this will increase the d.f. for $C*B'(A)$, which is the error term for C and $C*A$, whilst decreasing the d.f. for the residual variation, which is the error term only for random effects. The analysis will thereby have increased power to distinguish covariate effects (see worked example 3 on page 51).

The model describes a linear regression on C at each level of B nested in A. The variation in regression slopes among the levels of B is used as the error term to test the main-effect regression slope of the covariate, and also the $C|A$ interaction describing the difference in regression slopes between levels of A. Note that some packages will use the residual term (row **6** in the tables below) as the default error MS for testing the covariate main effect and its interaction with A, in effect ignoring the designation of B as a random factor for the purposes of the regressions.

The allocation table illustrates $b = 2$ samples nested in each of $a = 2$ levels of A, with each sample containing $n = 4$ subjects and each subject taking one of $c = 4$ values of covariate C. Note that analysis of main effects and interactions does not require replicate subjects for each level of factor B at each value of covariate C, nor does it require the same value of C to be sampled at each level of B. The assumption of a linear response can only be evaluated, however, if the covariate takes more than two values. Use adjusted SS rather than sequential SS if the design is not fully orthogonal. Non-orthogonality may arise from unequal replication or unequal sample sizes, or because each sampling unit takes a unique value of C (see page 237).

S'(C|B(A))	A_1		A_2	
	B_1	B_2	B_3	B_4
$C_1 \rightarrow$	S_1	...	...	...
$C_2 \rightarrow$	...	...	...	...
$C_3 \rightarrow$	...	...	...	...
$C_4 \rightarrow$	S_n	S_{nb}	...	S_{nba}

Model 3.3(v) *A is a fixed factor, B′ is a random factor, C is a covariate of the response:*

Mean square	d.f.	Components of variation estimated in population	F-ratio
1 A	$a-1$	$S'(C*B'(A)) + B'(A) + A$	**1/2**[a]
2 B′(A)	$(b-1)a$	$S'(C*B'(A)) + B'(A)$	**2/6**
3 C	1	$S'(C*B'(A)) + C*B'(A) + C$	**3/5**[b]
4 C*A	$(a-1)$	$S'(C*B'(A)) + C*B'(A) + C*A$	**4/5**[b]
5 C*B′(A)	$(b-1)a$	$S'(C*B'(A)) + C*B'(A)$	**5/6**
6 S′(C*B′(A))	$(n-2)ba$	$S'(C*B'(A))$	–
Total variation	$nba-1$		

[a] Planned *post hoc* pooling is permissible for A if B′(A) has $P > 0.25$. Use the pooled error mean square: $[SS\{B'(A)\} + SS\{S'(C*B'(A))\}]/[(b-1)a + (n-2)ba]$. See page 38.
[b] Planned *post hoc* pooling is permissible for C and C*A if C*B′(A) has $P > 0.25$. Use the pooled error mean square: $[SS\{C*B'(A)\} + SS\{S'(C*B'(A))\}]/[(b-1)a + (n-1)ba]$. See page 38.

Model 3.3(vi) *A′ and B′ are random factors, C is a covariate of the response:*

Mean square	d.f.	Components of variation estimated in population	F-ratio
1 A′	$a-1$	$S'(C*B'(A')) + B'(A') + A'$	**1/2**[a]
2 B′(A′)	$(b-1)a$	$S'(C*B'(A')) + B'(A')$	**2/6**
3 C	1	$S'(C*B'(A')) + C*B'(A') + C*A' + C$	**3/4**[b]
4 C*A′	$(a-1)$	$S'(C*B'(A')) + C*B'(A') + C*A'$	**4/5**[c]
5 C*B′(A′)	$(b-1)a$	$S'(C*B'(A')) + C*B'(A')$	**5/6**
6 S′(C*B′(A′))	$(n-2)ba$	$S'(C*B'(A'))$	–
Total variation	$nba-1$		

[a] Planned *post hoc* pooling is permissible for A′ if B′(A′) has $P > 0.25$. Use the pooled error mean square: $[SS\{B'(A')\} + SS\{S'(C*B'(A'))\}]/[(b-1)a + (n-2)ba]$. See page 38.
[b] Planned *post hoc* pooling is permissible for C if C*A′ has $P > 0.25$. Use the pooled error mean square: $[SS\{C*A'\} + SS\{C*B'(A')\}]/[(a-1) + (b-1)a]$. See page 38.
[c] Planned *post hoc* pooling is permissible for C*A′ if C*B′(A′) has $P > 0.25$. Use the pooled error mean square: $[SS\{C*B'(A')\} + SS\{S'(C*B'(A'))\}]/[(b-1)a + (n-2)ba]$. See page 38.

ANCOVA tables for analysis of terms C|A + C|B(A), with A as a covariate

Example 1 above could measure factor A as a covariate on a continuous scale. Alternatively, factor A may be treated as a covariate, for example in measuring the diversity of arboreal arthropods in relation to woodland area A and tree species C. The diversity response is measured by fumigating n trees of each of c species in each of b woods of different sizes.

The model describes c linear regressions on A of the mean response at each level of B. The allocation table illustrates samples of $n = 2$ replicate subjects in each of $c = 2$ levels of C for each of $b = 4$ levels of B each taking a unique value of covariate A. Note that a full analysis is possible with or without replicate observations (levels of B) for each value of A. The assumption of a linear response can only be evaluated, however, if the covariate takes more than two values.

Model 3.3(*vii*) *C is a fixed factor, B′ is a random factor, A is a covariate of the response:*

Mean square	d.f.	Components of variation estimated in population	F-ratio
1 A	1	$S'(C*B'(A)) + B'(A) + A$	$1/2^a$
2 B′(A)	$b - 2$	$S'(C*B'(A)) + B'(A)$	$2/6^c$
3 C	$c - 1$	$S'(C*B'(A)) + C*B'(A) + C$	$3/5^b$
4 C*A	$c - 1$	$S'(C*B'(A)) + C*B'(A) + C*A$	$4/5^b$
5 C*B′(A)	$(c-1)(b-2)$	$S'(C*B'(A)) + C*B'(A)$	5/6
6 S′(C*B′(A))	$(n-1)cb$	$S'(C*B'(A))$	–
Total variation	$ncb - 1$		

[a] Planned *post hoc* pooling is permissible for A if B′(A) has $P > 0.25$. Use the pooled error mean square: $[SS\{B'(A)\} + SS\{S'(C*B'(A))\}]/[(b-2) + (n-1)cb]$. See page 38.
[b] Planned *post hoc* pooling is permissible for C and C*A if C*B′(A) has $P > 0.25$. Use the pooled error mean square: $[SS\{C*B'(A)\} + SS\{S'(C*B'(A))\}]/[(c-1)(b-2) + (n-1)cb]$. See page 38.
[c] An unrestricted model tests the MS for B′(A) over the MS for its interaction with C (F-ratio = **2/5**). See page 242.

Model 3.3(*viii*) B' *and* C' *are random factors, and A is a covariate of the response:*

Mean square	d.f.	Components of variation estimated in population	F-ratio
1 A	1	$S'(C'*B'(A)) + C'*B'(A) + C'*A$ $+ B'(A) + A$	$1/(2 + 4 - 5)^a$
2 B'(A)	$b - 2$	$S'(C'*B'(A)) + C'*B'(A) + B'(A)$	$2/5^b$
3 C'	$c - 1$	$S'(C'*B'(A)) + C'*B'(A) + C'$	$3/5^b$
4 C'*A	$c - 1$	$S'(C'*B'(A)) + C'*B'(A) + C'*A$	$4/5^b$
5 C'*B'(A)	$(c - 1)(b - 2)$	$S'(C'*B'(A)) + C'*B'(A)$	5/6
6 S'(C'*B'(A))	$(n - 1)cb$	$S'(C'*B'(A))$	–
Total variation	$ncb - 1$		

[a] There is no exact denominator for this test (see page 40). If B'(A) and/or C'*A have $P > 0.25$, however, then *post hoc* pooling can be used to derive an exact denominator for A. If B'(A) has $P > 0.25$ (but C'*A has $P < 0.25$), then eliminate B'(A) from the mean square for A, making C'*A its error mean square. If C'*A has $P > 0.25$ (but B'(A) has $P < 0.25$), eliminate C'*A from the mean square for A, making B'(A) its error mean square. If both B'(A) and C'*A have $P > 0.25$, use the pooled error mean square: $[SS\{B'(A)\} + SS\{C'*A\} + SS\{C'*B'(A)\}]/[(b - 2) + (c - 1) + (c - 1)(b - 2)]$. Further pooling can be done if C'*B'(A) has $P > 0.25$. See page 38.

[b] Planned *post hoc* pooling is permissible for B'(A), C' and C'*A if C'*B'(A) has $P > 0.25$. Use the pooled error mean square: $[SS\{C'*B'(A)\} + SS\{S'(C'*B'(A))\}]/[(c - 1)(b - 2) + (n - 1)cb]$. See page 38.

ANCOVA table for analysis of terms C|A + C|B(A), with A and C as covariates

Example 1 above could measure factors A and C as covariates on continuous scales. Alternatively, factors A and C may be treated as covariates, for example in measuring the diversity of arboreal arthropods in relation to woodland area A and trunk girth C. The diversity response is measured by fumigating n trees of different girths in each of b woods of different sizes.

The model describes planes in the dimensions of Y, A and C at each level of B and all hinged on the regression of the mean response at each level of B on A. The planes may tilt with Y at their common hinge in the A dimension (significant A effect) and/or they may tilt with Y in the C dimension (significant C effect), and/or they may warp across their surfaces (significant C*A effect), and the tilts in the C dimension may differ according to the level of B (significant interaction with B).

   The allocation table illustrates b samples of $n = 4$ replicate subjects, with each subject taking a unique value of covariate C, and each of the $b = 4$ levels of B taking a unique value of covariate A. Note that analysis of main effects and interactions does not require replicate subjects for each value of covariate C at each level of factor B, nor does it require replicate levels of factor B at each value of covariate A. The assumption of linear responses can only be evaluated, however, if the covariates each take more than two values.

Model 3.3(ix) *A and C are covariates of the response, B' is a random factor:*

Mean square	d.f.	Components of variation estimated in population	F-ratio
1 A	1	$S'(C*B'(A)) + B'(A) + A$	**1/2**[a]
2 B'(A)	$b-2$	$S'(C*B'(A)) + B'(A)$	**2/6**
3 C	1	$S'(C*B'(A)) + C*B'(A) + C$	**3/5**[b]
4 C*A	1	$S'(C*B'(A)) + C*B'(A) + C*A$	**4/5**[b]
5 C*B'(A)	$b-2$	$S'(C*B'(A)) + C*B'(A)$	**5/6**
6 S'(C*B'(A))	$(n-2)b$	$S'(C*B'(A))$	–
Total variation	$nb-1$		

[a] Planned *post hoc* pooling is permissible for A if B'(A) has $P > 0.25$. Use the pooled error mean square: $[SS\{B'(A)\} + SS\{S'(C*B'(A))\}]/[(b-2) + (n-2)b]$. See page 38.

[b] Planned *post hoc* pooling is permissible for C and C*A if C*B'(A) has $P > 0.25$. Use the pooled error mean square: $[SS\{C*B'(A)\} + SS\{S'(C*B'(A))\}]/[(b-2) + (n-2)b]$. See page 38.

3.4 Nested cross-factored model

Model

$$Y = C(B|A) + \varepsilon$$

Test hypothesis

Variation in the response Y is explained by the combined effects of factors A and B. Subjects are nested in sampling groups (C'), which themselves are nested within A cross factored with B.

Description

Samples of n subjects or plots (S') are nested in each level of factor C, which is nested in each combination of levels of treatments B cross factored with A. Each subject is measured once.

Factors	Levels
A	a
B	b
C(B*A)	c

Allocation table

The table illustrates samples of $n = 4$ replicate subjects in each of $c = 2$ levels of C nested in each of $ba = 4$ levels of B*A.

S'(C(B|A))	A_1				A_2			
	B_1		B_2		B_1		B_2	
	C_1	C_2	C_3	C_4	C_5	C_6	C_7	C_8
S_1	...	...	...	...	...	...	...	
...	...	...	...	...	...	...	...	
...	...	...	...	...	...	...	...	
S_n	S_{nc}	...	S_{ncb}	...	...	...	S_{ncba}	

Examples

(1) H_1: Academic performance of students depends upon tutorial system (A) and gender (B), tested by assigning each of c randomly selected Tutors (C') of each Gender (B, with two levels: male and female) and each of a Systems (A) to n randomly selected Pupils (S').

(2) H_1: Fungal infection of horticultural plants depends upon fungicide, tested by measuring the number of fungal colonies per leaf for n Leaves (S') randomly selected from each of c Plants (C') subjected to one of ba levels of Fungicide treatment A and Light treatment B.

(3) H_1: Crop yield depends on a combination of Watering regime (A) and sowing Density (B) treatments, with ba combinations of levels randomly assigned amongst cba Plots (C'). Each plot contains n replicate Plants (S'). The response is the yield from each plant, measured at the end of the experiment.

(4) H_1: Plant growth depends on a combination of Temperature (A) and Light (B), with ba combinations of levels randomly assigned amongst cba Mesocosms (C'), each containing n replicate Trays of plants (S'). The response is the mean growth of plants in each of the $ncba$ trays.

Comparisons

Model 3.4 is an extension of model 3.1 to include sub-sampling of each sampling unit. If there is only one replicate observation for each level of C', then the model reverts to model 3.1.

The design is useful when sampling units (C') are costly or time consuming to set up, but collection of replicate observations (S') is relatively easy. If there is little variation among levels of C', C'(B*A) may be pooled into the residual error term, producing potentially substantial gains in power to test main effects A and B, and their interaction B*A.

If C' is a random factor that represents different locations or times then it may be regarded as a blocking factor, with subjects as plots nested within blocks. Applying levels of a third treatment factor to the plots within each block then yields split-plot model 5.9.

ANOVA tables for analysis of terms B|A + C(B A)

Model 3.4(i) A and B are both fixed, C' is a random factor:

Mean square	d.f.	Components of variation estimated in population	F-ratio
1 A	$a-1$	$S'(C'(B*A)) + C'(B*A) + A$	$1/4^a$
2 B	$b-1$	$S'(C'(B*A)) + C'(B*A) + B$	$2/4^a$
3 B*A	$(b-1)(a-1)$	$S'(C'(B*A)) + C'(B*A) + B*A$	$3/4^a$
4 C'(B*A)	$(c-1)ba$	$S'(C'(B*A)) + C'(B*A)$	4/5
5 S'(C'(B*A))	$(n-1)cba$	$S'(C'(B*A))$	–
Total variation	$ncba - 1$		

[a] Planned *post hoc* pooling is permissible for A, B and B*A if C'(B*A) has $P > 0.25$. Obtain the pooled error mean square from $[SS\{C'(B*A)\} + SS\{S'(C'(B*A))\}]/[(c-1)ba + (n-1)cba]$. See page 38.

Model 3.4(ii) A is fixed, B' and C' are random factors:

Mean square	d.f.	Components of variation estimated in population	F-ratio
1 A	$a-1$	$S'(C'(B'*A)) + C'(B'*A) + B'*A + A$	$1/3^a$
2 B'	$b-1$	$S'(C'(B'*A)) + C'(B'*A) + B'$	$2/4^{bc}$
3 B'*A	$(b-1)(a-1)$	$S'(C'(B'*A)) + C'(B'*A) + B'*A$	$3/4^b$
4 C'(B'*A)	$(c-1)ba$	$S'(C'(B'*A)) + C'(B'*A)$	4/5
5 S'(C'(B'*A))	$(n-1)cba$	$S'(C'(B'*A))$	–
Total variation	$ncba - 1$		

[a] Planned *post hoc* pooling is permissible for A if B'*A has $P > 0.25$. Obtain the pooled error mean square from $[SS\{B'*A\} + SS\{C'(B'*A)\}]/[(b-1)(a-1) + (c-1)ba]$. See page 38. Further pooling is possible if C'(B'*A) has $P > 0.25$.
[b] Planned *post hoc* pooling is permissible for B' and B'*A if C'(B'*A) has $P > 0.25$. Obtain the pooled error mean square from $[SS\{C'(B'*A)\} + SS\{S'(C'(B'*A))\}]/[(c-1)ba + (n-1)cba]$. See page 38.
[c] An unrestricted model tests the MS for B' over the MS for its interaction with A (F-ratio = **2/3**). See page 242.

Model 3.4(iii) A', B' and C' are all random factors:

Mean square	d.f.	Components of variation estimated in population	F-ratio
1 A'	$a-1$	$S'(C'(B'*A')) + C'(B'*A') + B'*A' + A'$	$1/3^a$
2 B'	$b-1$	$S'(C'(B'*A')) + C'(B'*A') + B'*A' + B'$	$2/3^a$
3 B'*A'	$(b-1)(a-1)$	$S'(C'(B'*A')) + C'(B'*A') + B'*A'$	$3/4^b$
4 C'(B'*A')	$(c-1)ba$	$S'(C'(B'*A')) + C'(B'*A')$	4/5
5 S'(C'(B'*A'))	$(n-1)cba$	$S'(C'(B'*A'))$	–
Total variation	$ncba - 1$		

[a] Planned *post hoc* pooling is permissible for A' and B' if B'*A' has $P > 0.25$. Obtain the pooled error mean square from $[SS\{B'*A'\} + SS\{C'(B'*A')\}]/[(b-1)(a-1) + (c-1)ba]$. See page 38. Further pooling is possible if C'(B'*A') has $P > 0.25$.
[b] Planned *post hoc* pooling is permissible for B'*A' if C'(B'*A') has $P > 0.25$. Obtain the pooled error mean square from $[SS\{C'(B'*A')\} + SS\{S'(C'(B'*A'))\}]/[(c-1)ba + (n-1)cba]$. See page 38.

ANCOVA tables for analysis of terms $B|A + C(B\,A)$, with B as a covariate

Examples 3 and 4 above could measure factor B as a covariate on a continuous scale. Alternatively, factor B may be treated as a covariate, for example in measuring the diversity of arboreal arthropods in relation to woodland isolation A and area B. The diversity response is measured by fumigating n trees in each of c woodland patches of different sizes at each of a levels of isolation from neighbouring woodland.

The model describes a linear regressions on B of the mean responses at each level of C. The allocation table illustrates samples of $n = 4$ replicate subjects in each of $c = 4$ levels of C each taking a unique value of covariate B and nested in $a = 2$ levels of factor A. Note that the analysis does not require replicate measures of C at each value of covariate B, or the same values of B at each level of A. The assumption of a linear response can only be evaluated, however, if the covariate takes more than two values.

S'(C(B|A))	A_1				A_2			
	B_1 ↓	B_2 ↓	B_3 ↓	B_4 ↓	B_1 ↓	B_2 ↓	B_3 ↓	B_4 ↓
	C_1	C_2	C_3	C_4	C_5	C_6	C_7	C_8
S_1	...	...	...	...	...	...	...	...
...	...	...	...	...	...	...	...	...
...	...	...	...	...	...	...	...	...
S_n	...	...	S_{nc}	...	...	...	...	S_{nca}

Model 3.4(*iv*) *A is a fixed factor, B is a covariate of the response, C' is a random factor:*

Mean square	d.f.	Components of variation estimated in population	F-ratio
1 A	$a-1$	$S'(C'(B*A)) + C'(B*A) + A$	$1/4^a$
2 B	1	$S'(C'(B*A)) + C'(B*A) + B$	$2/4^a$
3 B*A	$a-1$	$S'(C'(B*A)) + C'(B*A) + B*A$	$3/4^a$
4 C'(B*A)	$(c-2)a$	$S'(C'(B*A)) + C'(B*A)$	4/5
5 S'(C'(B*A))	$(n-1)ca$	$S'(C'(B*A))$	–
Total variation	$nca-1$		

[a] Planned *post hoc* pooling is permissible for A, B and B*A if C'(B*A) has $P > 0.25$. Obtain the pooled error mean square from $[\text{SS}\{C'(B*A)\} + \text{SS}\{S'(C'(B*A))\}]/[(c-2)a + (n-1)ca]$. See page 38.

Model 3.4(v) *A' and C' are random factors, B is a covariate of the response:*

Mean square	d.f.	Components of variation estimated in population	F-ratio
1 A'	$a-1$	$S'(C'(B*A')) + C'(B*A') + A'$	**1/4**[a]
2 B	1	$S'(C'(B*A')) + C'(B*A') + B*A' + B$	**2/3**[b]
3 B*A'	$a-1$	$S'(C'(B*A')) + C'(B*A') + B*A'$	**3/4**[a]
4 C'(B*A')	$(c-2)a$	$S'(C'(B*A')) + C'(B*A')$	**4/5**
5 S'(C'(B*A'))	$(n-1)ca$	$S'(C'(B*A'))$	**–**
Total variation	$nca-1$		

[a] Planned *post hoc* pooling is permissible for A' and B*A' if C'(B*A') has $P > 0.25$. Obtain the pooled error mean square from $[SS\{C'(B*A')\} + SS\{S'(C'(B*A'))\}]/[(c-2)a + (n-1)ca]$. See page 38.

[b] Planned *post hoc* pooling is permissible for B if B*A' has $P > 0.25$. Obtain the pooled error mean square from $[SS\{B*A'\} + SS\{C'(B*A')\}]/[(a-1) + (c-2)a]$. See page 38. Further pooling is possible if C'(B*A') has $P > 0.25$.

ANCOVA tables for analysis of terms B|A + C(B A), with A and B as covariates

Examples 3 and 4 above could measure factors A and B as covariates on continuous scales. Alternatively, factors A and B may be treated as covariates, for example in measuring the diversity of arboreal arthropods in relation to woodland isolation A and area B. The diversity response is measured by fumigating n trees in each of c woodland patches of b sizes at each of a levels of isolation from neighbouring woodland.

The model describes a plane in the dimensions of Y, A and B with tilt and warp determined by the mean responses at each level of C. The plane may tilt with Y in the A dimension (significant A effect) and/or in the B dimension (significant B effect), and/or may warp across its surface (significant B*A effect).

The model can be applied to a curvilinear relationship in one-dimension by requesting the covariates as a single polynomial predictor: A|A, and taking sequential SS.

The allocation table illustrates samples of $n = 4$ replicate subjects in each of $c = 8$ levels of C each taking a unique combination of values of covariates B*A. Note that the analysis does not require replicate measures of C at each value of B|A, or the same values of B at each level of A. The assumption of linear responses can only be evaluated, however, if the covariates each take more than two values.

Model 3.4*(vi)* *A and B are covariates of the response, C′ is a random factor:*

Mean square	d.f.	Components of variation estimated in population	F-ratio
1 A	1	$S'(C'(B*A)) + C'(B*A) + A$	**1/4**[a]
2 B	1	$S'(C'(B*A)) + C'(B*A) + B$	**2/4**[a]
3 B*A	1	$S'(C'(B*A)) + C'(B*A) + B*A$	**3/4**[a]
4 C′(B*A)	$c - 2^2$	$S'(C'(B*A)) + C'(B*A)$	**4/5**
5 S′(C′(B*A))	$(n-1)c$	$S'(C'(B*A))$	–
Total variation	$nc - 1$		

[a] Planned *post hoc* pooling is permissible for A, B and B*A if C′(B*A) has $P > 0.25$. Obtain the pooled error mean square from $[SS\{C'(B*A)\} + SS\{S'(C'(B*A))\}]/[(c-4) + (n-1)c]$. See page 38.

4
Randomised-block designs

Blocking is a method of partitioning out unwanted sources of variation that cannot otherwise be controlled for, in order to increase the power of an analysis to detect treatment effects. Blocking factors group sampling units or observations that are essentially homogeneous, leaving the full range of natural variation in the environment to be sampled between blocks. Blocks are therefore treated as random factors because they group together, and measure simultaneously, multiple sources of variation. Due to the origins of this experimental design in agricultural field trials, the sampling units or observations nested within each block are usually termed plots:

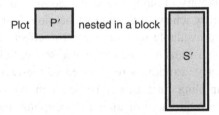

Blocks are often arbitrarily defined units of space or time. The characteristic feature of randomised-block designs is that treatment levels are randomly assigned to sampling units within each block. This distinguishes them from the fully replicated designs of Chapter 3 where treatment levels are randomly assigned across all sampling units. It also distinguishes them from repeated-measures designs, which use blocks, but assign treatment levels within each block in temporal or spatial sequence. Randomised-block models are otherwise conceptually similar to repeated-measures models of Chapter 6; taking repeated measurements on each block to control for spatial or temporal background variation is equivalent to taking repeated measurements on each subject to control for intrinsic variation between them.

115

We illustrate this similarity using S' to denote either blocks or subjects and P' to denote either plots nested in block or observations nested in subject.

Randomised-block designs are termed complete when every treatment level is present in every block. Incomplete block designs, in which every treatment level is not present in every block, present specific problems of analysis and interpretation that are summarised on pages 124 and 127.

Sampling units may be grouped into *spatial blocks* to control for known or suspected background variation from place to place. For example, in an experiment to compare the effectiveness of different fertiliser formulations on crop yield, experimental plots may be grouped into blocks to control for spatial variation in soil characteristics and microclimate across the field. Replicate pieces of field or laboratory equipment that group sampling units together spatially – such as buckets, mesocosms or PCR machines – may also be treated as blocks to control for variation among them.

Alternatively, sampling units may be grouped into *temporal blocks* to control for extraneous variables such as weather conditions, circadian cycles and drifts in calibration of equipment. For example, when sampling the densities of fish in replicate pools, runs and riffles over the course of three days, day could be included as a blocking factor to control for day-to-day variation in catch efficiency with water temperature, weather conditions and operator motivation. Temporal blocks are also used when limited availability of sampling units requires an experiment to be repeated over time to achieve adequate replication. For example, if only two mesocosms are available to investigate the effect of temperature on plant growth, pairs of trials may be conducted sequentially over time with temperature treatments randomly reallocated to the two mesocosms each time. If re-using sampling units, care must be taken to ensure that previous treatments do not contaminate or alter the sampling units in such a way that might affect the outcome of subsequent trials. Note that the identity of the sampling units is not considered as a factor in this design, and that each unit is not necessarily tested with every combination of treatments, in contrast to a subject-by-treatment repeated-measures design in which the identity of the sampling units (subjects) is considered as a factor and units are specifically tested in every level of the within-subject factor(s).

Blocks may also be discrete *biological units*, such as individual volunteers, trees or ponds. Each unit is tested in all levels of one or more treatment factors that can be randomly assigned within the unit. In a manipulative experiment, treatments are applied randomly to replicate parts of each unit; for example, the effect of ointment on acne may be tested by applying ointment to one cheek of each patient and a placebo to the other, the effect of herbivore attack on the production of trichomes may be tested by mechanically defoliating one branch on each sapling and leaving another branch intact as a control. In mensurative studies, the different levels of the within-block factor generally occur in a fixed sequence. For example, the manual dexterity of right and left hands of individual subjects, or the north and south sides of tree trunks cannot be randomly assigned, and are therefore more appropriately analysed as repeated-measures models (Chapter 6).

Randomised-block designs usually have just one observation of each treatment or treatment combination in each block, in which case the number of plots in each block equals the number of treatment combinations. The lack of within-block replication maximises the power of the experiment to detect treatment effects for a given availability of plots. It complicates the interpretation of results, however, because certain interactions between treatments and blocks cannot then be tested. Fully replicated randomised blocks, which have two or more observations of each treatment or treatment combination in each block, allow block-by-treatment interactions to be tested but often give relatively modest improvements in power for the extra resources invested (e.g., see meso-cosm example 4 on page 142). Blocked designs that have full replication are analysed by the models in Chapter 3 (further detailed in the section below on analysis of randomised-block designs).

For designs that block plots across some defined gradient (e.g., of soil moisture), the blocking factor could be substituted by a covariate measured in each plot, although there would then be little point in grouping the arrangement of plots. A more likely scenario is that a covariate is measured just once for each block, which yields an orthogonal design (modelled in Chapter 3). This approach of partitioning out sources of nuisance variation has two advantages over categorical blocks: (i) the interaction of the treatment with the covariate can be tested (unlike the interaction with a categorical block), and (ii) the covariate uses up just one d.f., so potentially leaving more error d.f. for testing the main treatment effect. These must be offset against two disadvantages: (i) the single measurement of the covariate per block makes an untested assumption that the value applies without error across the whole block, and (ii) the covariate will only increase the power of the test if it has a large, linear influence on the response. A covariate should never be used without satisfying its assumption of a linear response, because a non-significant result may mask real non-linear responses. Unless a gradient is well defined, it is often safer to partition out multiple sources of unknown random variation with a random blocking factor.

Assumptions

For models with more than two treatment levels, the restricted allocation of treatments to plots per block introduces an additional assumption of *homogeneity of covariances*. Unlike a completely randomised design, in which all sampling units are independent of each other, sampling units within a block are correlated with each other by virtue of being within the same block. This correlation does not present a problem, provided that the covariances (i.e., correlations) are the same between treatment levels within each block. This is an extension to the standard assumption of homogeneous variances that applies to all ANOVA (page 14), and it is relevant also to unreplicated split-plot (Chapter 5) and repeated-measures (Chapter 6) designs. In practice, these ANOVAs require only an additional homogeneity amongst the set of variances obtained from all pairs of treatment levels, where each variance is calculated from the differences in the response between the levels across blocks: known as the 'sphericity condition'. For a design with three levels of factor A each tested once in each of six blocks, one variance is calculated from the six differences in response between A_1 and A_2, another from the six for A_1–A_3, and the third from the six for A_2–A_3. Heterogeneity amongst these variances will result in a liberal test that inflates the Type I error rate. Kirk (1982), Winer *et al.* (1991) and Quinn and Keough (2002) suggest ways to adjust the ANOVA when this assumption is not met. If the design is fully replicated, then the assumption of homogeneity of covariances becomes subsumed within the standard assumption of homogeneity of variances between all samples.

With only one replicate sampling unit (plot) per combination of block and treatment levels, the requirement that it be drawn independently ceases to apply, but it must be representative of the block, level of A and level of B. Spatial non-independence of plots within blocks can be problematic when the sampling units are in close proximity, or when the block represents an indivisible biological unit. Care must be taken to ensure that the response of each plot is unaffected by the response of other plots in the same block. For example, in an agricultural field trial of an insecticide, plots within each block should be spaced far enough apart to ensure that insecticide concentrations applied to one plot do not contaminate neighbouring plots and that invertebrates cannot move easily from one plot to another. Similarly, an ointment applied to patients with acne should have only localised effects on the cheek to which it is applied, and not systemic effects on both control and treatment cheeks.

Despite the potential problem of non-independence among sampling units, the randomisation of treatment levels to plots within blocks ensures no systematic bias, in contrast to repeated-measures designs which are susceptible to bias from practice and carryover effects (see Chapter 6).

Unreplicated randomised-block designs generally cannot test for interactions of treatments with blocks, which must therefore be assumed to have negligible effect. Although full replication allows testing of these interactions, their interpretation remains problematic (see below).

Two approaches to analysis of randomised-block designs

Blocking factors are always random because they describe a randomly and independently drawn set of levels that group multiple sources of uncontrolled variation in a wider population (detailed on page 19). The precise identity of each block holds no value in itself and a subsequent analysis could use a different set of blocks drawn randomly from the population to re-test the same hypothesis. Random blocking factors differ from random treatment factors in two ways: they constrain the random allocation of other treatment factors to experimental units, and they measure multiple sources of variation. For example, variation among blocks of experimental plots in a field arises from sources such as soil moisture, shading, soil micro-nutrients and so on. Similarly, variation among randomly selected trees may comprise components due to individual genotype, local environmental conditions, age etc. Separating and testing these different sources of variation requires careful experimental design. For an illustration, see example 4 to model 3.1 on page 79.

Complete randomised-block experiments are analysed as factorial ANOVAs because every treatment level is present in every block. Textbooks prescribe two contrasting approaches to the analysis of randomised-block designs without full replication, which differ primarily in their a priori assumptions regarding the presence of the untestable block-by-treatment interactions. Following Newman *et al.* (1997), we term these approaches 'Model 1' and 'Model 2'. The *Model 1* approach assumes that block-by-treatment interactions are present and uses the relevant block-by-treatment MS as the *F*-ratio denominator to test treatment effects. The *Model 2* approach assumes that block-by-treatment interactions are absent and pools all block-by-treatment MS into the residual MS to test treatment effects. Be aware that textbooks and reports of analyses frequently omit to mention this assumption and give no indication in the ANOVA table that pooling has been carried out.

In practice, these two methods produce similar results for designs with a single treatment factor, but they can produce markedly different results for designs with two or more treatment factors. We illustrate both approaches for models 4.1 to 4.3 below. The Model-2 approach potentially provides a more powerful test of treatment effects but the assumption of no block-by-treatment interactions cannot be tested unless the design has replicate observations for each combination of treatments within each block to estimate the residual error term. Furthermore, Model 2 uses an error term for some treatment effects that comprises all block-by-treatment MS. For example, in model 4.2(i), A, B and their interactions are tested against the pooled error $MS[S'*A + S'*B + S'*B*A]$. Pooling in this manner assumes that these contributions to the error term have approximately equal MS values. Kirk (1982) recommends testing this assumption with an F_{max} test, and using the Model-1 approach in the event of heterogeneity of error MS contributions or significant block-by-treatment interactions.

Interpretation of non-significant treatment factors in randomised-block designs is problematic because they may indicate no treatment effect, or a treatment effect that has opposing effects in different blocks. The latter possibility often cannot be tested if the design is unreplicated. Full replication allows testing of the assumption of no significant block-by-treatment interactions and thereby – in the event of no significant interactions – validation of non-significant treatment effects. Fully replicated randomised-block designs can be analysed using equivalent completely randomised models in Chapters 1 to 3; if there is little evidence of block-by-treatment interactions (i.e., high P values), then those terms may be pooled into the residual MS to increase power to test treatment effects (see page 38). In the event of a significant block-by-treatment interaction, however, interpretation is problematic because the interaction with block means that the treatment effect may depend upon any of the multiple sources of variation encompassed by the blocking factor. Thus, the causal mechanisms giving rise to a significant block-by-treatment interaction cannot be interpreted without further experimentation. Significant treatment factors do not pose the same level of interpretative difficulty, because they are tested against interactions with the random block, and therefore report significance over and above any treatment-by-block interaction.

4.1 One-factor randomised-block model

Model

$$Y = S'|A$$

Test hypothesis

Variation in the response Y is explained by factor A.

Description

Each of a levels of treatment A is randomly assigned one of a plots (P') in each of n blocks (S'). This design is a complete randomised block because every treatment is represented in every block.

Factors	Levels	Repeated measures on S'
A	a	yes
S'	n	—

Allocation table

The table illustrates $a = 4$ levels of factor A assigned randomly amongst a plots (demarked by single lines) within each of $n = 4$ blocks (demarked by double lines). Note that the table does not indicate the spatial distribution of treatment combinations, which must be randomised within each block. For example, treatment level A_1 should not be assigned to the first plot in every block.

P'(S'|A)	S_1	S_2	S_3	S_4
A_1	P_1	...	...	P_n
A_2	...	...	...	...
A_3	...	...	...	...
A_4	...	...	...	P_{na}

Examples

(1) *Spatial block example*: H_1: Crop yield depends on sowing Density (A), with a densities randomly assigned amongst a Plots (P′) in each of n Blocks (S′). The blocks stratify a natural environmental gradient, such as soil moisture from top to bottom of a sloping field. The response is the yield from each plot, measured at the end of the experiment.

(2) *Temporal block example*: H_1: Plant growth depends on Temperature (A), with a temperatures randomly assigned amongst a Mesocosms (P′). The whole experiment is repeated with new plants n Times in sequence (S′), with temperatures randomly reassigned to mesocosms each time.

(3) *Spatial block example*: H_1: Acne is reduced by treatment with ointment, tested by applying the ointment to one cheek and a placebo to the other, with side randomised between subjects.

(4) *Spatial block example*: H_1: Barnacle settlement density on a rocky shore depends on rock-surface rugosity (A), with a roughness levels randomly assigned amongst a Plots (P′) at each of n Elevations (S′) up the shore.

Comparisons

This design can be extended to include a second crossed factor applied to whole blocks (model 5.6), to plots within blocks (model 4.2), or to replicate sub-plots within each plot (model 5.1).

When $a = 2$, model 4.1 is equivalent to a paired-sample t test. In testing the effect of a single treatment factor A, model 4.1 has similar objectives to completely randomised model 1.1 and repeated-measures model 6.1. It differs from model 1.1 in that a blocking factor (S′) partitions out unwanted sources of background variation among sampling units by grouping plots into blocks spatially or temporally. The random allocation of treatments to plots is then stratified so that each of the a levels of factor A is represented once in each block. Although the Model-1 analysis for model 4.1 is identical to that for repeated-measures model 6.1, with block corresponding with subject (S′), it escapes systematic bias from practice and carryover effects because the levels of A are randomised within each block rather than being tested sequentially on each subject.

Model 4.1 has a similar structure to model 3.1 (where S′ corresponds with B′) in that it tests the effect of two crossed factors. Indeed, the fully replicated version of model 4.1 is analysed with model 3.1. The design nevertheless differs from model 3.1 in that assignment of levels of A to sampling units is randomised only within blocks, and it is not fully replicated.

The Model-1 analysis is identical to the analysis of an unreplicated two-factor design with at least one random factor (model 7.1), except that it must meet the additional assumption of homogeneity of covariances across blocks.

Special assumptions (see also general assumptions on page 118)

The model cannot test the block-by-treatment interaction, because the lack of replication means that there is no residual error term (shaded grey in the ANOVA tables below). Interpretation of a non-significant A effect is therefore compromised by not knowing whether it arises from no effect or opposing effects in different blocks. The assumption of no significant block-by-treatment interaction can be tested if independent, replicate plots (P′) are used for each of the a treatments in each block. The design is then fully replicated and the analysis identical to that for model 3.1, with B′ substituting for S′. The interpretation of a significant block-by-treatment interaction is still problematic because the treatment effect may depend upon any of the multiple sources of variation encompassed by the blocking factor. Thus, the causal mechanisms underlying the significant interaction effect cannot be interpreted without further experimentation.

ANOVA tables for analysis of terms S + A

Model 4.1(*i*) A *is a fixed treatment,* S′ *is a random blocking factor:*

Mean square	d.f.	Components of variation estimated in population	F-ratio Model 1	F-ratio Model 2
Between n blocks				
1 S′	$n-1$	P′(S′*A) + S′	**No test**[a]	**1/3**
Between na plots				
2 A	$a-1$	P′(S′*A) + S′*A + A	**2/3**	**2/3**
3 S′*A	$(n-1)(a-1)$	P′(S′*A) + S′*A	**No test**	**No test**
4 P′(S′*A)	0	P′(S′*A)	**–**	**–**
Total variation	$na-1$			

[a] An unrestricted model tests the MS for S′ over the MS for its interaction with A (F-ratio = **1/3**). See page 242.

Model 4.1(*ii*) *A′ is a random factor, S′ is a random blocking factor*

Mean square	d.f.	Components of variation estimated in population	F-ratio Model 1	Model 2
Between n blocks				
1 S′	$b-1$	$P'(S'*A')+S'*A'+S'$	**1/3**	**1/3**
Between na plots				
2 A′	$a-1$	$P'(S'*A')+S'*A'+A'$	**2/3**	**2/3**
3 S′*A′	$(n-1)(a-1)$	$P'(S'*A')+S'*A'$	**No test**	**No test**
4 P′(S′*A′)	0	$P'(S'*A')$	–	–
Total variation	$na-1$			

Balanced incomplete-blocks variant

The randomised complete-block design has a reduced version known as a 'balanced incomplete block'. The design is incomplete because each of the n blocks tests only c levels of treatment A, where $c < a$.

The example allocation table shows four levels of treatment A tested in random pairs in each of six blocks (S′).

P′(S′|A)	S_1	S_2	S_3	S_4	S_5	S_6
A_1	P_1		P_2		P_3	
A_2	P_4			P_5		P_6
A_3		P_7	P_8			P_9
A_4		P_{10}		P_{11}	P_{12}	

This design is balanced provided that each treatment level is tested the same number of times, $r = nc/a$, and each pair of treatment levels appears in the same number of blocks, $\lambda = nc(c-1)/[a(a-1)]$. In the above example, $a = 4$, $n = 6$, $c = 2$, so $r = 3$ tests per treatment level, and $\lambda = 1$ block for each pair of treatment levels. The incomplete design means that factors A and S are not independent of each other, making it vital to randomly assign treatment levels to the c subjects (or plots) per block.

To analyse this design, request the model $Y = A + S$ in a GLM with adjusted SS (rather than sequential SS), so that the SS of A is calculated after partitioning out SS of S, and vice versa. The design assumes no interaction of S with A.

A further example of balanced incomplete blocks is the Youden square described on page 127.

Latin square variant

The 'Latin square' is an extension of a one-factor randomised-block design (model 4.1) to include a second blocking factor. The blocking factors may be both spatial, both temporal or a mixture. Its defining feature is that each blocking factor has the same number of blocks as there are levels of Factor A (treatments), and each treatment appears just once in each and every block. The design is conveniently represented as a square grid with as many columns and rows (the blocks) as treatment levels. The treatments are dispersed within the grid in such a way that they all appear once in each column (B) and once in each row (C).

Columns and rows may be treated as random blocks, or one of them may represent a fixed factor. They might account for unwanted variation in altitude or shading for example, or any unquantified spatial variation in two dimensions. Treating them as random factors means assuming that they representatively sample the true variation in the factors. The design is then a type of randomised complete block. The Latin-square design is required for crossover trials, in which treatment levels are assigned to different subjects for a given time period, after which the assignments are switched. The two blocking factors are then Subject (e.g., columns) and Time period (rows). The objective is for subjects to receive treatments in different sequences, always paying attention to the potential problem of carryover effects from one treatment into the next.

Below is an example of a Latin square layout for three treatment levels in a 3×3 grid of nine plots:

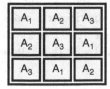

It is important that levels of the factors A, B and C are paired randomly. This can be assured for the 3×3 layout by beginning with the design above which has the levels of A in numerical order across the columns of row 1, starting with A_1 in column 1, and again in row 2 starting with A_2, etc. From this 'standard' form, randomly permute first rows and then columns of the matrix to obtain one of 12 possible Latin squares (including this one). Larger grids generate many more permutations. A 4×4 layout has 576 possible Latin squares, of which only 144 can be obtained by randomising from a standard form with the levels of A in numerical order. For these and larger squares, it is therefore recommended to ensure a truly random arrangement of treatment levels by using tables of Latin squares, or algorithms that are available on the web. Below is the design for ANOVA of the above layout.

The example allocation table shows three levels of treatment A dispersed across rows C and columns B in 3×3 standard form.

S'(C|B|A)	A_1			A_2			A_3		
	B_1	B_2	B_3	B_1	B_2	B_3	B_1	B_2	B_3
C_1	S_1				S_5				S_9
C_2			S_3	S_4				S_8	
C_3		S_2				S_6	S_7		

Regardless of whether B or C are treated as random or fixed, the design assumes no significant interactions. It is analysed with GLM, requesting the reduced model: $Y = A + B + C$. Each factor is then tested against a residual MS with $(a - 1)(a - 2)$ d.f., constructed from (SS[total] − SS[C] − SS[B] − SS[A])/($[a − 1][a − 2]$). More power can be achieved by replicating the Latin square, either in separate squares, or stacked in a single square. For example, a two-replicate stack of the 3×3 square would have six observations per treatment, distributed across three column blocks each with six plots and down six row blocks each with three plots. The increased size of the column block then allows testing of its interaction with the treatment.

The examples below are oppropriate for Latin Square designs.

(1) *Spatial example.* H_1: Crop yield in a sloping field depends on sowing Density (A). A square grid of a^2 Plots is used to control for spatial variation both down and across the slope. Within the grid, a Density treatments are randomly assigned to plots so that each treatment is tested once at each position down and across the slope.

(2) *Temporal example.* H_1: Plant growth depends on Temperature (A). Each of a ambient temperatures is randomly assigned to one of a Mesocosms (B') for a period sufficient for measuring plant growth. The whole experiment is then repeated over a Time periods (C'), each time with new plants and mesocosms reassigned to temperatures such that every mesocosm is tested at every temperature.

Youden square variant

The Youden square is a further reduction, in which a row or column has been removed from the Latin square (making it actually a rectangle). It is commonly used to balance out the effects of the position of a treatment in a repeated-measures sequence. For example, to test for predator aversion behaviour, each of b Mice (B) might be offered food tainted with a variety of predator Odours (A). Each mouse can be tested with one less than the total number of odour types, in Order (C) assigned by the Youden square.

Removing a row from the above design, we have treatment A with a levels compared across $b = a$ levels of a random block B', and $c = a - 1$ levels of a random block C'. This is one of many possible 'balanced incomplete-block' designs. The design is incomplete because it does not test each treatment level in each level of B and in each level of C (as the Latin square did). It is balanced because each treatment level is tested the same number of times, $r = bc/a$, and each pair of treatment levels appears in the same number of blocks, $\lambda = bc(c-1)/[a(a-1)]$. The design assumes no significant interactions. It is analysed with GLM, requesting the reduced model: $Y = A + B + C$. In this case, use adjusted SS in a GLM (rather than sequential, as in the Latin square), so that the SS of A is calculated after partitioning out SS of B, and vice versa.

4.2 Two-factor randomised-block model

Model
$$Y = S'|B|A$$

Test hypothesis

Variation in the response Y is explained by the combined effects of factor A and factor B.

Description

Each of ba combinations of crossed factors B and A is randomly assigned one of ba plots (P′) in each of n blocks (S′). This design is a complete randomised block because every treatment combination is represented in every block.

Factors	Levels	Repeated measures on S′
A	a	yes
B	b	yes
S′	n	–

Allocation table

The table shows $ba = 4$ combinations of levels of B*A assigned randomly amongst ba plots (demarked by single lines) within each of $n = 4$ blocks (demarked by double lines). Note that the table does not indicate the spatial distribution of treatment combinations, which must be randomised within each block. For example, treatment level B_1 should not be assigned to the first plot in every block.

Examples

(1) *Spatial block example*: H_1: Crop yield depends on a combination of sowing density (A) and Fertiliser (B) treatments, with *ba* combinations of levels randomly assigned amongst *ba* Plots (P′) in each of *n* Blocks (S′). The blocks stratify a natural environmental gradient, such as soil moisture from top to bottom of a sloping field. The response is the yield from each plot, measured at the end of the experiment.

(2) *Temporal block example*: H_1: Plant growth depends on a combination of Temperature (A) and Light (B), with *ba* combinations of levels randomly assigned amongst *ba* Mesocosms (P′). The whole experiment is repeated with new plants *n* Times in sequence (S′), with temperatures and light randomly reassigned to mesocosms each time.

Comparisons

Model 4.2 is an extension of a one-factor randomised-block model (model 4.1) to include a second crossed factor applied to plots. If A or B is random, then consider using the Latin or Youden Square variants of model 4.1 above (pages 125 to 127). The model can be extended to include a third crossed factor, which may be applied to whole blocks (model 5.7), to plots within blocks (model 4.3), or to replicate sub-plots within each plot (model 5.2).

In testing the combined effect of two crossed factors, model 4.2 has similar objectives to cross-factored models 3.1, 5.1, 5.6 and 6.2. Crucially, it differs from fully randomised model 3.1 in that the assignment of treatments to sampling units (plots) is randomised only within blocks, and it differs from split-plot models 5.1 and 5.6 in that both factors are applied to sampling units at the same scale. Although the Model 1 analysis for model 4.2 is identical to that for repeated-measures model 6.2, with block corresponding with subject (S′), it escapes systematic bias from practice and carryover effects because the levels of A and B are randomised within each block rather than being tested sequentially on each subject.

Model 4.2 has a similar structure to model 3.2 (where S′ corresponds with C′) in that it tests the effect of three crossed factors. Indeed, the fully replicated version of model 4.2 is analysed with model 3.2. The design nevertheless differs from model 3.2 in that assignment of the *ba* levels of factors A and B to sampling units is randomised only within blocks, and it is not fully replicated.

The Model-1 analysis is identical to the analysis of an unreplicated three-factor design with at least one random factor (model 7.2), except that it must meet the additional assumption of homogeneity of covariances across blocks.

Special assumptions (see also general assumptions on page 118)

The model assumes that some or all block-by-treatment interactions are absent or not significant, many of which cannot be tested anyway because the lack of replication means that there is no residual error term (shaded grey in the ANOVA tables below). Interpretation of non-significant A, B or A*B is compromised because it could result either from no effect, or from opposing effects in different blocks. The assumption of no significant block-by-treatment interactions can be tested if independent, replicate plots (P′) are used for each of the *ab* treatment combinations in each block. The design is then fully replicated and the analysis identical to that for model 3.2, with C′ substituting for S′. The interpretation of a significant block-by-treatment interaction is nevertheless problematic because the treatment effect may depend upon any of the multiple sources of variation encompassed by the blocking factor. Thus, the causal mechanisms underlying the significant interaction effect cannot be interpreted without further experimentation.

If all block-by-treatment interactions are assumed to be absent, the error term for some treatment effects may comprise all block-by-treatment MS (Model 2, Newman *et al.* 1997). For example, in model 4.2 (*i*), A, B and B*A are tested against the pooled error MS[S′*A + S′*B + S′*B*A]. Pooling in this manner assumes that these contributions to the error term have approximately equal MS values (see page 120).

ANOVA tables for analysis of terms S|B|A – S*B*A (Model 1) or S + B|A (Model 2)

Model 4.2(i) A and B are fixed treatments, S' is a random blocking factor:

Mean square	d.f.	Components of variation estimated in population	F-ratio Model 1	F-ratio Model 2
Between n blocks				
1 S'	$n-1$	P'(S'*B*A)+S'	No test[a]	1/p[5+6+7]
Between nba plots				
2 A	$a-1$	P'(S'*B*A)+S'*A+A	2/5	2/p[5+6+7]
3 B	$b-1$	P'(S'*B*A)+S'*B+B	3/6	3/p[5+6+7]
4 B*A	$(b-1)(a-1)$	P'(S'*B*A)+S'*B*A+B*A	4/7	4/p[5+6+7]
5 S'*A	$(n-1)(a-1)$	P'(S'*B*A)+S'*A	No test	No test
6 S'*B	$(n-1)(b-1)$	P'(S'*B*A)+S'*B	No test	No test
7 S'*B*A	$(n-1)(b-1)(a-1)$	P'(S'*B*A)+S'*B*A	No test	No test
8 P'(S'*B*A)	0	P'(S'*B*A)	–	–
Total variation	$nba-1$			

[a] An unrestricted model has an inexact F-ratio denominator (see page 242).

131

Model 4.2(*ii*) *A is a fixed treatment, B' is a random factor, S' is a random blocking factor:*

Mean square	d.f.	Components of variation estimated in population	F-ratio Model 1	F-ratio Model 2
Between *n* blocks				
1 S'	$n-1$	$P'(S'*B'*A)+S'*B'+S'$	1/6[b]	1/p[5+6+7]
Between *nba* plots				
2 A	$a-1$	$P'(S'*B'*A)+S'*B'*A+S'*A+B'*A+A$	2/(4+5−7)[ab]	2/4
3 B'	$b-1$	$P'(S'*B'*A)+S'*B'+B'$	3/6[b]	3/p[5+6+7][c]
4 B'*A	$(b-1)(a-1)$	$P'(S'*B'*A)+S'*B'*A+B'*A$	4/7	4/p[5+6+7]
5 S'*A	$(n-1)(a-1)$	$P'(S'*B'*A)+S'*B'*A+S'*A$	5/7	Not tested
6 S'*B'	$(n-1)(b-1)$	$P'(S'*B'*A)+S'*B'$	No test	No test
7 S'*B'*A	$(n-1)(b-1)(a-1)$	$P'(S'*B'*A)+S'*B'*A$	No test	No test
8 P'(S'*B'*A)	0	$P'(S'*B'*A)$	–	–
Total variation	$nba-1$			

[a] There is no exact denominator for this test (see page 40). If B'*A and/or S'*A have $P>0.25$, however, then *post hoc* pooling can be used to derive an exact denominator for A. If B'*A has $P>0.25$ (but S'*A has $P<0.25$), eliminate B'*A from the mean square for A, making S'*A its error mean square. If S'*A has $P>0.25$ (but B'*A has $P<0.25$), then eliminate S'*A from the mean square for A, making B'*A its error mean square. If both B'*A and S'*A have $P>0.25$, use the pooled error mean square: [SS{B'*A}+ SS{S'*A}+SS{S'*B'*A}]/[(b−1)(a−1)+(n−1)(a−1)+(n−1)(b−1)(a−1)]. See page 38.

[b] An unrestricted model has an inexact F-ratio denominator (see page 242).

[c] An unrestricted model tests B' over the MS for its interaction with A (F-ratio = **3/4**). See page 242.

Model 4.2(iii) A' and B' are random factors, S' is a random blocking factor:

Mean square	d.f.	Components of variation estimated in population	F-ratio Model 1	F-ratio Model 2
Between n blocks				
1 S'	$n-1$	$P'(S'*B'*A') + S'*B'*A' + S'*B' + S'*A' + S'$	$1/(5+6-7)$[a]	$1/p[5+6+7]$
Between nba plots				
2 A'	$a-1$	$P'(S'*B'*A') + S'*B'*A' + S'*A' + B'*A' + A'$	$2(4+5-7)$[a]	2/4
3 B'	$b-1$	$P'(S'*B'*A') + S'*B'*A' + S'*B' + B'*A' + B'$	$3(4+6-7)$[a]	3/4
4 B'*A'	$(b-1)(a-1)$	$P'(S'*B'*A') + S'*B'*A' + B'*A'$	4/7	$4/p[5+6+7]$
5 S'*A'	$(n-1)(a-1)$	$P'(S'*B'*A') + S'*B'*A' + S'*A'$	5/7	Not tested
6 S'*B'	$(n-1)(b-1)$	$P'(S'*B'*A') + S'*B'*A' + S'*B'$	6/7	Not tested
7 S'*B'*A'	$(n-1)(b-1)(a-1)$	$P'(S'*B'*A') + S'*B'*A'$	No test	No test
8 P'(S'*B'*A')	0	$P'(S'*B'*A')$	–	–
Total variation	$nba-1$			

[a] There is no exact denominator for this test (see page 40). If higher-order interactions contributing to the mean square have $P > 0.25$, however, then they can be removed from the mean square in *post hoc* pooling to derive an exact denominator (applying the same technique as for A in model (*ii*) above).

133

4.3 Three-factor randomised-block model

Model

$$Y = S'|C|B|A$$

Test hypothesis

Variation in the response Y is explained by the combined effects of factor A, factor B and factor C.

Description

Each of *cba* combinations of crossed factors C, B and A is randomly assigned one of *cba* plots (P') in each of *n* blocks (S'). This design is a complete randomised block because every treatment combination is represented in every block.

Factors	Levels	Repeated measures on S'
A	*a*	yes
B	*b*	yes
C	*c*	yes
S'	*n*	–

Allocation table

The table shows *cba* = 8 combinations of levels of C*B*A assigned randomly amongst *cba* plots (demarked by single lines) within each of *n* = 4 blocks (demarked by double lines). Note that the table does not indicate the spatial distribution of treatment combinations, which must be randomised within each block. For example, treatment level C_1 should not be assigned to the first plot in every block.

P'(S'|C|B|A)			S_1	S_2	S_3	S_4
A_1	B_1	C_1	P_1	...	...	P_n
		C_2	...	...	...	P_{nc}
	B_2	C_1	...	...	...	...
		C_2	...	...	...	P_{ncb}
A_2	B_1	C_1	...	...	...	...
		C_2	...	...	...	...
	B_2	C_1	...	...	...	...
		C_2	...	...	...	P_{ncba}

Examples

(1) *Spatial block example*: H_1: Crop yield depends on a combination of Herbicide (A), sowing Density (B) and Fertiliser (C) treatments, with *cba* combinations of levels randomly assigned amongst *cba* Plots (P') in each of *n* Blocks (S'). The blocks stratify a natural environmental gradient, such as soil moisture from top to bottom of a sloping field. The response is the yield from each Plot, measured at the end of the experiment.

(2) *Temporal block example*: H_1: Plant growth depends on a combination of Temperature (A), Light (B) and Fertiliser (C), with *cba* combinations of levels randomly assigned amongst *cba* Mesocosms (P'). The whole experiment is repeated with new plants *n* Times in sequence (S'), with temperatures, light levels and fertiliser type randomly reassigned to mesocosms each time. It is likely that different fertiliser treatments can be applied within each mesocosm, in which case use model 5.2, which uses only *ba* mesocosms.

Comparisons

Model 4.3 is an extension of a two-factor randomised-block model (model 4.2) to include a third crossed factor applied to plots. In testing the combined effect of three crossed factors, model 4.3 has similar objectives to completely randomised model 3.2, split-plot models 5.2, 5.3, 5.4, 5.5, 5.7, 5.9 and repeated-measures models 6.5 and 6.7. Crucially, it differs from model 3.2 in that the assignment of treatments to sampling units (plots) is not completely randomised. It differs from the various split-plot models in that factors A, B and C are assigned to sampling units at the same scale, and from the repeated-measures models in that factor levels are randomly assigned within blocks rather than being applied in sequence.

Special assumptions (see also general assumptions on page 118)

The model assumes that some or all block-by-treatment interactions are absent or not significant, many of which cannot be tested anyway because the lack of replication means that there is no residual error term (shaded grey in the ANOVA tables below). Interpretation of non-significant effects amongst A, B, C and their interactions is compromised because the result could mean either no effect, or opposing effects in different blocks. The assumption of no significant block-by-treatment interactions can be tested if independent, replicate plots (P') are used for each of the *cba* treatment combinations in each block. The interpretation of a significant block-by-treatment interaction is nevertheless problematic because the treatment effect may depend upon any of the multiple sources of variation encompassed by the blocking factor. Thus, the causal mechanisms underlying the significant interaction effect cannot be interpreted without further experimentation.

If all block-by-treatment interactions are assumed to be absent, the error term for some treatment effects may comprise all block-by-treatment MS (Model 2, Newman *et al.* 1997). For example, in model 4.3(*i*), A, B, C and their interactions are tested against the pooled error MS $[S'*A + S'*B + S'*C + S'*B*A + S'*C*A + S'*C*B + S'*C*B*A]$. Pooling in this manner assumes that these contributions to the error term have approximately equal MS values (see page 120).

ANOVA tables for analysis of terms S|C|B|A – S*C*B*A (Model 1) or S+C|B|A (Model 2)

Model 4.3(i) A, B and C are fixed treatments, S' is a random blocking factor:

Mean square	d.f.	Components of variation estimated in population	F-ratio Model 1	F-ratio Model 2
Between n blocks				
1 S'	$n-1$	P'(S'*C*B*A)+S'	No test[a]	1/p[9+10+11+12+13+14+15]
Between ncba plots				
2 A	$a-1$	P'(S'*C*B*A)+S'*A+A	2/9	2/p[9+10+11+12+13+14+15]
3 B	$b-1$	P'(S'*C*B*A)+S'*B+B	3/10	3/p[9+10+11+12+13+14+15]
4 C	$c-1$	P'(S'*C*B*A)+S'*C+C	4/11	4/p[9+10+11+12+13+14+15]
5 B*A	$(b-1)(a-1)$	P'(S'*C*B*A)+S'*B*A+B*A	5/12	5/p[9+10+11+12+13+14+15]
6 C*A	$(c-1)(a-1)$	P'(S'*C*B*A)+S'*C*A+C*A	6/13	6/p[9+10+11+12+13+14+15]
7 C*B	$(c-1)(b-1)$	P'(S'*C*B*A)+S'*C*B+C*B	7/14	7/p[9+10+11+12+13+14+15]
8 C*B*A	$(c-1)(b-1)(a-1)$	P'(S'*C*B*A)+S'*C*B*A+C*B*A	8/15	8/p[9+10+11+12+13+14+15]
9 S'*A	$(n-1)(a-1)$	P'(S'*C*B*A)+S'*A	No test[a]	No test
10 S'*B	$(n-1)(b-1)$	P'(S'*C*B*A)+S'*B	No test[a]	No test
11 S'*C	$(n-1)(c-1)$	P'(S'*C*B*A)+S'*C	No test[a]	No test
12 S'*B*A	$(n-1)(b-1)(a-1)$	P'(S'*C*B*A)+S'*B*A	No test	No test
13 S'*C*A	$(n-1)(c-1)(a-1)$	P'(S'*C*B*A)+S'*C*A	No test	No test
14 S'*C*B	$(n-1)(c-1)(b-1)$	P'(S'*C*B*A)+S'*C*B	No test	No test
15 S'*C*B*A	$(n-1)(c-1)(b-1)(a-1)$	P'(S'*C*B*A)+S'*C*B*A	No test	No test
16 P'(S'*C*B*A)	0	P'(S'*C*B*A)	–	–
Total variation	$ncba-1$			

[a] An unrestricted model has an inexact F-ratio denominator (see page 242).

137

Model 4.3(ii) A, B are fixed treatments, C' is a random factor, S' is a random blocking factor:

Mean square	d.f.	Components of variation estimated in population	F-ratio Model 1	F-ratio Model 2
Between n blocks				
1 S'	$n-1$	$P'(S'*C'*B*A)+S'*C'+S'$	$1/11^b$	$1/p[9+10+11+12+13+14+15]$
Between $ncba$ plots				
2 A	$a-1$	$P'(S'*C'*B*A)+S'*C'*A+S'*A+C'*A+A$	$2/(6+9-13)^{ab}$	$2/6$
3 B	$b-1$	$P'(S'*C'*B*A)+S'*C'*B+S'*B+C'*B+B$	$3/(7+10-14)^{ab}$	$3/7$
4 C'	$c-1$	$P'(S'*C'*B*A)+S'*C'+C'$	$4/11^b$	$4/p[9+10+11+12+13+14+15]^b$
5 B*A	$(b-1)(a-1)$	$P'(S'*C'*B*A)+S'*C'*B*A+S'*B*A+C'*B*A+B*A$	$5/(8+12-15)^{ab}$	$5/8$
6 C'*A	$(c-1)(a-1)$	$P'(S'*C'*B*A)+S'*C'*A+C'*A$	$6/13^b$	$6/p[9+10+11+12+13+14+15]^c$
7 C'*B	$(c-1)(b-1)$	$P'(S'*C'*B*A)+S'*C'*B+C'*B$	$7/14^b$	$7/p[9+10+11+12+13+14+15]^c$
8 C'*B*A	$(c-1)(b-1)(a-1)$	$P'(S'*C'*B*A)+S'*C'*B*A+C'*B*A$	$8/15$	$8/p[9+10+11+12+13+14+15]$
9 S'*A	$(n-1)(a-1)$	$P'(S'*C'*B*A)+S'*C'*A+S'*A$	$9/13^b$	Not tested
10 S'*B	$(n-1)(b-1)$	$P'(S'*C'*B*A)+S'*C'*B+S'*B$	$10/14^b$	Not tested
11 S'*C'	$(n-1)(c-1)$	$P'(S'*C'*B*A)+S'*C'$	No test^b	No test
12 S'*B*A	$(n-1)(b-1)(a-1)$	$P'(S'*C'*B*A)+S'*C'*B*A+S'*B*A$	$12/15$	Not tested
13 S'*C'*A	$(n-1)(c-1)(a-1)$	$P'(S'*C'*B*A)+S'*C'*A$	No test	No test
14 S'*C'*B	$(n-1)(c-1)(b-1)$	$P'(S'*C'*B*A)+S'*C'*B$	No test	No test
15 S'*C'*B*A	$(n-1)(c-1)(b-1)(a-1)$	$P'(S'*C'*B*A)+S'*C'*B*A$	No test	No test
16 P'(S'*C'*B*A)	0	$P'(S'*C'*B*A)$	–	–
Total variation	$ncba-1$			

[a] There is no exact denominator for this test (see page 40). If certain terms have $P > 0.25$, however, then *post hoc* pooling can be used to derive an exact denominator for A, B and B*A (see page 38 for details and model 4.2(ii) for a similar example).

[b] An unrestricted model has an inexact F-ratio denominator (see page 242).

[c] An unrestricted model tests the two-way interactions over the MS for the three-way interaction C'*B*A (see page 242).

Model 4.3(iii) A is a fixed treatment, B' and C' are random factors, S' is a random blocking factor:

Mean square	d.f.	Components of variation estimated in population	F-ratio Model 1	F-ratio Model 2
Between n blocks				
1 S'	$n-1$	P'(S'*C*B'*A)+S'*C*B'+S'*C'+S'*B'+S'	$1/(10+11-14)^{ab}$	$1/p[9+10+11+12+13+14+15]$
Between ncba plots				
2 A	$a-1$	P'(S'*C*B'*A)+S'*C*B'*A+S'*C'*A+S'*B'*A+S'*A+C'*B'*A+C'*A+B'*A+A	$2/(5+6+9-8-12-13+15)^{ab}$	$2/(5+6-8)^{ab}$
3 B'	$b-1$	P'(S'*C*B'*A)+S'*C*B'+S'*B'+C'*B'+B'	$3/(7+10-14)^{ab}$	$3/7^{b}$
4 C'	$c-1$	P'(S'*C*B'*A)+S'*C*B'+S'*C'+C'*B'+C'	$4/(7+11-14)^{ab}$	$4/7^{b}$
5 B'*A	$(b-1)(a-1)$	P'(S'*C*B'*A)+S'*C*B'*A+S'*B'*A+C'*B'*A+B'*A	$5/(8+12-15)^{ab}$	5/8
6 C'*A	$(c-1)(a-1)$	P'(S'*C*B'*A)+S'*C*B'*A+S'*C'*A+C'*B'*A+C'*A	$6/(8+13-15)^{ab}$	6/8
7 C'*B'	$(c-1)(b-1)$	P'(S'*C*B'*A)+S'*C*B'+C'*B'	$7/14^{b}$	$7/p[9+10+11+12+13+14+15]^{c}$
8 C'*B'*A	$(c-1)(b-1)(a-1)$	P'(S'*C*B'*A)+S'*C*B'*A+C'*B'*A	8/15	$8/p[9+10+11+12+13+14+15]$
9 S'*A	$(n-1)(a-1)$	P'(S'*C*B'*A)+S'*C*B'*A+S'*C'*A+S'*B'*A+S'*A	$9/(12+13-15)^{ab}$	Not tested
10 S'*B'	$(n-1)(b-1)$	P'(S'*C*B'*A)+S'*C*B'+S'*B'	$10/14^{b}$	Not tested
11 S'*C'	$(n-1)(c-1)$	P'(S'*C*B'*A)+S'*C*B'+S'*C'	$11/14^{b}$	Not tested
12 S'*B'*A	$(n-1)(b-1)(a-1)$	P'(S'*C*B'*A)+S'*C*B'*A+S'*B'*A	12/15	Not tested
13 S'*C'*A	$(n-1)(c-1)(a-1)$	P'(S'*C*B'*A)+S'*C*B'*A+S'*C'*A	13/15	Not tested
14 S'*C'*B'	$(n-1)(c-1)(b-1)$	P'(S'*C*B'*A)+S'*C*B'	No test	No test
15 S'*C'*B'*A	$(n-1)(c-1)(b-1)(a-1)$	P'(S'*C*B'*A)+S'*C*B'*A	No test	No test
16 P'(S'*C*B'*A)	0	P'(S'*C*B'*A)	–	–
Total variation	$ncba-1$			

[a] There is no exact denominator for this test (see page 40). If certain terms have $P > 0.25$, however, then *post hoc* pooling can be used to derive an exact denominator (see page 38 for details and model 4.2(ii) for a similar example).

[b] An unrestricted model has an inexact F-ratio denominator (see page 242).

[c] An unrestricted model tests C'*B' over the MS for its interaction with A (F-ratio = **7/8**). See page 242.

Model 4.3(iv) A', B' and C' are random factors, S' is a random blocking factor:

Mean square	d.f.	Components of variation estimated in population	F-ratio Model 1	F-ratio Model 2
Between n blocks				
1 S'	$n-1$	$P'(S'*C'*B'*A') + S'*C'*B'*A' + S'*C'*A' + S'*B'*A' + S'*C' + S'*B' + S'*A' + S'$	$1/(9+10+11-12-13-14+15)^a$	$1/p[9+10+11+12+13+14+15]$
Between ncba plots				
2 A'	$a-1$	$P'(S'*C'*B'*A') + S'*C'*B'*A' + S'*C'*A' + S'*B'*A' + S'*A' + C'*B'*A' + B'*A' + A'$	$2/(5+6+9-8-12-13+15)^a$	$2/(5+6-8)^a$
3 B'	$b-1$	$P'(S'*C'*B'*A') + S'*C'*B'*A' + S'*C'*B' + S'*B'*A' + S'*B' + C'*B'*A' + C'*B' + B'*A' + B'$	$3/(5+7+10-8-12-14+15)^a$	$3/(5+7-8)^a$
4 C'	$c-1$	$P'(S'*C'*B'*A') + S'*C'*B'*A' + S'*C'*B' + S'*C'*A' + S'*C' + C'*B'*A' + C'*B' + C'*A' + C'$	$4/(6+7+11-8-13-14+15)^a$	$4/(6+7-8)^a$
5 B'*A'	$(b-1)(a-1)$	$P'(S'*C'*B'*A') + S'*C'*B'*A' + S'*B'*A' + C'*B'*A' + B'*A'$	$5/(8+12-15)^a$	5/8
6 C'*A'	$(c-1)(a-1)$	$P'(S'*C'*B'*A') + S'*C'*B'*A' + S'*C'*A' + C'*B'*A' + C'*A'$	$6/(8+13-15)^a$	6/8
7 C'*B'	$(c-1)(b-1)$	$P'(S'*C'*B'*A') + S'*C'*B'*A' + S'*C'*B' + C'*B'*A' + C'*B'$	$7/(8+14-15)^a$	7/8
8 C'*B'*A'	$(c-1)(b-1)(a-1)$	$P'(S'*C'*B'*A') + S'*C'*B'*A' + C'*B'*A'$	$8/15$	$8/p[9+10+11+12+13+14+15]$
9 S'*A'	$(n-1)(a-1)$	$P'(S'*C'*B'*A') + S'*C'*B'*A' + S'*C'*A' + S'*B'*A' + S'*A'$	$9/(12+13-15)^a$	Not tested
10 S'*B'	$(n-1)(b-1)$	$P'(S'*C'*B'*A') + S'*C'*B'*A' + S'*C'*B' + S'*B'*A' + S'*B'$	$10/(12+14-15)^a$	Not tested
11 S'*C'	$(n-1)(c-1)$	$P'(S'*C'*B'*A') + S'*C'*B'*A' + S'*C'*B' + S'*C'*A' + S'*C'$	$11/(13+14-15)^a$	Not tested
12 S'*B'*A'	$(n-1)(b-1)(a-1)$	$P'(S'*C'*B'*A') + S'*C'*B'*A' + S'*B'*A'$	12/15	Not tested
13 S'*C'*A'	$(n-1)(c-1)(a-1)$	$P'(S'*C'*B'*A') + S'*C'*B'*A' + S'*C'*A'$	13/15	Not tested
14 S'*C'*B'	$(n-1)(c-1)(b-1)$	$P'(S'*C'*B'*A') + S'*C'*B'*A' + S'*C'*B'$	14/15	Not tested
15 S'*C'*B'*A'	$(n-1)(c-1)(b-1)(a-1)$	$P'(S'*C'*B'*A') + S'*C'*B'*A'$	No test	No test
16 P'(S'*C'*B'*A')	0	$P'(S'*C'*B'*A')$	–	–
Total variation	$ncba-1$			

[a] There is no exact denominator for this test (see page 40). If certain terms have $P > 0.25$, however, then *post hoc* pooling can be used to derive an exact denominator (see page 38 for details and model 4.2(ii) for a similar example).

5

Split-plot designs

Split-plot models extend the randomised-block designs of Chapter 4 to situations in which different treatments are assigned to sampling units at different scales. In addition to one or more treatments being assigned at random to plots within each block, further treatments are assigned at random to whole blocks and/or to sub-plots nested in plots (and even to sub-sub-plots nested within each sub-plot). Cross-factored treatments are therefore applied to a hierarchy of nested sampling units: sub-sub-plots in sub-plots in plots in blocks. Further details of split-plot designs are given on page 25.

These are the four scales of sampling unit to which a given treatment level may be assigned in the models described in this chapter:

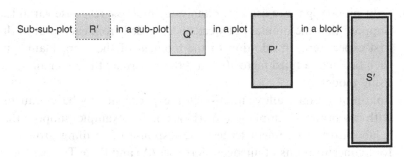

As with randomised-block designs, randomisation of treatments to sampling units occurs only within each block, plot or sub-plot. Split-plot designs are usually unreplicated, with just one observation of each treatment or combination of treatments within a particular block, plot, sub-plot or sub-sub-plot. This lack of replication complicates the interpretation of results, because it precludes testing of certain interactions between treatment factors and sampling units. Full replication allows

141

testing of these interactions, but often gives relatively modest improvements in power for the extra resources invested.

The application of treatments at more than one (usually spatial) scale has a number of practical advantages.

(1) In multi-factor experiments it may be impractical to apply some treatments to very large or very small sampling units. For example, in a field trial to test the response of crop yield to watering regime (A) and fertiliser concentration (B), neighbouring small plots cannot receive different watering regimes because the water will leach across plot boundaries. One solution is to apply different watering regimes to replicate groups of plots (blocks, S′) and to apply different fertiliser concentrations to plots (P′) within each block, resulting in split-plot model 5.6.

(2) Split-plot designs allow new treatment factors to be introduced into an experiment already in progress. Each of the smallest existing sampling units can be split into yet smaller units, to which the levels of the new factor are applied. Suppose, for example, that an investigator decides to incorporate a third treatment, pesticide (C), into the above experiment. As the experiment is already in progress and no more plots of land are available, each plot is further subdivided into c sub-plots (Q′) and one concentration of pesticide is applied to each sub-plot. The experiment is then analysed using model 5.5.

(3) Split-plot designs are useful for analysing multiple response variables. Suppose that the biomass of weeds is recorded from each plot in the first experiment, in addition to the biomass of the crop. Plant type then becomes a third factor (C) and the experiment is again analysed using model 5.5.

(4) Split-plot designs allow multi-factor experiments to be conducted with few primary sampling units (blocks). For example, suppose that a laboratory experiment to test the response of seedling growth to four concentrations of nitrogen Fertiliser (A) and three Temperatures (B) has available only six mesocosms (S′). The investigator wants to test for interacting effects of fertiliser and temperature, but cannot do this in a fully replicated two-factor design without having at least 24 mesocosms – one for each of two replicates at each of the 12 combinations of levels of A and B. However, all treatment effects may be tested with just six mesocosms if each of high, medium and low temperature are allocated to two mesocosms and all four

concentrations of fertiliser are then tested in each mesocosm, one per tray of seedlings (P'). As more than one observation is made in each mesocosm, the analysis must now declare Mesocosm as a random blocking factor (S') to account for variation between mesocosms. Since each mesocosm has its own temperature setting but all levels of fertiliser, the factor Mesocosm is nested in Temperature and cross factored with Fertiliser, giving model 5.6. Note that having just three mesocosms will not suffice, because the effect of temperature is then entirely confounded with unmeasured differences between the mesocosms.

Assumptions

Split-plot models involve repeated measurements on blocks (and on plots if sub-plots are present, and on sub-plots if sub-sub-plots are present), which introduces an additional assumption of *homogeneity of covariances*. Because blocks group plots (which in turn group sub-plots, which in turn group sub-sub-plots), any observations made on factors within these blocks (or plots or sub-plots) are not independent of each other. This source of correlation between levels of within-block (or plot or sub-plot) factors is not a problem provided that the covariances (i.e., correlations) are the same between treatment levels within each block (or plot or sub-plot). This is an extension to the standard assumption of homogeneous variances, which applies to all ANOVA (page 14). In practice, these ANOVAs require only an additional homogeneity amongst the set of variances obtained from all pairs of treatment levels, where each variance is calculated from the differences in response between the levels across blocks (or plots or sub-plots): known as the 'sphericity condition'. Heterogeneity amongst these variances will result in a liberal test that inflates the Type I error rate. Kirk (1982), Winer *et al.* (1991) and Quinn and Keough (2002) suggest ways to adjust the ANOVA when this assumption is not met. If the design is fully replicated, then the assumption of homogeneity of covariances becomes subsumed within the standard assumption of homogeneity of variances between all samples.

With only one replicate observation per combination of sampling unit and treatment levels, the requirement that it be drawn independently ceases to apply, but it must be representative of the sampling and treatment level. Spatial non-independence of sampling units can be a problem if they are in close proximity. To avoid this problem, replicate plots (or sub-plots or sub-sub-plots) should be spaced apart such that treatments applied to one sampling unit do not influence measurements taken from its neighbours. Despite the potential for non-independence among sampling units, the randomisation of treatment levels to sampling units ensures no systematic bias, in contrast to repeated-measures designs which are susceptible to bias from practice and carryover effects (see Chapter 6).

Unreplicated split-plot designs generally cannot test for interactions of within-block treatments with blocks, which must therefore be assumed to have negligible effect. Although full replication would allow testing of these interactions, their interpretation remains problematic (see below).

Analysis

Split-plot designs are analysed as unreplicated factorial models with nesting. They are factorial because each level of each treatment factor is tested in combination with each level of the other treatment factors, and nested because the sampling units (blocks, plots, sub-plots and sub-sub-plots) to which the treatments are applied are hierarchical. The nesting of sampling units means that each sampling scale has its own ANOVA table.

Analysis follows the Model-2 approach used for randomised-block designs (page 119). If the design is unreplicated then it is not possible to test for interactions of treatment factors with blocks, plots, sub-plots or sub-sub-plots because the relevant error terms cannot be estimated. These interaction terms are assumed to be zero and pooled together in order to test treatment effects. The error term for a particular treatment effect is then the interaction between blocks and all treatments that are applied to that sampling unit or larger. Pooling assumes that the MS contributions to the pooled error term have approximately equal MS values. Kirk (1994) recommends an F_{max} test of this assumption, and using the less powerful unpooled test in the event of heterogeneous variances.

Interpretation of non-significant results is problematic because they may indicate no treatment effect, or a treatment effect that has opposing effects in different sampling units. Full replication allows testing of the assumption of no sampling unit-by-treatment interactions and thereby – in the event of no significant interactions – validation of non-significant treatment effects. Interpretation of significant interactions is nevertheless problematic because the treatment effect may depend upon any of the multiple sources of variation encompassed by the blocking factor. Thus, the causal mechanisms giving rise to a significant sampling unit-by-treatment interaction cannot be interpreted without further experimentation. Significant treatment factors do not pose the same level of interpretative difficulty, because they are tested against interactions with the random sampling units, and therefore report significance over and above any interactions with them.

Types of split-plot model

Textbooks vary in the terminology used to describe the nested sampling units in split-plot designs. For consistency with the randomised-block models in Chapter 4, we refer to the top level in the hierarchy as blocks, and subsequent levels in the hierarchy as plots, sub-plots and sub-sub-plots (see also Underwood 1997; Crawley 2002; Quinn and Keough 2002). However, other books refer to the top level in the hierarchy as plots and term the lower levels accordingly (for example, Winer *et al.* 1991).

Split-plot models are similar in concept to repeated-measures models. Repeated observations are taken on each block in the same way that repeated measurements are taken on each subject. We illustrate this similarity using S' to denote both blocks and subjects and P' to denote both plots nested in blocks and observations nested in subject. Split-plot models differ from repeated-measures models, however, in that treatment levels are randomly assigned within blocks (subjects), rather than being applied in spatial or temporal sequence. Split-plot designs therefore do not suffer systematic bias from practice and carryover effects, which are unique to repeated-measures designs. Care must be taken, nevertheless, to ensure that treatments applied to one part of a sampling unit do not affect other treatments applied to other parts of the sampling unit.

In this chapter, we describe nine common split-plot designs, listed in Table 5. Because split-plot designs have been developed specifically for multiple treatments, we detail all models with up to three fixed factors having categorical levels. Models 5.1 to 5.5 have no equivalent amongst standard repeated-measures models. They may be used as repeated-measures models, however, if the factor applied at the lowest level in the hierarchy is a temporal or spatial sequence. For example, model 5.1 could be a one-factor (A) randomised-block model with each plot repeatedly sampled over time (B). Models 5.6 to 5.9 are directly equivalent to

Table 5 *Split-plot designs with up to three fixed treatments factors (A, B, C) allocated to blocks, plots within blocks, sub-plots within plots and sub-sub plots within sub-plots. Any corresponding repeated-measures models are identified in the first column.*

| Model Number | Model | Treatments applied to | | | |
		Sub-sub-plots (R')	Sub-plots (Q')	Plots (P')	Blocks (S')
5.1	$Y = B\|P'(S'\|A)$		B	A	–
5.2	$Y = C\|P'(S'\|B\|A)$		C	B|A	–
5.3	$Y = C\|B\|P'(S'\|A)$		C|B	A	–
5.4	$Y = C\|Q'(B\|P'(S'\|A))$	C	B	A	–
5.5	$Y = C\|P'(B\|S'(A))$		C	B	A
5.6 = 6.3	$Y = B\|S'(A)$			B	A
5.7 = 6.5	$Y = C\|B\|S'(A)$			C|B	A
5.8 = 6.6	$Y = C\|S'(B(A))$			C	B(A)
5.9 = 6.7	$Y = C\|S'(B\|A)$			C	B|A

standard repeated-measures models 6.3 and 6.5 to 6.7. As the analysis of equivalent split-plot and repeated-measures models is identical, we refer readers to the ANOVA tables in Chapter 6 to avoid unnecessary replication.

5.1 Two-factor split-plot model (i)

Model

$$Y = B|P'(S'|A)$$

Test hypothesis

Variation in the response Y is explained by the combined effects of factor A and factor B.

Description

Each of *a* levels of treatment A is randomly assigned one of *a* plots (P') in each of *n* blocks (S'), and each of *b* levels of treatment B is randomly assigned one of *b* sub-plots (Q') in each plot.

Factors	Levels	Repeated measures on S'
A	a	yes
B	b	yes
S'	n	–

Allocation table

The table shows $a = 2$ levels of factor A allocated amongst a plots P' in each of $n = 4$ blocks S', and $b = 2$ levels of factor B allocated amongst b sub-plots Q' in each plot. Note that the table does not indicate the spatial distribution of treatment combinations, which must be randomised within each sampling unit. For example, treatment level B_1 should not be assigned to the first sub-plot in every plot.

Q'(B|P'(S'|A))		S_1	S_2	S_3	S_4
A_1	B_1	Q_1	...	...	Q_n
	B_2	...	...	...	Q_{nb}
A_2	B_1	...	...	...	...
	B_2	...	...	...	Q_{nba}

Examples

(1) *Spatial block example:* H_1: Crop yield depends on a combination of Watering regime (A) and sowing Density (B) treatments. The a levels of watering are randomly assigned amongst a Plots (P') in each of n Blocks (S'), and the b sowing densities are randomly assigned amongst b Sub-plots (Q') within each Plot. The response is the yield from each sub-plot, measured at the end of the experiment.

(2) *Temporal block example*: H_1: Plant growth depends on a combination of Temperature (A) and Fertiliser (B). The a temperatures are randomly assigned amongst a Mesocosms (P') and b levels of fertiliser are randomly assigned amongst b Trays of plants (Q') within each mesocosm. The whole experiment is repeated with new plants n Times in sequence (S'), with temperatures randomly reassigned to mesocosms and fertiliser treatment randomly reassigned to trays within mesocosms each Time.

Comparisons

Model 5.1 is an extension of a one-factor randomised-block model 4.1 to include a second crossed factor applied to sub-plots nested within plots.

Model 5.1 can be extended to include a third, crossed treatment factor applied to whole blocks (model 5.5), plots (model 5.2), sub-plots (model 5.3) or sub-sub-plots (model 5.4).

In testing the combined effect of two crossed factors, model 5.1 has similar objectives to cross-factored models 3.1, 4.2, 5.6, 6.2 and 6.3. Crucially, it differs from fully randomised model 3.1 in that the assignment of treatments to sampling units (plots) is not completely randomised, and from randomised-block model 4.2 in that factors A and B are assigned to sampling units at different scales. Model 5.1 differs from split-plot model 5.6 only in the way treatment factors are applied to sampling units. In contrast to repeated-measures models 6.2 and 6.3, model 5.1 randomly assigns levels of both treatment factors within blocks rather than applying them sequentially.

Special assumptions (see also general assumptions on page 143)

The model assumes no interactions of sampling units with treatments, which cannot be tested anyway because the lack of replication means that there is no residual error term (shaded grey in the ANOVA table below). Interpretation of non-significant A, B or A*B is compromised because the result could mean either no effect, or opposing effects in different sampling units. The assumption of no sampling unit-by-treatment interactions can be tested if independent, replicate plots (P') are used for each level of A in each block and independent, replicate sub-plots (Q') are used for each level of B in each plot. The interpretation of a significant sampling unit-by-treatment interaction is nevertheless problematic because the treatment effect may depend upon any of the multiple sources of variation encompassed by the blocking factor. Thus, the causal mechanisms underlying a significant interaction cannot be interpreted without further experimentation.

The nesting of Sub-plot'(Plot'(Block')) means that the error term for each fixed main effect or main-effect interaction comprises the interaction between the block and all factors applied to that sampling unit or larger. Thus, A is tested against the error MS[S'*A], while B and B*A are tested against the pooled error MS[B*S' + B*S'*A]. Pooling terms in this manner assumes that these contributions to the error term have approximately equal MS values (see page 144).

ANOVA table for analysis of terms B|A + S|A

Model 5.1(i) A in plots and B in sub-plots are fixed factors, S' is a random blocking factor:

Mean square	d.f.	Components of variation estimated in population	F-ratio
Between n blocks			
1 S'	$n-1$	Q'(B*P'(S'*A)) + P'(S'*A) + S'	No test[a]
Between na plots			
2 A	$a-1$	Q'(B*P'(S'*A)) + P'(S'*A) + S'*A + A	2/3
3 S'*A	$(n-1)(a-1)$	Q'(B*P'(S'*A)) + P'(S'*A) + S'*A	No test
4 P'(S'*A)	0	Q'(B*P'(S'*A)) + P'(S'*A)	No test
Between nba sub-plots			
5 B	$b-1$	Q'(B*P'(S'*A)) + B*P'(S'*A) + B*S' + B	5/p[7 + 8]
6 B*A	$(b-1)(a-1)$	Q'(B*P'(S'*A)) + B*P'(S'*A) + B*S'*A + B*A	6/p[7 + 8]
7 B*S'	$(b-1)(n-1)$	Q'(B*P'(S'*A)) + B*P'(S'*A) + B*S'	No test
8 B*S'*A	$(b-1)(n-1)(a-1)$	Q'(B*P'(S'*A)) + B*P'(S'*A) + B*S'*A	No test
9 B*P'(S'*A)	0	Q'(B*P'(S'*A)) + B*P'(S'*A)	No test
10 Q'(B*P'(S'*A))	0	Q'(B*P'(S'*A))	–
Total variation	$nba-1$		

[a] An unrestricted model tests S' over the MS for its interaction with A (F-ratio = **1/3**). See page 242.

5.2 Three-factor split-plot model (i)

Model

$$Y = C|P'(S'|B|A)$$

Test hypothesis

Variation in the response Y is explained by the combined effects of factors A, B and C.

Description

Each of *ba* combinations of levels of A*B is randomly assigned one of *ba* plots (P') in each of *n* blocks (S'), and each of *c* levels of treatment C is randomly assigned one of *c* sub-plots (Q') in each plot.

Factors	Levels	Repeated measures on S'
A	*a*	yes
B	*b*	yes
C	*c*	yes
S'	*n*	–

Allocation table

The table shows *ba* = 4 combinations of levels of factors B and A allocated amongst *ba* plots P' in each of *n* = 4 blocks S', and *c* = 2 levels of factor C allocated amongst *c* sub-plots Q' in each plot. Note that the table does not indicate the spatial distribution of treatment combinations, which must be randomised within each sampling unit. For example, treatment level C_1 should not be assigned to the first sub-plot in every plot.

Q'(C|P'(S'|B|A))			S$_1$	S$_2$	S$_3$	S$_4$
A$_1$	B$_1$	C$_1$	Q$_1$	...	...	Q$_n$
		C$_2$	...	...	...	Q$_{nc}$
	B$_2$	C$_1$	...	...	...	...
		C$_2$	...	...	...	Q$_{ncb}$
A$_2$	B$_1$	C$_1$	...	...	...	...
		C$_2$	...	...	...	...
	B$_2$	C$_1$	...	...	...	...
		C$_2$	...	...	...	Q$_{ncba}$

Examples

(1) *Spatial block example:* H_1: Crop yield depends on a combination of Watering regime (A), sowing Density (B) and Fertiliser (C) treatments. The *ba* combinations of watering and density are randomly assigned amongst *ba* Plots (P') in each of *n* Blocks (S'), and the *c* levels of fertiliser are randomly assigned amongst *c* Sub-plots (Q') within each Plot. The response is the yield from each sub-plot, measured at the end of the experiment.

(2) *Temporal block example*: H_1: Plant growth depends on a combination of Temperature (A), Light (B) and Fertiliser (C). The *ba* combinations of temperature and light are randomly assigned amongst *ba* Mesocosms (P'), and the *c* fertiliser concentrations are randomly assigned amongst *c* Trays of plants (Q') within each mesocosm. The whole experiment is repeated with new plants *n* Times in sequence (S'), with temperatures and light levels randomly reassigned to mesocosms and fertiliser levels randomly reassigned to trays within mesocosms each time.

Comparisons

Model 5.2 is an extension of two-factor randomised-block model 4.2 to include a third, crossed factor, applied to sub-plots within each plot, and an extension of split-plot model 5.1 to include a third crossed factor applied to plots.

In testing the combined effect of three crossed factors, model 5.2 has similar objectives to cross-factored models 3.2, 4.3, 5.3, 5.4, 5.5, 5.7, 5.9, 6.5 and 6.7. Crucially, it differs from fully randomised model 3.2 in that the assignment of treatments to sampling units is not completely randomised, and from randomised-block model 4.3 in that factors A, B and C are assigned to sampling units at different scales. Model 5.2 differs from the other three-factor split-plot models only in the way treatment factors are applied to sampling units. In contrast to repeated-measures models 6.5 and 6.7, model 5.2 randomly assigns treatment levels rather than applying them sequentially.

Special assumptions (see also general assumptions on page 143)

The model assumes no interactions of sampling units with treatments, which cannot be tested anyway because the lack of replication means that there is no residual error term (shaded grey in the ANOVA table below). Interpretation of any non-significant main effects and interactions is compromised because the result could mean either no effect, or opposing effects in different sampling units. The assumption of no sampling unit-by-treatment interactions can be tested if independent, replicate plots (P′) are used for each of the *ba* levels of factors B and A in each block and independent, replicate sub-plots (Q′) are used for each level of C in each plot. The interpretation of a significant sampling unit-by-treatment interaction is nevertheless problematic because the treatment effect may depend upon any of the multiple sources of variation encompassed by the blocking factor. Thus, the causal mechanisms underlying a significant interaction cannot be interpreted without further experimentation.

The nesting of Sub-Plot′(Plot′(Block′)) means that the error term for each fixed main effect or main-effect interaction comprises the interaction between the block and all factors applied to that sampling unit or larger. Pooling terms in this manner assumes that these contributions to the error term have approximately equal MS values (see page 144).

ANOVA table for analysis of terms S|B|A + C|B|A

Model 5.2(i) *A and B in plots and C in sub-plots are fixed factors, S' is a random blocking factor:*

Mean square	d.f.	Components of variation estimated in population	F-ratio
Between n blocks			
1 S'	$n-1$	Q'(C*P'(S'*B*A)) + P'(S'*B*A)) + S'	No test[a]
Between nba plots			
2 A	$a-1$	Q'(C*P'(S'*B*A)) + P'(S'*B*A)) + S'*A + A	2/p[5+6+7]
3 B	$b-1$	Q'(C*P'(S'*B*A)) + P'(S'*B*A)) + S'*B + B	3/p[5+6+7]
4 B*A	$(b-1)(a-1)$	Q'(C*P'(S'*B*A)) + P'(S'*B*A)) + S'*B*A + B*A	4/p[5+6+7]
5 S'*A	$(n-1)(a-1)$	Q'(C*P'(S'*B*A)) + P'(S'*B*A)) + S'*A	No test
6 S'*B	$(n-1)(b-1)$	Q'(C*P'(S'*B*A)) + P'(S'*B*A)) + S'*B	No test
7 S'*B*A	$(n-1)(b-1)(a-1)$	Q'(C*P'(S'*B*A)) + P'(S'*B*A)) + S'*B*A	No test
8 P'(S'*B*A)	0	Q'(C*P'(S'*B*A)) + P'(S'*B*A))	No test
Between ncba sub-plots			
9 C	$c-1$	Q'(C*P'(S'*B*A)) + C*P'(S'*B*A)) + C*S' + C	9/p[13+14+15+16]
10 C*A	$(c-1)(a-1)$	Q'(C*P'(S'*B*A)) + C*P'(S'*B*A)) + C*S'*A + C*A	10/p[13+14+15+16]
11 C*B	$(c-1)(b-1)$	Q'(C*P'(S'*B*A)) + C*P'(S'*B*A)) + C*S'*B + C*B	11/p[13+14+15+16]
12 C*B*A	$(c-1)(b-1)(a-1)$	Q'(C*P'(S'*B*A)) + C*P'(S'*B*A)) + C*S'*B*A + C*B*A	12/p[13+14+15+16]
13 C*S'	$(c-1)(n-1)$	Q'(C*P'(S'*B*A)) + C*P'(S'*B*A)) + C*S'	No test
14 C*S'*A	$(c-1)(n-1)(a-1)$	Q'(C*P'(S'*B*A)) + C*P'(S'*B*A)) + C*S'*A	No test
15 C*S'*B	$(c-1)(n-1)(b-1)$	Q'(C*P'(S'*B*A)) + C*P'(S'*B*A)) + C*S'*B	No test
16 C*S'*B*A	$(c-1)(n-1)(b-1)(a-1)$	Q'(C*P'(S'*B*A)) + C*P'(S'*B*A)) + C*S'*B*A	No test
17 C*P'(S'*B*A)	0	Q'(C*P'(S'*B*A)) + C*P'(S'*B*A))	No test
18 Q'(C*P'(S'*B*A))	0	Q'(C*P'(S'*B*A))	–
Total variation	$ncba-1$		

[a] An unrestricted model has an inexact F-ratio denominator (see page 242).

5.3 Three-factor split-plot model (ii)

Model

$$Y = C|B|P'(S'|A)$$

Test hypothesis

Variation in the response Y is explained by the combined effects of factors A, B and C.

Description

Each of a levels of treatment A is randomly assigned one of a plots (P') in each of n blocks (S'), and each of cb combinations of levels of treatments C and B is randomly assigned one of cb sub-plots (Q') in each plot.

Factors	Levels	Repeated measures on S'
A	a	yes
B	b	yes
C	c	yes
S'	n	–

Allocation table

The table shows $a = 2$ levels of factor A allocated amongst a plots P' in each of $n = 4$ blocks S', and $cb = 4$ combinations of levels of factors C and B allocated amongst cb sub-plots Q' in each plot. Note that the table does not indicate the spatial distribution of treatment combinations, which must be randomised within each sampling unit. For example, treatment level C_1 should not be assigned to the first sub-plot in every plot.

Q'(C|B|P'(S'|A))			S_1	S_2	S_3	S_4
A_1	B_1	C_1	Q_1	...	...	Q_n
		C_2	...	...	...	Q_{nc}
	B_2	C_1	...	...	...	...
		C_2	...	...	...	Q_{ncb}
A_2	B_1	C_1	...	...	...	...
		C_2	...	...	...	...
	B_2	C_1	...	...	...	...
		C_2	...	...	...	Q_{ncba}

Examples

(1) *Spatial block example:* H_1: Crop yield depends on a combination of Watering regime (A), sowing Density (B) and Fertiliser (C) treatments. The a levels of watering are randomly assigned amongst a Plots (P') in each of n Blocks (S'), and the cb combinations of sowing density and fertiliser are randomly assigned amongst cb Sub-plots (Q') within each Plot. The response is the yield from each sub-plot, measured at the end of the experiment.

(2) *Temporal block example*: H_1: Plant growth depends on a combination of Temperature (A), Light (B) and Fertiliser (C). The a temperatures are randomly assigned amongst a Mesocosms (P'), and the cb combinations of light and fertiliser are randomly assigned amongst cb Trays of plants (Q') within each Mesocosm. The whole experiment is repeated with new plants n Times in sequence (S'), with temperatures randomly reassigned to mesocosms and light and fertiliser levels randomly reassigned to trays within mesocosms each time.

Comparisons

Model 5.3 is an extension of split-plot model 5.1 to include a third crossed factor applied to sub-plots.

In testing the combined effect of three crossed factors, model 5.3 has similar objectives to cross-factored models 3.2, 4.3, 5.2, 5.4, 5.5, 5.7, 5.9, 6.5 and 6.7. Crucially, it differs from fully randomised model 3.2

in that the assignment of treatments to sampling units is not completely randomised, and from randomised-block model 4.3 in that factors A, B and C are assigned to sampling units at different scales. Model 5.3 differs from the other three-factor split-plot models only in the way treatment factors are applied to sampling units. In contrast to repeated-measures models 6.5 and 6.7, model 5.3 randomly assigns treatment levels rather than applying them sequentially.

Special assumptions (see also general assumptions on page 143)

The model assumes no interactions of sampling units with treatments, which cannot be tested anyway because the lack of replication means that there is no residual error term (shaded grey in the ANOVA table below). Interpretation of any non-significant main effects and interactions is compromised because the result could mean either no effect, or opposing effects in different sampling units. The assumption of no sampling unit-by-treatment interactions can be tested if independent, replicate plots (P′) are used for each of the a levels of factor A in each block and indepen-dent, replicate sub-plots (Q′) are used for each of the cb levels of factors B and C in each plot. The interpretation of a significant sampling unit-by-treatment interaction is nevertheless problematic because the treatment effect may depend upon any of the multiple sources of variation encompassed by the blocking factor. Thus, the causal mechanisms underlying a significant interaction cannot be interpreted without further experimentation.

The nesting of Sub-Plot′(Plot′(Block′)) means that the error term for each fixed main effect or main-effect interaction comprises the interaction between the block and all factors applied to that sampling unit or larger. Pooling terms in this manner assumes that these contributions to the error term have approximately equal MS values (see page 144).

ANOVA table for analysis of terms C|B|A + S|A

Model 5.3(i) *A in plots and B and C in sub-plots are fixed factors, S' is a random blocking factor:*

Mean square	d.f.	Components of variation estimated in population	F-ratio
Between n blocks			
1 S'	$n-1$	Q'(C*B*P'(S*A)) + P'(S*A)) + S'	No test[a]
Between na plots			
2 A	$a-1$	Q'(C*B*P'(S*A)) + P'(S*A)) + S'*A + A	2/3
3 S'*A	$(n-1)(a-1)$	Q'(C*B*P'(S*A)) + P'(S*A)) + S'*A	No test
4 P'(S*A))	0	Q'(C*B*P'(S*A)) + P'(S*A))	No test
Between ncba sub-plots			
5 B	$b-1$	Q'(C*B*P'(S*A)) + B*P'(S*A)) + B*S' + B	5/p[11+12+14+15+17+18]
6 B*A	$(b-1)(a-1)$	Q'(C*B*P'(S*A)) + B*P'(S*A)) + B*S'*A + B*A	6/p[11+12+14+15+17+18]
7 C	$c-1$	Q'(C*B*P'(S*A)) + C*P'(S*A)) + C*S' + C	7/p[11+12+14+15+17+18]
8 C*A	$(c-1)(a-1)$	Q'(C*B*P'(S*A)) + C*P'(S*A)) + C*S'*A + C*A	8/p[11+12+14+15+17+18]
9 C*B	$(c-1)(b-1)$	Q'(C*B*P'(S*A)) + C*B*P'(S*A)) + C*B*S' + C*B	9/p[11+12+14+15+17+18]
10 C*B*A	$(c-1)(b-1)(a-1)$	Q'(C*B*P'(S*A)) + C*B*P'(S*A)) + C*B*S'*A + C*B*A	10/p[11+12+14+15+17+18]
11 B*S'	$(b-1)(n-1)$	Q'(C*B*P'(S*A)) + B*P'(S*A)) + B*S'	No test
12 B*S'*A	$(b-1)(n-1)(a-1)$	Q'(C*B*P'(S*A)) + B*P'(S*A)) + B*S'*A	No test
13 B*P'(S*A))	0	Q'(C*B*P'(S*A)) + B*P'(S*A))	No test
14 C*S'	$(c-1)(n-1)$	Q'(C*B*P'(S*A)) + C*P'(S*A)) + C*S'	No test
15 C*S'*A	$(c-1)(n-1)(a-1)$	Q'(C*B*P'(S*A)) + C*P'(S*A)) + C*S'*A	No test
16 C*P'(S*A))	0	Q'(C*B*P'(S*A)) + C*P'(S*A))	No test
17 C*B*S'	$(c-1)(b-1)(n-1)$	Q'(C*B*P'(S*A)) + C*B*P'(S*A)) + C*B*S'	No test
18 C*B*S'*A	$(c-1)(b-1)(n-1)(a-1)$	Q'(C*B*P'(S*A)) + C*B*P'(S*A)) + C*B*S'*A	No test
19 C*B*P'(S*A))	0	Q'(C*B*P'(S*A)) + C*B*P'(S*A))	
20 Q'(C*B*P'(S*A))	0	Q'(C*B*P'(S*A))	–
Total variation	$ncba-1$		

[a] An unrestricted model tests S' over the MS for its interaction with A (*F*-ratio = 1/3). See page 242.

5.4 Split-split-plot model (i)

Model

$$Y = C|Q'(B|P'(S'|A))$$

Test hypothesis

Variation in the response Y is explained by the combined effects of factors A, B and C.

Description

Each of a levels of treatment A is randomly assigned one of a plots (P') in each of n blocks (S'), and each of b levels of treatment B is randomly assigned one of b sub-plots (Q') in each plot, and each of c levels of treatment C is randomly assigned one of c sub-sub-plots (R') in each plot.

Factors	Levels	Repeated measures on S'
A	a	yes
B	b	yes
C	c	yes
S'	n	–

Allocation table

The table shows $a = 2$ levels of factor A allocated amongst a plots P' in each of $n = 4$ blocks S', and $b = 2$ levels of factor B allocated amongst b sub-plots Q' in each plot, and $c = 2$ levels of factor C allocated amongst c sub-sub-plots R' in each sub-plot. Note that the table does not indicate the spatial distribution of treatment combinations, which must be randomised within each sampling unit. For example, treatment level B_1 should not be assigned to the first sub-plot in every plot.

R'(C|Q'(B|P'(S'|A)))			S_1	S_2	S_3	S_4
A_1	B_1	C_1	R_1	...	...	R_n
		C_2	...	...	...	R_{nc}
	B_2	C_1	...	...	...	...
		C_2	...	...	...	R_{ncb}
A_2	B_1	C_1	...	...	...	...
		C_2	...	...	...	...
	B_2	C_1	...	...	...	...
		C_2	...	...	...	R_{ncba}

Examples

(1) *Spatial block example: H_1:* Crop yield depends on a combination of Watering regime (A), sowing Density (B) and Fertiliser (C) treatments. The *a* levels of watering are randomly assigned amongst *a* Plots (P') in each of *n* Blocks (S'), the *b* levels of sowing density are randomly assigned amongst *b* Sub-plots (Q') within each Plot, and the *c* levels of fertiliser are randomly assigned amongst *c* Sub-sub-plots (R') within each Sub-plot. The response is the yield from each sub-sub-plot, measured at the end of the experiment.

(2) *Temporal block example*: H_1: Plant growth depends on a combination of Temperature (A), Light (B) and Fertiliser (C). The *a* temperatures are randomly assigned amongst *a* Mesocosms (P'), the *b* levels of light are randomly assigned amongst *b* Shelves (Q') within each mesocosm, and the *c* levels of fertiliser are randomly assigned amongst *c* Trays (R') on each shelf. The whole experiment is repeated with new plants *n* Times in sequence (S'), each time with a random reassignment of temperatures to mesocosms, light levels to shelves within mesocosms, and fertiliser levels to trays on each shelf.

Comparisons

Model 5.4 is an extension of split-plot model 5.1 to include a third crossed factor applied to sub-sub-plots within each sub-plot.

In testing the combined effect of three crossed factors, model 5.4 has similar objectives to cross-factored models 3.2, 4.3, 5.2, 5.3, 5.5, 5.7, 5.9,

6.5 and 6.7. Crucially, it differs from fully randomised model 3.2 in that the assignment of treatments to sampling units is not completely randomised, and from randomised-block model 4.3 in that factors A, B and C are assigned to sampling units at different scales. Model 5.4 differs from the other three-factor split-plot models only in the way treatment factors are applied to sampling units. In contrast to repeated-measures models 6.5 and 6.7, model 5.4 randomly assigns treatment levels rather than applying them sequentially.

Special assumptions (see also general assumptions on page 143)

The model assumes no interactions of sampling units with treatments, which cannot be tested anyway because the lack of replication means that there is no residual error term (shaded grey in the ANOVA table below). Interpretation of any non-significant main effects and interactions is compromised because the result could mean either no effect, or opposing effects in different sampling units. The assumption of no sampling unit-by-treatment interactions can be tested if independent, replicate plots (P′) are used for each level of factor A in each block, independent replicate sub-plots (Q′) are used for each level of factor B in each plot, and independent replicate sub-sub-plots (R′) are used for each level of factor C in each sub-plot. The interpretation of a significant sampling unit-by-treatment interaction is nevertheless problematic because the treatment effect may depend upon any of the multiple sources of variation encompassed by the blocking factor. Thus, the causal mechanisms underlying a significant interaction cannot be interpreted without further experimentation.

The nesting of Sub-sub-plot′(Sub-plot′(Plot′(Block′))) means that the error term for each fixed main effect or main-effect interaction comprises the interaction between the block and all factors applied to that sampling unit or larger. Pooling terms in this manner assumes that these contributions to the error term have approximately equal MS values (see page 144).

ANOVA table for analysis of terms C|B|A + B|S|A

Model 5.4(i) A in plots, B in sub-plots and C in sub-sub-plots *are fixed factors; S' is a random block:*

Mean square	d.f.	Components of variation estimated in population	F-ratio
Between n blocks			
1 S'	$n-1$	R'(C*Q'(B*P'(S'*A))) + Q'(B*P'(S'*A)) + P'(S'*A) + S'	No test[a]
Between na plots			
2 A	$a-1$	R'(C*Q'(B*P'(S'*A))) + Q'(B*P'(S'*A)) + P'(S'*A) + S'*A + A	2/3
3 S'*A	$(n-1)(a-1)$	R'(C*Q'(B*P'(S'*A))) + Q'(B*P'(S'*A)) + P'(S'*A) + S'*A	No test
4 P'(S'*A)	0	R'(C*Q'(B*P'(S'*A))) + Q'(B*P'(S'*A)) + P'(S'*A)	No test
Between nba sub-plots			
5 B	$b-1$	R'(C*Q'(B*P'(S'*A))) + Q'(B*P'(S'*A)) + B*P'(S'*A) + B*S' + B	5/p[7+8]
6 B*A	$(b-1)(a-1)$	R'(C*Q'(B*P'(S'*A))) + Q'(B*P'(S'*A)) + B*P'(S'*A) + B*S'*A + B*A	6/p[7+8]
7 B*S'	$(b-1)(n-1)$	R'(C*Q'(B*P'(S'*A))) + Q'(B*P'(S'*A)) + B*P'(S'*A) + B*S'	No test
8 B*S'*A	$(b-1)(n-1)(a-1)$	R'(C*Q'(B*P'(S'*A))) + Q'(B*P'(S'*A)) + B*P'(S'*A) + B*S'*A	No test
9 B*P'(S'*A)	0	R'(C*Q'(B*P'(S'*A))) + Q'(B*P'(S'*A)) + B*P'(S'*A)	No test
10 Q'(B*P'(S'*A))	0	R'(C*Q'(B*P'(S'*A))) + Q'(B*P'(S'*A))	No test
Between $ncba$ sub-sub-plots			
11 C	$c-1$	R'(C*Q'(B*P'(S'*A))) + C*Q'(B*P'(S'*A)) + C*P'(S'*A) + C*S' + C	11/p[15+16+18+19]
12 C*A	$(c-1)(a-1)$	R'(C*Q'(B*P'(S'*A))) + C*Q'(B*P'(S'*A)) + C*P'(S'*A) + C*S'*A + C*A	12/p[15+16+18+19]

Model 5.4(i) (cont.)

Mean square	d.f.	Components of variation estimated in population	F-ratio
13 C*B	$(c-1)(b-1)$	R'(C*Q(B*P'(S'*A))) + C*Q'(B*P'(S'*A)) + C*B*P'(S'*A) + C*B*S' + C*B	13/p[15 + 16 + 18 + 19]
14 C*B*A	$(c-1)(b-1)(a-1)$	R'(C*Q(B*P'(S'*A))) + C*Q'(B*P'(S'*A)) + C*B*P'(S'*A) + S'*C*B*A + C*B*A	14/p[15 + 16 + 18 + 19]
15 C*S'	$(c-1)(n-1)$	R'(C*Q(B*P'(S'*A))) + C*Q'(B*P'(S'*A)) + C*P'(S'*A) + C*S'	No test
16 C*S'*A	$(c-1)(n-1)(a-1)$	R'(C*Q(B*P'(S'*A))) + C*Q'(B*P'(S'*A)) + C*P'(S'*A) + C*A*S'	No test
17 C*P'(S'*A)	0	R'(C*Q(B*P'(S'*A))) + C*Q'(B*P'(S'*A)) + C*P'(S'*A)	No test
18 C*B*S'	$(c-1)(b-1)(n-1)$	R'(C*Q(B*P'(S'*A))) + C*Q'(B*P'(S'*A)) + C*B*P'(S'*A) + C*B*S'	No test
19 C*B*S'*A	$(c-1)(b-1)(n-1)(a-1)$	R'(C*Q(B*P'(S'*A))) + C*Q'(B*P'(S'*A)) + C*B*P'(S'*A) + C*B*S'*A	No test
20 C*B*P'(S'*A)	0	R'(C*Q(B*P'(S'*A))) + C*Q'(B*P'(S'*A)) + C*B*P'(S'*A)	No test
21 C*Q'(B*P'(S'*A))	0	R'(C*Q(B*P'(S'*A))) + C*Q'(B*P'(S'*A))	No test
22 R'(C*Q(B*P'(S'*A)))	0	R'(C*Q(B*P'(S'*A)))	–
Total variation	$ncba - 1$		

^{a} An unrestricted model tests S' over the MS for its interaction with A (F-ratio = 1/3). See page 242.

5.5 Split-split-plot model (ii)

Model

$$Y = C|P'(B|S'(A))$$

Test hypothesis

Variation in the response Y is explained by the combined effects of factors A, B and C.

Description

Replicate whole blocks (S') are assigned to each level of treatment A, and each of b levels of treatment B is randomly assigned one of b plots (P') in each block, and each of c levels of treatment C is randomly assigned one of c sub-plots (Q') in each plot.

Factors	Levels	Repeated measures on S'
A	a	no
B	b	yes
C	c	yes
S'	n	–

Allocation table

The table shows $n = 2$ replicate blocks S' nested in each of $a = 2$ levels of factor A, and $b = 2$ levels of factor B allocated amongst b plots P' in each block, and $c = 2$ levels of factor C allocated amongst c sub-plots Q' in each plot. Note that the table does not indicate the spatial distribution of treatment combinations, which must be randomised within each sampling unit. For example, treatment level C_1 should not be assigned to the first sub-plot in every plot.

Q'(C|P'(B|S'(A)))		A₁		A₂	
		S_1	S_2	S_3	S_4
B_1	C_1	Q_1	Q_n	...	Q_{na}
	C_2	...	...	...	Q_{nca}
B_2	C_1	...	...	...	...
	C_2	...	...	...	Q_{ncba}

Examples

(1) *Spatial block example:* H_1: Crop yield depends on a combination of Watering regime (A), sowing Density (B) and Fertiliser (C) treatments. The *a* levels of watering are randomly assigned amongst *na* Blocks (S'), the *b* levels of sowing density are randomly assigned amongst *b* Plots (P') within each block, and the *c* levels of fertiliser are randomly assigned amongst *c* Sub-plots (Q') within each Plot. The response is the yield from each sub-plot, measured at the end of the experiment.

(2) *Temporal block example*: H_1: Plant growth depends on a combination of Temperature (A), Light (B) and Fertiliser (C). The *a* temperatures are randomly assigned amongst a series of *na* Trials (S') conducted sequentially. In each trial, *b* light levels are randomly assigned amongst *b* Mesocosms (P') all held at the same temperature, and the *c* levels of fertiliser are randomly assigned amongst *c* Trays of plants (Q') within each mesocosm. For each trial, new plants are used, light levels are randomly reassigned to mesocosms, and fertiliser levels are randomly reassigned to trays within mesocosms.

Comparisons

Model 5.5 is an extension of split-plot model 5.6 to include a third crossed factor applied to sub-plots within each plot.

In testing the combined effect of three crossed factors, model 5.5 has similar objectives to cross-factored models 3.2, 4.3, 5.2, 5.3, 5.4, 5.7, 5.9, 6.5 and 6.7. Crucially, it differs from fully randomised model 3.2 in that the assignment of treatments to sampling units is not completely randomised, and from randomised-block model 4.3 in that factors A, B and C are assigned to sampling units at different scales. Model 5.5

differs from the other three-factor split-plot models only in the way treatment factors are applied to sampling units. In contrast to repeated-measures models 6.5 and 6.7, model 5.5 randomly assigns treatment levels rather than applying them sequentially.

Special assumptions (see also general assumptions on page 143)

The model assumes no interactions of sampling units with treatments, which cannot be tested anyway because the lack of replication means that there is no residual error term (shaded grey in the ANOVA table below). Interpretation of any non-significant main effects and interactions is compromised because the result could mean either no effect, or opposing effects in different sampling units. The assumption of no sampling unit-by-treatment interactions can be tested if independent, replicate plots (P') are used for each level of factor B in each block, and if replicate sub-plots (Q') are used for each level of factor C in each plot. The interpretation of a significant sampling unit-by-treatment interaction is nevertheless problematic because the treatment effect may depend upon any of the multiple sources of variation encompassed by the blocking factor. Thus, the causal mechanisms underlying a significant interaction cannot be interpreted without further experimentation.

The nested structure of Sub-plot'(Plot'(Block')) means that the error terms for B, C and all their interactions comprise the interaction between the block and all factors applied to that sampling unit or larger. Pooling terms in this manner assumes that these contributions to the error term have approximately equal MS values (see page 144).

ANOVA table for analysis of terms C|B|A + B|S(A)

Model 5.5(i) A in blocks, B in plots and C in sub-plots are fixed factors, S' is a random blocking factor:

Mean square	d.f.	Components of variation estimated in population	F-ratio
Between *na* blocks			
1 A	$a-1$	Q'(C*P'(B*S'(A))) + P'(B*S'(A)) + S'(A) + A	1/2
2 S'(A)	$(n-1)a$	Q'(C*P'(B*S'(A))) + P'(B*S'(A)) + S'(A)	No test[a]
Between *nba* plots			
3 B	$b-1$	Q'(C*P'(B*S'(A))) + P'(B*S'(A)) + B*S'(A) + B	3/5
4 B*A	$(b-1)(a-1)$	Q'(C*P'(B*S'(A))) + P'(B*S'(A)) + B*S'(A) + B*A	4/5
5 B*S'(A)	$(b-1)(n-1)a$	Q'(C*P'(B*S'(A))) + P'(B*S'(A)) + B*S'(A)	No test
6 P'(B*S'(A))	0	Q'(C*P'(B*S'(A))) + P'(B*S'(A))	No test
Between *ncba* sub-plots			
7 C	$c-1$	Q'(C*P'(B*S'(A))) + C*P'(B*S'(A)) + C*S'(A) + C	7/p[11+12]
8 C*A	$(c-1)(a-1)$	Q'(C*P'(B*S'(A))) + C*P'(B*S'(A)) + C*S'(A) + C*A	8/p[11+12]
9 C*B	$(c-1)(b-1)$	Q'(C*P'(B*S'(A))) + C*P'(B*S'(A)) + C*B*S'(A) + C*B	9/p[11+12]
10 C*B*A	$(c-1)(b-1)(a-1)$	Q'(C*P'(B*S'(A))) + C*P'(B*S'(A)) + C*B*S'(A) + C*B*A	10/p[11+12]
11 C*S'(A)	$(c-1)(n-1)a$	Q'(C*P'(B*S'(A))) + C*P'(B*S'(A)) + C*S'(A)	No test
12 C*B*S'(A)	$(c-1)(b-1)(n-1)a$	Q'(C*P'(B*S'(A))) + C*P'(B*S'(A)) + C*B*S'(A)	No test
13 C*P'(B*S'(A))	0	Q'(C*P'(B*S'(A))) + C*P'(B*S'(A))	No test
14 Q'(C*P'(B*S'(A)))	0	Q'(C*P'(B*S'(A)))	–
Total variation	$ncba-1$		

[a] An unrestricted model tests the MS for S'(A) over the MS for its interaction with B (*F*-ratio = **2/5**). See page 242.

5.6 Two-factor split-plot model (ii)

Model

$$Y = B|S'(A)$$

Test hypothesis

Variation in the response Y is explained by the combined effects of factor A and factor B.

Description

Replicate whole blocks (S′) are assigned to each level of treatment A, and each of b levels of treatment B is randomly assigned one of b plots (P′) in each block.

Factors	Levels	Repeated measures on S′
A	a	no
B	b	yes
S′	n	–

Allocation table

The table shows $n = 2$ replicate blocks S′ nested in each of $a = 2$ levels of factor A, and $b = 4$ levels of factor B allocated amongst b plots P′ in each block. Note that the table does not indicate the spatial distribution of treatment combinations, which must be randomised within each sampling unit. For example, treatment level B_1 should not be assigned to the first plot in every block.

P′(B|S′(A))	A$_1$		A$_2$	
	S$_1$	S$_2$	S$_3$	S$_4$
B$_1$	P$_1$	P$_n$	...	P$_{na}$
B$_2$	...	...	...	...
B$_3$	...	...	...	...
B$_4$	...	...	...	P$_{nba}$

Examples

(1) S*patial block example:* H_1: Crop yield depends on a combination of Watering regime (A) and sowing Density (B) treatments. The *a* concentrations of watering are randomly assigned amongst *na* Blocks (S'), and the *b* sowing densities are randomly assigned amongst *b* Plots (P') in each block. The response is the yield from each plot, measured at the end of the experiment.

(2) *Temporal block example*: H_1: Plant growth depends on a combination of Temperature (A) and Light (B). The *a* temperatures are randomly assigned amongst a series of *na* Trials (S') conducted sequentially. In each trial, *b* light levels are randomly assigned amongst *b* Mesocosms (P'), which are all held at the same temperature. For each trial, new plants are used and light levels are randomly reassigned to Mesocosms.

(3) *Spatial block example*: H_1: Barnacle settlement depends upon background rate of recruitment and resident adult cluster size, tested by measuring barnacle density on *b* Patches (P') of rock subjected to different cluster-size Treatments (B) on Shores (S') nested in background rate of Recruitment (A). See worked example 3 on page 51 for a fully replicated version of this design.

(4) *Temporal block example*: A local environmental disturbance Event (A, with two levels: before and after) is monitored at random Times (S') and random Locations (B'), with impact gauged by B'*A. The unbalanced version of this 'before-after-control-impact' design is described in Underwood (1994).

Comparisons

Model 5.6 is an extension of model 1.1 to include a second crossed factor applied to plots nested within each block, and is an extension of randomised-block model 4.1 to include a second crossed factor applied to whole blocks. It can be extended to include a third crossed factor applied to blocks (model 5.9), to plots within blocks (model 5.7) or to sub-plots within plots (model 5.5).

The test for the main effect of A is identical to a fully replicated one-factor ANOVA (model 1.1) on the mean value of the response for each block pooled across levels of B. When $b = 2$, the test for the interaction B*A is identical to a fully replicated one-factor ANOVA on *a* treatment levels, tested with one response per block comprising the value of B_2 subtracted from B_1.

In testing the combined effect of two crossed factors, model 5.6 has similar objectives to cross-factored models 3.1, 4.2, 5.1 and 6.2. Crucially, it differs from fully randomised model 3.1 in that the assignment of treatments to sampling units (plots) is not completely randomised, and from randomised-block model 4.2 in that factors A and B are assigned to sampling units at different scales. Model 5.6 differs from split-plot model 5.1 only in the way treatment factors are applied to sampling units. In contrast to repeated-measures model 6.2, model 5.6 randomly assigns treatment levels within blocks rather than applying them sequentially.

Model 5.6 has a similar structure to completely randomised model 3.3 (where S' corresponds with B', and B corresponds with C) in that it tests the effect of one factor nested in another and crossed with a third factor. It differs from model 3.3, however, in two important respects: the assignment of treatments to sampling units is constrained because S' groups plots spatially or temporally, and the interaction of treatment B with blocks S' is not replicated. The interpretation of the analysis is influenced by the fact that the allocation of factor levels is constrained to be randomised only within each block (see special assumptions below), and the lack of full replication is acceptable only under the assumption of homogeneity of covariances (see the general assumptions of split plots on page 143).

Model 5.6 is equivalent to repeated-measures model 6.3, where block corresponds with subject (S'), except that levels of factor B are randomly assigned to plots within each block rather than being tested sequentially on each subject. It therefore escapes systematic bias from practice and carryover effects, which are unique to the sequential application of treatments.

Special assumptions (see also general assumptions on page 143)

The model assumes no $B*S'$ interaction, which cannot be tested because lack of replication means that there is no residual error term. Interpretation of non-significant B or $B*A$ is compromised because the result could mean either no effect, or opposing effects in different blocks. This problem is not resolved by excising the lack of replication with a response variable that measures the difference between $b = 2$ levels of factor B. The assumption of no $B*S'$ interaction can be tested if independent, replicate plots (P') are used for each of b levels of factor B in each of n

blocks (S'). The design is then fully replicated and can be analysed using model 3.3, with B' substituting for S' and C substituting for B. The interpretation of a significant treatment-by-block interaction is nevertheless problematic because the treatment effect may depend upon any of the multiple sources of variation encompassed by the blocking factor. Thus, the causal mechanisms underlying a significant interaction cannot be interpreted without further experimentation.

ANOVA tables

Use tables for model 6.3 on page 198, where 'Subjects' denotes 'Blocks'.

5.7 Three-factor split-plot model (iii)

Model
$$Y = C|B|S'(A)$$

Test hypothesis

Variation in the response Y is explained by the combined effects of factors A, B and C.

Description

Replicate whole blocks (S') are assigned to each level of treatment A, and each of cb combinations of levels of treatments C and B is randomly assigned one of cb plots (P') in each block.

Factors	Levels	Repeated measures on S'
A	a	no
B	b	yes
C	c	yes
S'	n	–

Allocation table

The table shows $n = 2$ replicate blocks S′ nested in each of $a = 2$ levels of factor A, and $cb = 4$ combinations of levels of factors C and B allocated amongst cb plots P′ in each block. Note that the table does not indicate the spatial distribution of treatment combinations, which must be randomised within each sampling unit. For example, treatment level C_1 should not be assigned to the first plot in every block.

P′(C|B|S′(A))		A_1		A_2	
		S_1	S_2	S_3	S_4
B_1	C_1	P_1	P_n	...	P_{na}
	C_2	...	...	...	P_{nca}
B_2	C_1	...	...	...	...
	C_2	...	...	...	P_{ncba}

Examples

(1) *Spatial block example: H_1:* Crop yield depends on a combination of Watering regime (A), sowing Density (B) and Fertiliser (C) treatments. The a levels of watering are randomly assigned amongst na Blocks (S′), and cb combinations of sowing density and fertiliser are randomly assigned amongst cb Plots (P′) in each block. The response is the yield from each plot, measured at the end of the experiment.

(2) *Temporal block example*: H_1: Plant growth depends on a combination of Temperature (A), Light (B) and Fertiliser (C). The a temperatures are randomly assigned amongst a series of na Trials (S′) conducted sequentially. In each trial, cb combinations of light and fertiliser are randomly assigned amongst cb Mesocosms (P′). For each trial, new plants are used and light and fertiliser treatments are randomly reassigned to mesocosms.

(3) *Spatial block example*: H_1: Barnacle settlement depends upon background recruitment, rock type and resident adult cluster size, tested by measuring barnacle density on cb Boulders (P′) randomly selected from b available Rock types (B′), and subjected to c different cluster-size Treatments (C) on n Shores (S′) nested in a background rates of Recruitment (A). This design is a variant of the design for worked example 3 on page 51, with stratified random sampling of rock

types, which assumes that the boulders of different rock types are distributed independently, not grouped together.

Comparisons

Model 5.7 is an extension of randomised-block model 4.2 to include a third crossed factor applied to blocks, and an extension of split-plot model 5.6 to include a third crossed factor applied to plots.

The test for the main effect of A is identical to a fully replicated one-factor ANOVA (model 1.1) on the mean value of the response for each block pooled across levels of B and C. When $c = 2$, the interaction of C with $B|S'(A)$ is identical to split-plot model 5.6 on a treatments, tested with b responses per block each comprising the value of C_2 subtracted from C_1. When both c and $b = 2$, the interaction of C*B with A is identical to a fully replicated one-factor ANOVA on a treatments (model 1.1), tested with one response per block comprising the value of $[(C_2 - C_1)$ at $B_2] - [(C_2 - C_1)$ at $B_1]$.

Model 5.7 is equivalent to repeated-measures model 6.5, where block corresponds with subject (S'), except that the cb levels of factors B and C are randomly assigned to plots within each block rather than being tested sequentially on each subject. It therefore escapes systematic bias from practice and carryover effects, which are unique to the sequential application of treatments in repeated-measures.

In testing the combined effect of three crossed factors, model 5.7 has similar objectives to cross-factored models 3.2, 4.3, 5.2, 5.3, 5.4, 5.5, 5.9 and 6.7. Crucially, it differs from fully randomised model 3.2 in that the assignment of treatments to sampling units (plots) is not completely randomised, and from randomised-block model 4.3 in that factors A, B and C are assigned to sampling units at different scales. Model 5.7 differs from the other three-factor split-plot models only in the way treatment factors are applied to sampling units. In contrast to repeated-measures model 6.7, model 5.7 randomly assigns treatment levels within blocks rather than applying them sequentially.

Special assumptions (see also general assumptions on page 143)

The model assumes no interactions of B and C with S', which cannot be tested because the lack of replication means that there is no residual error term. Interpretation of any non-significant terms amongst B, C, C*B and their interactions with A is compromised because the result could mean either no effect, or opposing effects in different blocks. The assumption of no treatment-by-block interactions can be tested if independent, replicate plots (P′) are used for each of the bc combinations of factors B and C in each block. The interpretation of a significant treatment-by-block interaction is nevertheless problematic because the treatment effect may depend upon any of the multiple sources of variation encompassed by the blocking factor. Thus, the causal mechanisms underlying a significant treatment-by-block effect cannot be interpreted without further experimentation.

ANOVA tables

Use tables for model 6.5 on page 208, where 'Subjects' denotes 'Blocks'.

5.8 Split-plot model with nesting

Model
$$Y = C|S'(B(A))$$

Test hypothesis

Variation in the response Y is explained by the combined effects of factors A, B nested in A, and C.

Description

Replicate blocks (S′) are nested in super-blocks (B′) which are themselves nested in levels of treatment A, and each of c levels of treatment C is randomly assigned one of c plots in each block.

Factors	Levels	Repeated measures on S′
A	a	no
B(A)	b	no
C	c	yes
S′	n	–

Allocation table

The table shows $n = 2$ replicate blocks S$'$ nested in each of $b = 2$ levels of super-blocks B$'$ nested in each of $a = 2$ levels of treatment A, and $c = 4$ levels of factor C allocated amongst c plots P$'$ in each block. The a temperatures are randomly assigned amongst a series of nba Trials (S$'$) conducted sequentially, with a randomly selected Mesocosm (B$'$) used for each trial. In each trial, c levels of fertiliser are randomly assigned amongst c Trays of plants (P$'$).

P$'$(C|S$'$(B(A)))	A_1				A_2			
	B_1		B_2		B_3		B_4	
	S_1	S_2	S_3	S_4	S_5	S_6	S_7	S_8
C_1	P_1	P_n	...	P_{nb}	...	...	...	P_{nba}
C_2	...	...	...	...	...	...	...	...
C_3	...	...	...	...	...	...	...	...
C_4	...	...	...	...	...	...	...	P_{ncba}

Examples

(1) *Spatial block example:* H_1: Crop yield depends on a combination of Watering regime (A) and sowing Density (C). The a watering regimes are randomly assigned amongst ba Fields (B$'$) sampled at random across a region, and the c levels of sowing density are randomly assigned amongst c Plots (P$'$) in each of n Blocks (S$'$) per field. The response is the yield from each plot, measured at the end of the experiment.

(2) *Temporal block example*: H_1: Plant growth depends on a combination of Temperature (A) and Fertiliser (C). The a temperatures are randomly assigned amongst a series of ba Trials (B$'$) conducted sequentially, with n Mesocosms (S$'$) used for each trial. In each mesocosm, c levels of fertiliser are randomly assigned amongst c Trays of plants (P$'$). For each trial, new plants are used and fertiliser treatments are randomly reassigned to trays.

(3) *Spatial block example*: H_1: Barnacle settlement depends upon background rate of recruitment, shore and resident adult cluster size, tested by measuring barnacle density on c Boulders (P$'$) randomly

subjected to different cluster-size Treatments (C) in n randomly selected Patches (S') on each of b randomly-selected Shores (B') in each of a background rates of Recruitment (A).

Comparisons

Model 5.8 is an extension of model 2.1, in which each subject (S') is tested in every level of a third factor C. If $c = 2$, tests for interactions with C are numerically equivalent to nested model 2.1 using a response of $C_2 - C_1$.

Model 5.8 is equivalent to repeated-measures model 6.6, where block corresponds with subject (S'), except that levels of factor C are randomly assigned to plots within each block rather than being applied sequentially on each subject. It therefore escapes systematic bias from practice and carryover effects, which are unique to the sequential application of treatments in repeated measures.

Special assumptions (see also general assumptions on page 143)

The model assumes no C*S' interaction, which cannot be tested because the lack of replication means that there is no residual error term. Interpretation of a non-significant C or C*A is compromised because the result could mean either no effect or opposing effects in different blocks. The assumption of no C*S' interaction can be tested if independent, replicate plots (P') are used for each of the c levels of factor C in each block. The interpretation of a significant C*S' is nevertheless problematic because the treatment effect may depend upon any of the multiple sources of variation encompassed by the blocking factor. Thus, the causal mechanisms underlying a significant treatment-by-block effect cannot be interpreted without further experimentation.

ANOVA tables

Use tables for model 6.6 on page 216, where 'Subjects' denotes 'Blocks'.

5.9 Three-factor split-plot model (iv)

Model
$$Y = C|S'(B|A)$$

Test hypothesis

Variation in the response Y is explained by the combined effects of treatments A, B and C.

Description

Each of ba combinations of levels of treatments B and A is randomly allocated to n whole blocks (S'), and each of c levels of treatment C is randomly assigned one of c plots (P') in each block.

Factors	Levels	Repeated measures on S'
A	a	no
B	b	no
C	c	yes
S'	n	–

Allocation table

The table shows $n = 2$ replicate blocks S' nested in each of $ba = 4$ combinations of levels of factors B and A, and $c = 4$ levels of factor C allocated amongst c plots P' in each block. Note that the table does not indicate the spatial distribution of treatment combinations, which must be randomised within each sampling unit. For example, treatment level C_1 should not be assigned to the first plot in every block.

P'(C|S'(B|A))	A_1				A_2			
	B_1		B_2		B_1		B_2	
	S_1	S_2	S_3	S_4	S_5	S_6	S_7	S_8
C_1	P_1	P_n	...	P_{nb}	...	...	...	P_{nba}
C_2	...	...	...	...	...	...	...	...
C_3	...	...	...	...	...	...	...	...
C_4	...	...	...	...	...	...	...	P_{ncba}

Examples

(1) *Spatial block example:* H_1: Crop yield depends on a combination of Watering regime (A), sowing Density (B) and Fertiliser (C) treatments. The *ba* combinations of watering and sowing density are randomly assigned amongst *nba* Blocks (S'), and the *c* levels of fertiliser are randomly assigned amongst *c* Plots (P') within each block. The response is the yield from each plot, measured at the end of the experiment.

(2) *Temporal block example*: H_1: Plant growth depends on a combination of Temperature (A), Light (B) and CO_2 concentration (C). The *ba* combinations of temperature and light are randomly assigned amongst a series of *nba* Trials (S') conducted sequentially. In each trial, *c* concentrations of CO_2 are randomly assigned amongst *c* Mesocosms (P'). For each trial, new plants are used and CO_2 concentrations are randomly reassigned to mesocosms.

Comparisons

Model 5.9 is an extension of completely randomised two-factor model 3.1 in which each subject (S') is tested in every level of an extra cross factor (C), and also an extension of split-plot model 5.6 to include a third crossed factor applied to blocks. If $c = 2$, tests for interactions with C are numerically equivalent to fully replicated two-factor model 3.1 using a response of $C_2 - C_1$.

Model 5.9 is equivalent to repeated-measures model 6.7, where block corresponds with subject (S'), except that levels of factor C are randomly assigned to plots within each block rather than being applied sequentially on each subject. It therefore escapes systematic bias from practice and carryover effects, which are unique to the sequential application of treatments in repeated measures.

In testing the combined effect of three crossed factors, model 5.9 has similar objectives to cross-factored models 3.2, 4.3, 5.2, 5.3, 5.4, 5.5, 5.7 and 6.5. Crucially, it differs from fully randomised model 3.2 in that the assignment of treatments to sampling units (plots) is not completely randomised, and from randomised-block model 4.3 in that factors A, B and C are assigned to sampling units at different scales. Model 5.9 differs from the other three-factor split-plot models only in the way treatment factors are applied to sampling units. In contrast to repeated-measures model 6.5, model 5.9 randomly assigns levels of treatment factors rather than applying them sequentially.

Special assumptions (see also general assumptions on page 143)

The model assumes no C*S′ interaction, which cannot be tested because the lack of replication means that there is no residual error term. Interpretation of non-significant terms amongst C and its interactions with A and B is compromised because the result could mean either no effect, or opposing effects in different blocks. The assumption of no C*S′ interaction can be tested if independent, replicate plots (P′) are used for each of the c levels of factor C in each block. The interpretation of a significant C*S′ is nevertheless problematic because the treatment effect may depend upon any of the multiple sources of variation encompassed by the blocking factor. Thus, the causal mechanisms underlying a significant treatment-by-block effect cannot be interpreted without further experimentation.

ANOVA tables

Use tables for model 6.7 on page 223, where 'Subjects' denotes 'Blocks'.

6

Repeated-measures designs

Repeated-measures designs involve measuring each sampling unit repeatedly over time or applying treatment levels in temporal or spatial sequence to each sampling unit. Because these designs were developed primarily for use in medical research, sampling units are often referred to as subjects. Those factors for which each subject participates in every level are termed 'within-subject' or 'repeated-measures' factors; levels of the within-subject factor are applied in sequence to each subject. Conversely, 'between-subjects' factors are grouping factors, for which each subject participates in only one level. Repeated-measures models are classified into two types, subject-by-trial and subject-by-treatment models, according to the nature of the within-subject factors (Kirk 1994).

Subject-by-trial designs apply the levels of the within-subject factor to each subject in an order that cannot be randomised, because time or space is an inherent component of the factor. Subjects (sampling units) may be measured repeatedly over time to track natural temporal changes in some measurable trait – for example, blood pressure of patients at age 40, 50 and 60, biomass of plants in plots at fixed times after planting, build-up of lactic acid in muscle during exercise. Likewise, subjects may be measured repeatedly through space to determine how the response varies with position – for example barnacle density in plots at different shore elevations, or lichen diversity on the north and south sides of trees. Alternatively, subjects may be measured before and after an experimental manipulation or specific event – for example, blood pressure of patients before and after taking a drug, biomass of plants in plots before and after a fire, lactic acid concentration in muscles before, during and after a race. At each sampling occasion, either the whole subject is sampled non-destructively (for example, the blood pressure of a patient), or a part of each subject is removed for measurement (for example, one randomly

179

selected plant from each plot, on the assumption that this will not affect subsequent growth of remaining plants).

When assessing the effect of a natural event or experimental manipulation occurring at a particular point in time, a control treatment level is required to ensure that the effect of the event or manipulation is not confounded by time or by factors that co-vary with time such as the state of the environment or the condition of the subjects. For example, to study the effect of fire on plant biomass, replicate plots susceptible to burning should be compared to a control set of unburned plots measured at the same times. In medicinal trials, the control treatment may take the form of a placebo. Consider an experiment in which a new drug to lower blood pressure is given to a randomly selected group of patients. The blood pressure of each patient is measured before, and again eight hours after, administering the drug in the form of an oral pill. Any statistically significant difference in mean activity level over time cannot be attributed unambiguously to the effect of the drug, because a whole range of confounding influences could have influenced the change, such as time of day, temperature or hunger level, or the psychological boost to the patient resulting simply from believing in the treatment. No logically valid conclusion can be drawn from the experiment without including a placebo treatment to control for these confounding influences. The treatment levels of drug and placebo are randomly assigned to patients, with the placebo taking the form of a pill that is identical in all respects to the drug pill except that it does not contain the drug. The drug and placebo treatments will need administering in a 'double blind' process for any trial involving human subjects. This means coding the doses in such a way that neither the patient nor the doctor are aware of which treatment level is being administered, in order to minimise bias in the results due to prior beliefs or desires about the effectiveness of the drug. Some form of blinding should be considered in any experimental manipulation that risks bias in the recording or analysis of results.

Treatments with a control or placebo always introduce a between-subject grouping factor to the design. Further between-subject factors may be used to compare the effect of the treatment among different populations of subjects. Isolated, one-off events, such as pollution incidents or hurricanes, which cannot be replicated in space, require more specialised asymmetrical designs (see Underwood 1994).

The same hypotheses are often testable using a completely randomised model, with separate sets of subjects measured on each occasion or subjects measured only after the event. However, repeatedly measuring the same subjects can increase the power to detect treatment effects because the repeated measures control for inherent differences among subjects, for example in blood pressure among patients, in plant biomass among plots or in fitness among athletes.

Subject-by-treatment designs apply the sequential levels of the within-subject factor (treatments) in an order that is randomised in time. For example, the performance-enhancing effects of drinking a specially formulated isotonic glucose electrolyte may be tested by clocking athletes' times over a 10 km course after drinking either the electrolyte or water, and clocking them again after swapping their treatments. The order in which each athlete receives the two treatments is randomised. Similarly, the palatability of three types of seeds may be tested by presenting the seeds, one type at a time, to individual mice and measuring the mass of seeds consumed in two minutes. Again, the treatments are applied to each subject in a random order. Testing all levels of a within-subject factor on each subject increases the power of the experiment to detect an effect of the within-subject factor by controlling for inherent differences among subjects – in fitness among athletes, or in body size among mice. Thus, a repeated-measures design requires fewer subjects to achieve the same power and precision as a completely randomised design, in which each subject is tested in just one level of an experimental factor.

Subject-by-treatment designs may have between-subject factors, just as the subject-by-trial designs group subjects by treatment versus control. For example, athletes could be classified according to their level of fitness to test the hypothesis that the type of fluid intake affects the performance of elite athletes more than that of recreational joggers; similarly, mice could be classified according to body size to test the hypothesis that larger mice prefer larger seeds.

The disadvantage of the subject-by-treatment design is its inherent susceptibility to *practice effects* and *carryover effects*. Practice effects arise when the condition of the subjects changes systematically during the course of the experiment. For example, athletes could be more tired in the second trial than the first due to their exertions in the first trial; the appetite of the mice might decrease over time as they become satiated. Carryover effects arise when exposure to one experimental treatment influences the effect of one or more subsequent treatments. For example, athletes that receive the electrolyte drink in the first trial may still derive some benefit from it during the second trial; mice may be more likely to consume a particular type of seed if it looks or smells like one they have been presented with previously. In statistical terms, practice effects are an effect of time since the start of the study, whilst carryover effects are an interaction between a treatment factor and the order or sequence of application of its levels. Both effects can potentially increase the variation within each subject and thereby reduce the power of the experiment to test treatment effects.

Practice effects and carryover effects may be reduced or eliminated by providing rest periods between successive treatments, for example by conducting trials on successive days to allow athletes sufficient rest for their fluid levels to return to normal between trials. However, this may not be an effective solution to carryover effects that arise from subjects remembering or learning from previous treatments. For example, the behaviour of mice may be modified by their memory of previously encountered seed types even after a rest period of several days or weeks.

Alternatively, practice effects and carryover effects can be controlled for by systematically varying the presentation order of the treatments, a process known as 'counterbalancing' or 'switching'. For example, if half the athletes drink water first and electrolyte second and the other half drink electrolyte first and water second, then the order of the treatments will be balanced across all the subjects and any difference between the treatments will not be confounded by practice or carryover effects. The advantage of counterbalancing is that the existence of a carryover effect can then be tested by seeking an interaction between the treatment and its order of application. For example, we could test whether any benefit of the electrolyte drink depends on the fatigue of the athlete, or whether the palatability of seeds is affected by prior experience of other seed types. The disadvantage of counterbalancing is that it may require large numbers of subjects for factors with three or more levels. For example, controlling for all carryover effects in the seed palatability study requires testing at least two mice in each of the six permutations of order, and then cross factoring order with seed type ($a = 6$ levels of Order, $b = 3$ levels of Seed type in model 6.3). However, since this design requires at least 12 subjects, seed preference could have been tested more efficiently with a fully replicated one-factor ANOVA in which 12 mice are each tested with just one seed type, assigned to them at random (model 1.1). Alternatively, the Latin square variant of one-factor randomised blocks provides a design that uses just three mice as levels of a Subject block, which are cross factored with three levels of an Order block (detailed on page 125). Although this kind of 'crossover' design only samples the variation in order, it can be replicated to improve power (see examples in Ratkowski *et al.* 1993; Crawley 2002; Quinn and Keough 2002).

Repeated-measures models are similar in concept to randomised-block and split-plot models (see Chapters 4 and 5): taking repeated measurements on each subject to control for intrinsic variation between them is equivalent to taking repeated measurements on each block to control for inherent spatial or temporal background variation. We illustrate this similarity using S' to denote both subjects and blocks and P' to denote both observations nested in subject and plots nested in blocks. Repeated-measures models differ from randomised-block and split-plot models, however, in that the within-subject (block) treatment levels are assigned in spatial or temporal sequence rather than being randomly assigned within each block. Practice and carryover effects are therefore unique to repeated-measures designs.

The sampling unit for a given treatment level or combination in repeated-measures designs is the observation:

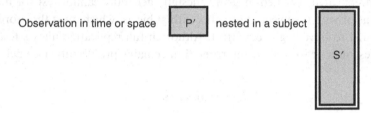

Observation in time or space P' nested in a subject S'

Assumptions

As with randomised-block and split-plot models, repeated measures designs make an assumption of *homogeneity of covariances* because the repeated measurements on each subject from different levels of the within-subject factor are not independent of each other. This source of correlation between levels of the within-subject factor is not a problem provided that the covariances (i.e., correlations) are the same between treatment levels within each subject. This is an extension to the standard assumption of homogeneous variances, which applies to all ANOVA (page 14). In practice, the assumption requires only an additional homogeneity amongst the set of variances obtained from all pairs of within-subject treatment levels, where each variance is calculated from the differences in response between the levels across subjects: known as the 'sphericity condition'. Thus, in the design for model 6.1 below, with $a = 3$ levels of factor A and $n = 6$ subjects, one variance is calculated from the six differences in response between A_1 and A_2, another from the six for A_1 and A_3, and the third from the six for A_2 and A_3. Heterogeneity amongst these variances will result in a liberal test that inflates the Type I error rate. Kirk (1982), Winer *et al.* (1991) and Quinn and Keough (2002) suggest methods of dealing with this problem. Note that a model that has a single within-subject factor with just two levels has only one covariance, and is therefore not subject to the sphericity condition. If the design is fully replicated, then the assumption of homogeneity of covariances becomes subsumed within the standard assumption of homogeneity of variances between all samples.

With only one replicate observation made per subject on each level of the within-subject factor(s), the requirement that it be drawn independently ceases to apply, but it must be representative of the subject, and of that level of the within-subject factor(s). Unlike randomised-block designs, which randomise the assignment of treatment levels within each block, repeated-measures designs are constrained by a sequential assignment of levels. They must therefore assume no practice or carryover effects.

Unreplicated repeated-measures designs generally cannot test for interactions of within-subject treatments with subjects, which must therefore be assumed to have negligible effect. Although full replication allows testing of these interactions, their interpretation remains problematic (see below).

Analysis

Repeated measurement of the same subject over time or of the same subject in spatial sequence will give rise to non-independent observations. Treating these observations as independent replicates constitutes pseudoreplication (Hurlbert 1984), which can increase the probability of a Type I error (rejection of a true null hypothesis) by inflating the denominator degrees of freedom for tests of treatment effects. This non-independence is explicitly accounted for in repeated-measures models by including Subject as a random factor (S').

Subjects are always crossed with within-subject factors and nested in between-subject factors. Subject-by-trial designs have the sequential factor Time or Location as the within-subject factor. When measurements are taken on each subject three or more times, *post hoc* tests or orthogonal contrasts (page 245) may be used to compare measurements. For example, a study of lactic acid concentrations in muscles before, during and after exercise could use Dunnett's test to specifically compare the during and after measurements with the before measurements. Alternatively, repeated measurements that track natural changes in the subjects can model time as a covariate to compare regression slopes among subjects.

Repeated-measures models usually test every subject just once in each level of the within-subject factor, as this maximises the power of the experiment to detect treatment effects. The lack of replication has a serious shortcoming, common to all unreplicated models. Specifically, interactions between subjects and within-subject factors generally cannot be tested, which thereby increases the likelihood of a Type II error (acceptance of a false null hypothesis) when interpreting lower-order effects (Underwood 1997). In other words, an apparently non-significant within-subject factor may have a real influence on the response that varies by subject. However, the existence of within-subject effects can retain interest regardless of interactions with subject, if the priority is to avoid Type I errors.

A number of approaches overcome or avoid the problem of incomplete replication:

- The possiblity that subjects have opposing responses to a treatment can be excluded *post hoc* by finding positive correlations of equal magnitude between all pairs of levels of the within-subject factor.
- Obtain full replication by repeatedly testing every subject in each level of the within-subject factor. In some cases, the design can then be analysed using equivalent models in Chapter 3. Although this allows all subject-by-treatment interactions to be tested, full replication may provide relatively little improvement in power for the extra resources invested and may be impossible in subject-by-trial designs.
- Eliminate the repeated measures altogether by redefining the response as a single summary statistic per subject that encapsulates the information on the within-subject factor of interest (Grafen and Hails 2002). For example, to compare the biomass of plants in plots at fixed times after planting, one could take a response variable from the last observation only, or from the difference between the first and the last, or from the slope of the regression of biomass against time.
- Employ a multivariate approach, such as discriminant function analysis or MANOVA (see, for example, Underwood 1997; Grafen and Hails 2002).

All of the repeated-measures designs described in this chapter have an equivalent randomised-block or split-plot model in which levels of the within-subject factor are applied to different parts of each subject (block) rather than in sequence. This is reflected in the allocation tables for this chapter, which denote subjects by S' to illustrate their similarity with blocks, and the replicate observations on each subject by P' to illustrate their similarity with plots nested in blocks. The randomised-block and split-plot designs are analysed and interpreted in exactly the same way as repeated measures, except that they do not suffer the inherent biases of practice and carryover effects. In order to appreciate the fundamental differences between these types of model, consider variations on an agricultural experiment to test the effect of a fertiliser Treatment (A) on crop yield. Imagine that the experiment requires a random factor Block with eight levels to group unmeasured environmental heterogeneity. The experiment could be designed with various levels of replication and randomisation, and these considerations will determine which of Chapters 1 to 6 provide the appropriate ANOVA tables.

Chapter 1. Fully replicated one-factor model 1.1. Treatment levels are randomly assigned to whole blocks (S′) and one response measured per block.

Chapter 2. Fully replicated nested model 2.1. The response is measured as the yield per plot (S′) nested in blocks (B′).

Chapter 3. Fully replicated cross-factored model 3.1(ii). Each treatment level is randomly assigned to replicate plots (S′) within each block (B′).

Chapter 4. Randomised-block model 4.1. Each treatment level is randomly assigned to one plot (P′) within each block (S′).

Chapter 5. Split-plot model 5.6. Treatment levels are randomly assigned to whole blocks (S′), and tested against a sowing Density cross factor (B, with two levels: high and low) randomly assigned to plots (P′) within blocks.

Chapter 6(a). Repeated measures in time (subject-by-trial) model 6.3. Treatment levels are randomly assigned to whole blocks (S′), and tested against a Time cross factor (B′, with two levels: before and after fertiliser application).

Chapter 6(b). Repeated measures in space (subject-by-trial) model 6.3. Treatments level are randomly assigned to whole blocks (S′), and tested against a cross factor Sector (B, with two levels: north and south end of block).

Chapter 6(c). Repeated measures in time (subject-by-treatment) model 6.3. Whole blocks (S′) are allocated at random to fertiliser treatments of phosphate then nitrogen, or nitrogen then phosphate. This design has two cross factors: Order (A, with two levels: earlier and later application of phosphate) in which the blocks are nested, and the repeated-measures factor of Fertiliser (B, with two levels: phosphate and nitrogen). Although the Order factor could be ignored, since it is randomised, the testable Order*Treatment interaction would likely be of interest if significant.

Chapter 6(d). Repeated measures in space (subject-by-treatment) model 6.3. Whole blocks (S′) are allocated at random to phosphate and nitrogen in north and south ends respectively, or in south and north ends respectively. This design has two cross-factors: Sector (A, with two levels: north and south end for phosphate) in which the blocks are nested, and the repeated-measures factor of fertiliser (B, with two levels: phosphate and nitrogen). Although the Sector factor could be ignored, since it is randomised, the testable Sector*Treatment interaction would likely be of interest if significant.

6.1 One-factor repeated-measures model

Model

$$Y = S'|A$$

Test hypothesis

Variation in the response Y is explained by repeated-measures factor A.

Description

Repeated observations (P') are taken on n subjects (S'), once at each level of factor A.

Factors	Levels	Repeated measures on S'
A	a	yes
S'	n	–

Allocation table

The table illustrates $n = 4$ subjects S' each observed once at a sequence of $a = 4$ levels of factor A. Unlike the allocation table for randomised-block model 4.1, this table does indicate the spatial or temporal sequence of treatment combinations.

P'(S'|A)	S_1	S_2	S_3	S_4
A_1	P_1	...	...	P_n
A_2	...	...	...	...
A_3	...	...	...	...
A_4	...	...	...	P_{na}

Examples

(1) *Subject-by-trial design*: H_1: Barnacle settlement density on Shores (S′) varies with elevation (A), tested by sampling one Plot (P′) at each of *a* elevations on each of *n* shores.

(2) *Subject-by-trial design*: H_1: Species diversity of lichens on Trees (S′) changes with tree Aspect (A), tested by sampling once on each of north and south sides of each tree.

(3) *Subject-by-treatment design*: H_1: Performance of *n* Athletes (S′) depends on Drink treatment (A with two levels: isotonic glucose electrolyte and water). Performance is measured by clocking the running times of athletes over a 10 km course after drinking either electrolyte or water, and clocking them again after swapping their treatments. The order in which each athlete receives the two treatments is randomised.

(4) *Subject-by-treatment design*: H_1: Social interactions in *n* captive lemur Groups (S′) depend on public Viewing (A with two levels: open and closed to view). The order in which each group of lemurs is opened and closed to view is randomised.

Comparisons

Model 6.1 can be extended to include a second crossed factor applied to subjects (model 6.3) or tested sequentially on each subject (model 6.2).

When $a = 2$, the test is equivalent to a paired-sample *t* test, which itself is equivalent to testing the mean difference in response between two times against the null hypothesis of zero difference.

In testing the effect of a single treatment factor A, model 6.1 has similar objectives to completely randomised model 1.1 and randomised-block model 4.1. It differs from model 1.1 in that each subject (S′) is tested in each level of factor A to partition out unwanted sources of background variation among subjects. Although the analysis for model 6.1 is identical to model 4.1 (Model 1), with subject corresponding with block (S′), the levels of A are tested sequentially on each subject rather than being randomised within each block. Model 6.1 is therefore inherently susceptible to practice and carryover effects from the sequential application of treatments in repeated measures.

The analysis of model 6.1 is identical to the analysis of an unreplicated two-factor design with at least one random factor (model 7.1), except that it must meet the additional assumptions of homogeneity of covariances across subjects and no practice and carryover effects.

Special assumptions (see also general assumptions of repeated measures on page 183)

The model cannot test the subject-by-treatment interaction, because the lack of replication means that there is no residual error term (shaded grey in the ANOVA tables below). Interpretation of a non-significant A is compromised because the result could mean either no effect, or opposing effects on different subjects. The assumption of no significant subject-by-treatment interaction can be tested if independent, replicate observations (P′) are made for each of the *a* treatments on each subject. The design is then fully replicated and the analysis identical to that for model 3.1, with B′ substituting for S′. The interpretation of a significant block-by-treatment interaction is nevertheless problematic because the treatment effect may depend upon any of the multiple sources of variation encompassed by the subject factor. In Example 1 above, a significant S′*A interaction would mean that the effect of shore elevation on barnacle settlement varies spatially, due to differences among shores in geology, microclimate, human impact and so on. Thus, the causal mechanisms underlying a significant subject-by-treatment effect cannot be interpreted without further experimentation.

Notes

Model 6.1 is suitable only for detecting changes over time (or across space), and not for attributing causality to the change. It cannot analyse treatments in 'before–after' experiments because it has no control for the numerous factors that co-vary with time. For some studies, the confounding influence of time can be avoided by cross factoring it with a between-subject treatment, using model 6.3. For example, subjects may be tested before and after ingesting a medical treatment, with one group given a drug and another a placebo. Causality can then be inferred from a significant treatment-by-time interaction.

ANOVA tables for analysis of terms S + A

Model 6.1(*i*) *A is a fixed factor, S' is a random subject:*

Mean square	d.f.	Components of variation estimated in population	*F*-ratio
Between subjects			
1 S'	$n-1$	$P'(S'*A) + S'$	No test[a]
Within subjects			
2 A	$a-1$	$P'(S'*A) + S'*A + A$	2/3
3 S'*A	$(n-1)(a-1)$	$P'(S'*A) + S'*A$	No test
4 P'(S'*A)	0	$P'(S'*A)$	–
Total variation	$na-1$		

[a] An unrestricted model tests the MS for S' over the MS for its interaction with A (*F*-ratio = **1/3**). See page 242.

Model 6.1(*ii*) *A' is a random factor, S' is a random subject:*

Mean square	d.f.	Components of variation estimated in population	*F*-ratio
Between subjects			
1 S'	$n-1$	$P'(S'*A') + S'*A' + S'$	1/3
Within subjects			
2 A'	$a-1$	$P'(S'*A') + S'*A' + A'$	2/3
3 S'*A'	$(n-1)(a-1)$	$P'(S'*A') + S'*A'$	No test
4 P'(S'*A')	0	$P'(S'*A')$	–
Total variation	$na-1$		

6.2 Two-factor repeated-measures model

Model

$$Y = S'|B|A$$

Test hypothesis

Variation in the response Y is explained by the combined effects of factor A and factor B.

Description

Repeated observations (P′) are taken on n subjects (S′), once at each combination of levels of cross factors B and A.

Factors	Levels	Repeated measures on S′
A	a	yes
B	b	yes
S′	n	–

Allocation table

The table illustrates $n = 4$ subjects S′, each observed once at each of $ba = 4$ combinations of levels of factors B and A.

P′(S′|B|A)		S_1	S_2	S_3	S_4
A1	B_1	P_1	...	...	P_n
	B_2	...	...	...	P_{nb}
A2	B_1	...	...	...	...
	B_2	...	...	...	P_{nba}

Examples

(1) *Subject-by-trial design*: H_1: Barnacle settlement density on Shores (S′) varies with Elevation (A) and Surface rugosity (B), tested by allocating one Plot (P′) to each of b levels of rugosity at each of a elevations on each of n shores.

(2) *Subject-by-trial design*: H_1: Species diversity of lichens on Trees (S′) changes with Aspect (A with two levels: north or south side) and Age (B with three levels: 5, 10 and 20 years) of tree. Both sides of n trees are sampled repeatedly at ages 5, 10 and 20 years.

(3) *Subject-by-treatment design*: H_1: Performance of Athletes (S′) depends on Drink treatment (A with two levels: isotonic glucose electrolyte and water) and Vitamin supplement (B, vitamin tablet, placebo control). Performance is measured by clocking the running times of athletes (S′) over a 10km course after taking each combination of drink and

vitamin supplement. The order in which each athlete receives the four treatment combinations is randomised.

Comparisons

Model 6.2 is an extension of model 6.1 to include a second crossed factor (B). It can be extended to include a third crossed factor applied to subjects (model 6.5).

In testing the combined effect of two crossed factors, model 6.2 has similar objectives to cross-factored models 3.1, 4.2, 5.1, 5.6 and 6.3. Crucially, it differs from fully randomised model 3.1 in that each subject (S′) is tested in all levels of factors A and B to partition out unwanted sources of background variation among subjects. Although the analysis of model 6.2 is identical to randomised-block model 4.2 (Model 1), with subject corresponding with block (S′), the *ba* levels of factors A and B are tested sequentially on each subject rather than being randomised within each block. Model 6.2 is therefore inherently susceptible to practice and carryover effects from the sequential application of treatments in repeated measures. Similarly, model 6.2 is distinguished from split-plot models 5.1 and 5.6 by the sequential application of treatments to sampling units. Finally, model 6.2 differs from repeated-measures model 6.3 in that A is a within-subjects factor rather than a between-subjects factor.

The analysis of model 6.2 is identical to the analysis of an unreplicated three-factor design with at least one random factor (model 7.2), except that it must meet the additional assumptions of homogeneity of covariances across subjects and no practice and carryover effects.

Special assumptions (see also general assumptions of repeated measures on page 183)

Model 6.2 cannot test subject-by-treatment interactions, because the lack of replication means that there is no residual error term (shaded grey in the ANOVA tables below). Interpretation of non-significant A, B or B*A is compromised because the result could mean either no effect, or opposing effects on different subjects. The assumption of no significant subject-by-treatment interaction can be tested if independent, replicate observations (P′) are made on each subject for each of the *ba* levels of factors A and B. The design is then fully replicated and the analysis identical to that for model 3.2, with C′ substituting for S′. The interpretation of a significant block-by-treatment interaction is nevertheless problematic because the treatment effect may depend upon any of the multiple sources of variation encompassed by the subject factor.

In example 2 above, the slow growth rates of lichens provides little opportunity to take independent replicate observations on a tree within each aspect and age group. An alternative fully replicated design would involve measuring simultaneously many trees of different ages and aspects. The test hypothesis for such a two-factor ANOVA would be that lichen diversity varies with tree age and aspect, as opposed to changing with tree age according to aspect, which is the question directly tested by the repeated-measures design.

Notes

Model 6.2 is suitable only for detecting changes over time, and not for attributing causality to the change. It cannot analyse treatments in 'before–after' experiments because it has no control for the numerous factors that co-vary with time. For some studies, the confounding influence of time can be avoided by cross factoring it with between-subject treatments, using model 6.7. For example, male and female subjects may be tested before and after ingesting a medical treatment, with one group of each sex given a drug and another a placebo. Causality can then be inferred from a significant treatment-by-time interaction.

ANOVA tables for analysis of terms S|B|A − S*B*A

Model 6.2(i) *A and B are fixed factors, S′ is a random subject:*

Mean square	d.f.	Components of variation estimated in population	F-ratio
Between subjects			
1 S′	$n-1$	$P'(S'*B*A) + S'$	No test[a]
Within subjects			
2 A	$a-1$	$P'(S'*B*A) + S'*A + A$	2/5
3 B	$b-1$	$P'(S'*B*A) + S'*B + B$	3/6
4 B*A	$(b-1)(a-1)$	$P'(S'*B*A) + S'*B*A + B*A$	4/7
5 S′*A	$(n-1)(a-1)$	$P'(S'*B*A) + S'*A$	No test
6 S′*B	$(n-1)(b-1)$	$P'(S'*B*A) + S'*B$	No test
7 S′*B*A	$(n-1)(b-1)(a-1)$	$P'(S'*B*A) + S'*B*A$	No test
8 P′(S′*B*A)	0	$P'(S'*B*A)$	–
Total variation	$nba - 1$		

[a] An unrestricted model has an inexact F-ratio denominator (see page 242).

Model 6.2(ii) A *is a fixed factor,* B' *is a random factor,* S' *is a random subject:*

Mean square	d.f.	Components of variation estimated in population	F-ratio
Between subjects			
1 S'	$n-1$	$P'(S'*B'*A) + S'*B' + S'$	$1/6^b$
Within subjects			
2 A	$a-1$	$P'(S'*B'*A) + S'*B'*A + S'*A + B'*A$ $+ A$	$2/(4+5-7)^{ab}$
3 B'	$b-1$	$P'(S'*B'*A) + S'*B' + B'$	$3/6^b$
4 $B'*A$	$(b-1)(a-1)$	$P'(S'*B'*A) + S'*B'*A + B'*A$	$4/7$
5 $S'*A$	$(n-1)(a-1)$	$P'(S'*B'*A) + S'*B'*A + S'*A$	$5/7$
6 $S'*B'$	$(n-1)(b-1)$	$P'(S'*B'*A) + S'*B'$	No test
7 $S'*B'*A$	$(n-1)(b-1)(a-1)$	$P'(S'*B'*A) + S'*B'*A$	No test
8 $P'(S'*B'*A)$	0	$P'(S'*B'*A)$	–
Total variation	$nba - 1$		

[a] There is no exact denominator for this test (see page 40). If $B'*A$ and/or $S'*A$ have $P > 0.25$, however, then *post hoc* pooling can be used to derive an exact denominator for A. If $B'*A$ has $P > 0.25$ (but $S'*A$ has $P < 0.25$), eliminate $B'*A$ from the mean square for A, making $S'*A$ its error mean square. If $S'*A$ has $P > 0.25$ (but $B'*A$ has $P < 0.25$), then eliminate $S'*A$ from the mean square for A, making $B'*A$ its error mean square. If both $B'*A$ and $S'*A$ have $P > 0.25$, use the pooled error mean square: [SS $\{B'*A\} + SS\{S'*A\} + SS\{S'*B'*A\}]/[(b-1)(a-1) + (n-1)(a-1) + (n-1)(b-1)(a-1)]$. Further pooling can be done if $S'*B'*A$ has $P > 0.25$. See page 38.
[b] An unrestricted model has an inexact F-ratio denominator (see page 242).

Model 6.2(iii) A' *and* B' *are random factors,* S' *is a random subject:*

Mean square	d.f.	Components of variation estimated in population	F-ratio
Between subjects			
1 S'	$n-1$	$P'(S'*B'*A') + S'*B'*A' + S'*B' + S'*A' + S'$	$1/(5+6-7)^a$
Within subjects			
2 A'	$a-1$	$P'(S'*B'*A') + S'*B'*A' + S'*A' + B'*A' + A'$	$2/(4+5-7)^a$
3 B'	$b-1$	$P'(S'*B'*A') + S'*B'*A' + S'*B' + B'*A' + B'$	$3/(4+6-7)^a$
4 $B'*A'$	$(b-1)(a-1)$	$P'(S'*B'*A') + S'*B'*A' + B'*A'$	$4/7$
5 $S'*A'$	$(n-1)(a-1)$	$P'(S'*B'*A') + S'*B'*A' + S'*A'$	$5/7$
6 $S'*B'$	$(n-1)(b-1)$	$P'(S'*B'*A') + S'*B'*A' + S'*B'$	$6/7$
7 $S'*B'*A'$	$(n-1)(b-1)(a-1)$	$P'(S'*B'*A') + S'*B'*A'$	No test
8 $P'(S'*B'*A')$	0	$P'(S'*B'*A')$	–
Total variation	$nba - 1$		

[a] There is no exact denominator for this test (see page 40). If higher-order interactions contributing to the mean square have $P > 0.25$, however, then they can be removed from the mean square in *post hoc* pooling to derive an exact denominator (applying the same technique as for A in model (ii) above).

6.3 Two-factor model with repeated measures on one cross factor

Model

$$Y = B|S'(A)$$

Test hypothesis

Variation in the response Y is explained by the combined effects of factor A and factor B.

Description

Replicate subjects (S') are assigned to each level of treatment A, and repeated observations (P') are taken on each subject, once at each level of factor B.

Factors	Levels	Repeated measures on S'
A	a	no
B	b	yes
S'	n	–

Allocation table

The table shows $n = 2$ replicate subjects S' nested in each of $a = 2$ levels of factor A, and each subject observed once at each of $b = 4$ levels of factor B.

Examples

(1) *Subject-by-trial design*: H_1: Blood pressure of Patients (S′) responds to Ingestion (B with two levels: before and after) of Medicine (A with two levels: drug and placebo).

(2) *Subject-by-trial design*: H_1: Visual acuity varies between left and right Eye (B) of each Subject (S′) according to their Handedness (A).

(3) *Subject-by-trial design*: Barnacle settlement density is measured on Patches (P′) of rock at different Elevations (B) on Shores (S′) nested in background rate of Recruitment (A).

(4) *Subject-by-treatment design*: H_1: Performance of Athletes (S′) depends on Drink treatment (B with two levels: isotonic glucose electrolyte and water). Performance is measured by clocking the running times of athletes over a 10 km course after drinking either electrolyte or water, and clocking them again after swapping their treatments. Each athlete receives the two treatments in a particular Order (A with two levels: electrolyte first and water first).

(5) *Subject-by-treatment design*: H_1: Social interactions in Groups of captive lemurs (S′) depend on public Viewing (B with two levels: open and closed to view) and Management regime (A with two levels: single-species cages and mixed-species cages). n groups of lemurs are studied in each of a management regimes. The order in which each group of lemurs is opened and closed to view is randomised. This analysis assumes that the effect of management is not confounded by other factors, such as number of individuals per cage.

Comparisons

Model 6.3 is an extension of model 1.1 in which each subject is tested sequentially in every level of a second, crossed factor B, and it is an extension of repeated-measures model 6.1 to include a between-subjects factor. It can be further extended to include an additional between-subjects factor (model 6.7) or an additional within-subjects factor (model 6.5).

The test for the main effect of A is identical to a fully replicated one-factor ANOVA on the mean value of the response for each subject pooled across levels of B. When $b = 2$, the test for the interaction B*A is identical to a fully replicated one-factor ANOVA on a treatments (model 1.1), tested with one response per subject comprising the value of B_2 subtracted from B_1.

Model 6.3 is equivalent to split-plot model 5.6, where subject corresponds with block (S′), except that levels of factor B are tested sequentially on each subject rather than being randomly assigned within each block. It is therefore inherently susceptible to practice and carryover effects from the sequential application of treatments in repeated measures.

In testing the combined effect of two crossed-factors, model 6.3 has similar objectives to cross factored models 3.1, 4.2, 5.1 and 6.2. Crucially, it differs from fully randomised model 3.1, randomised-block model 4.2 and split-plot model 5.1 in that the *b* levels of factor B are tested sequentially on each subject. Finally, model 6.3 differs from repeated-measures model 6.2 in that A is a between-subjects factor rather than a within-subjects factor.

Special assumptions (see also general assumptions of repeated measures on page 183)

Model 6.3 cannot test the B*S′ interaction, because lack of replication means that there is no residual error term (shaded grey in the ANOVA tables below). Interpretation of non-significant B or B*A is compromised because the result could mean either no effect, or opposing effects on different subjects. This problem is not resolved by excising the lack of replication with a response variable that measures the difference between $b = 2$ levels of factor B. The assumption of no significant B*S′ interaction can be tested if independent, replicate observations (P′) are made for each of *b* levels of factor B in each of *n* subjects (S′). The design is then fully replicated and can be analysed using model 3.3, with B′ substituting for S′ and C substituting for B. The interpretation of a significant treatment-by-subject interaction is nevertheless problematic because the treatment effect may depend upon any of the multiple sources of variation encompassed by the subject factor. If treatment effects may be subject-dependent, one should consider what aspect of the subject may be influencing the treatment effect and include it as an additional between-subjects factor (using model 6.7).

For instance, Example 1 above tests particularly for a significant B*A interaction, which indicates an effective drug. The model cannot test whether this effect depends on subject, however, and a non-significant interaction could mean either that the drug has no effect, or that it has opposing effects on different subjects. These questions of causality are not resolved by applying a one-factor ANOVA between the drug and placebo to a response variable that compares change in blood pressure

(B_2 subtracted from B_1). Testing for a subject-dependent effect requires taking random and independent observations within each subject and level of the crossfactor and using model 3.3 (with factor B' coding for subjects in both cases, and S' for observations). The interpretation of a significant interaction with subject is nevertheless problematic because the random subject factor encompasses multiple sources of variation. Thus, the causal mechanisms underlying a significant interaction with subject cannot be interpreted without further experimentation.

ANOVA tables for analysis of terms $B|A + B|S(A) - B*S(A)$

Model 6.3(i) *A and B are fixed factors, S' is a random subject:*

Mean square	d.f.	Components of variation estimated in population	F-ratio
Between subjects			
1 A	$a-1$	$P'(B*S'(A)) + S'(A) + A$	**1/2**
2 S'(A)	$(n-1)a$	$P'(B*S'(A)) + S'(A)$	No test[a]
Within subjects			
3 B	$b-1$	$P'(B*S'(A)) + B*S'(A) + B$	**3/5**
4 B*A	$(b-1)(a-1)$	$P'(B*S'(A)) + B*S'(A) + B*A$	**4/5**
5 B*S'(A)	$(b-1)(n-1)a$	$P'(B*S'(A)) + B*S'(A)$	No test
6 P'(B*S'(A))	0	$P'(B*S'(A))$	–
Total variation	$nba-1$		

[a] An unrestricted model tests the MS for $S'(A)$ over the MS for its interaction with B (F-ratio = **2/5**). See page 242.

Model 6.3(ii) *A is a fixed factors, B' is a random factor, S' is a random subject:*

Mean square	d.f.	Components of variation estimated in population	F-ratio
Between subjects			
1 A	$a-1$	$P'(B'*S'(A)) + B'*S'(A) + B'*A + S'(A) + A$	$1/(2+4-5)$[a]
2 S'(A)	$(n-1)a$	$P'(B'*S'(A)) + B'*S'(A) + S'(A)$	**2/5**
Within subjects			
3 B'	$b-1$	$P'(B'*S'(A)) + B'*S'(A) + B'$	**3/5**[b]
4 B'*A	$(b-1)(a-1)$	$P'(B'*S'(A)) + B'*S'(A) + B'*A$	**4/5**
5 B'*S'(A)	$(b-1)(n-1)a$	$P'(B'*S'(A)) + B'*S'(A)$	No test
6 P'(B'*S'(A))	0	$P'(B'*S'(A))$	–
Total variation	$nba-1$		

[a] There is no exact denominator for this test (see page 40). If $S'(A)$ and/or $B'*A$ have $P > 0.25$, however, then *post hoc* pooling can be used to derive an exact denominator for A. If $S'(A)$ has $P > 0.25$ (but $B'*A$ has $P < 0.25$), then eliminate $S'(A)$ from the mean square for A, making $B'*A$ its error mean square. If $B'*A$ has $P > 0.25$ (but $S'(A)$ has $P < 0.25$), eliminate $B'*A$ from the mean square for A, making $S'(A)$ its error mean square. If both $S'(A)$ and $B'*A$ have $P > 0.25$, use the pooled error mean square: $[SS\{S'(A)\} + SS\{B'*A\} + SS\{B'*S'(A)\}]/[(n-1)a + (b-1)(a-1) + (b-1)(n-1)a]$. See page 38.
[b] An unrestricted model tests the MS for B' over the MS for its interaction with A (F-ratio = **3/4**). See page 242.

Model 6.3(*iii*) A' *is a random factor, B is a fixed factor, S' is a random subject:*

Mean square	d.f.	Components of variation estimated in population	F-ratio
Between subjects			
1 A'	$a-1$	$P'(B*S'(A')) + S'(A') + A'$	$1/2^a$
2 $S'(A')$	$(n-1)a$	$P'(B*S'(A')) + S'(A')$	No test[b]
Within subjects			
3 B	$b-1$	$P'(B*S'(A')) + B*S'(A') + B*A' + B$	$3/4^c$
4 $B*A'$	$(b-1)(a-1)$	$P'(B*S'(A')) + B*S'(A') + B*A'$	4/5
5 $B*S'(A')$	$(b-1)(n-1)a$	$P'(B*S'(A')) + B*S'(A')$	No test
6 $P'(B*S'(A'))$	0	$P'(B*S'(A'))$	–
Total variation	$nba-1$		

[a] An unrestricted model has an inexact F-ratio denominator (see page 242).
[b] An unrestricted model tests the MS for $S'(A')$ over the MS for its interaction with B (F-ratio $= 2/5$). See page 242.
[c] Planned *post hoc* pooling is permissible for B if $B*A'$ has $P > 0.25$. Use the pooled error mean square: $[SS\{B*A'\} + SS\{B*S'(A')\}]/[(b-1)(a-1) + (b-1)(n-1)a]$. See page 38.

Model 6.3(*iv*) A' *and B' are random factors, S' is a random subject:*

Mean square	d.f.	Components of variation estimated in population	F-ratio
Between subjects			
1 A'	$a-1$	$P'(B'*S'(A')) + B'*S'(A') + B'*A'$ $+ S'(A') + A'$	$1/(2+4-5)^a$
2 $S'(A')$	$(n-1)a$	$P'(B'*S'(A')) + B'*S'(A') + S'(A')$	2/5
Within subjects			
3 B'	$b-1$	$P'(B'*S'(A')) + B'*S'(A') + B'*A' + B'$	$3/4^b$
4 $B'*A'$	$(b-1)(a-1)$	$P'(B'*S'(A')) + B'*S'(A') + B'*A'$	4/5
5 $B'*S'(A')$	$(b-1)(n-1)a$	$P'(B'*S'(A')) + B'*S'(A')$	No test
6 $P'(B'*S'(A'))$	0	$P'(B'*S'(A'))$	–
Total variation	$nba-1$		

[a] There is no exact denominator for this test (see page 40). If $S'(A')$ and/or $B'*A'$ have $P > 0.25$, however, then *post hoc* pooling can be used to derive an exact denominator for A'. If $S'(A')$ has $P > 0.25$ (but $B'*A'$ has $P < 0.25$), then eliminate $S'(A')$ from the mean square for A', making $B'*A'$ its error mean square. If $B'*A'$ has $P > 0.25$ (but $S'(A')$ has $P < 0.25$), eliminate $B'*A'$ from the mean square for A', making $S'(A')$ its error mean square. If both $S'(A')$ and $B'*A'$ have $P > 0.25$, use the pooled error mean square: $[SS\{S'(A')\} + SS\{B'*A'\} + SS\{B'*S'(A')\}]/[(n-1)a + (b-1)(a-1) + (b-1)(n-1)a]$. See page 38.
[b] Planned *post hoc* pooling is permissible for B' if $B'*A'$ has $P > 0.25$. Use the pooled error mean square: $[SS\{B'*A'\} + SS\{B'*S'(A')\}]/[(b-1)(a-1) + (b-1)(n-1)a]$. See page 38.

6.4 Three-factor model with repeated measures on nested cross factors

Model

$$Y = C(B)|S'(A)$$

Test hypothesis

Variation in the response Y is explained by A cross factored with repeated measures on B and C nested in B.

Description

Replicate subjects (S') are assigned to each level of treatment A, and repeated observations (P') are taken on each subject, once at each level of factor C nested in levels of treatment B.

Factors	Levels	Repeated measures on S'
A	a	no
B	b	yes
C(B)	c	yes
S'	n	–

Allocation table

The table shows $n = 2$ replicate subjects S' nested in each of $a = 2$ levels of treatment A, and each subject observed once at each of $c = 2$ levels of factor C nested in each of $b = 2$ levels of treatment B.

P'(C(B)|S'(A))		A_1		A_2	
		S_1	S_2	S_3	S_4
B_1	C_1	P_1	P_n	...	P_{na}
	C_2	...	...	...	P_{nca}
B_2	C_3	...	...	...	...
	C_4	...	...	...	P_{ncba}

Examples

(1) *Subject-by-trial design*: H_1: Blood pressure of Patients (S') responds to Ingestion (B with two levels: before and after) of Medicine (A with two levels: drug and placebo). The blood pressure of each patient is monitored at random Times (C') before and after taking the medicine.

(2) *Subject-by-trial design*: The effect of a local environmental disturbance Event (B, with two levels: before and after) is monitored by repeated measures of stress levels at random Times C' in Subjects (S') occupying different Locations (A'), with impact gauged by B*A'. This is a variation on the 'before-and-after-control-impact' design given by model 5.6.

Comparisons

Model 6.4 is an extension of model 6.3 to include an extra nested factor (C').

The test for the main effect of A is identical to a fully replicated one-factor ANOVA (model 1.1) on the mean value of the response for each subject pooled across levels of C.

Special assumptions (see also general assumptions of repeated measures on page 183)

The model cannot test the C'*S' interaction, because the lack of replication means that there is no residual error term (shaded grey in the ANOVA tables below). If independent, replicate observations (P') are made for each of the *cb* levels of factor C nested in B in each subject, then the design is fully replicated. The principal advantage of full replication is that it allows testing of the assumption of no significant interaction of C' with S' and thereby – in the event of no significant S'*C' – validation of a non-significant main effect C. The interpretation of a significant treatment-by-subject interaction is nevertheless problematic because the treatment effect may depend upon any of the multiple sources of variation encompassed by the subject factor. Thus, the causal mechanisms underlying a significant treatment-by-subject effect cannot be interpreted without further experimentation.

ANOVA tables for analysis of terms B|A + B|S(A) + A|C(B)

Model 6.4(i) *A and B are fixed factors, C is a random factor, S' is a random subject:*

Mean square	d.f.	Components of variation estimated in population	F-ratio
Between subjects			
1 A	$a-1$	P'(C'(B)*S'(A)) + C'(B)*S'(A) + C'(B)*A + S'(A) + A	1/(2+7−8)[a]
2 S'(A)	$(n-1)a$	P'(C'(B)*S'(A)) + C'(B)*S'(A) + S'(A)	2/8[c]
Within subjects			
3 B	$b-1$	P'(C'(B)*S'(A)) + C'(B)*S'(A) + C'(B) + B*S'(A) + B	3/(5+6−8)[b]
4 B*A	$(b-1)(a-1)$	P'(C'(B)*S'(A)) + C'(B)*S'(A) + C'(B)*A + B*S'(A) + B*A	4/(5+7−8)[b]
5 B*S'(A)	$(b-1)(n-1)a$	P'(C'(B)*S'(A)) + C'(B)*S'(A) + B*S'(A)	5/8
6 C'(B)	$(c-1)b$	P'(C'(B)*S'(A)) + C'(B)*S'(A) + C'(B)	6/8[d]
7 C'(B)*A	$(c-1)b(a-1)$	P'(C'(B)*S'(A)) + C'(B)*S'(A) + C'(B)*A	7/8
8 C'(B)*S'(A)	$(c-1)b(n-1)a$	P'(C'(B)*S'(A)) + C'(B)*S'(A)	No test
9 P'(C'(B)*S'(A))	0	P'(C'(B)*S'(A))	–
Total variation	$ncba-1$		

[a] There is no exact denominator for this test (see page 40). If S'(A) and/or C'(B)*A have $P > 0.25$, however, then *post hoc* pooling can be used to derive an exact denominator for A. If S'(A) has $P > 0.25$ (but C'(B)*A has $P < 0.25$), then eliminate S'(A) from the mean square for A, making C'(B)*A its error mean square. If C'(B)*A has $P > 0.25$ (but S'(A) has $P < 0.25$), eliminate C'(B)*A from the mean square for A, making S'(A) its error mean square. If both S'(A) and C'(B)*A have $P > 0.25$, use the pooled error mean square: [SS{S'(A)} + SS{C'(B)*A} + SS{C'(B)*S'(A)}]/[(n−1)a + (c−1)b(a−1) + (c−1)b(n−1)a]. See page 38.

[b] There is no exact denominator for this test (see page 40). If higher-order interactions contributing to the mean square have $P > 0.25$, however, then they can be removed from the mean square in *post hoc* pooling to derive an exact denominator (applying the same technique as for A above; see page 38).

[c] An unrestricted model tests the MS for S'(A) over the MS for its interaction with B (*F*-ratio = **2/5**). See page 242.

[d] An unrestricted model tests the MS for C'(B) over the MS for its interaction with A (*F*-ratio = **6/7**). See page 242.

Model 6.4(ii) A is a fixed factor, B' and C' are random factors, S' is a random subject:

Mean square	d.f.	Components of variation estimated in population	F-ratio
Between subjects			
1 A	$a-1$	$P'(C'(B')'S'(A)) + C'(B')'S'(A) + C'(B')*A + B'*S'(A) + B'*A + S'(A) + A$	$1/(2 + 4 - 5)^a$
2 S'(A)	$(n-1)a$	$P'(C'(B')'S'(A)) + C'(B')'S'(A) + B'*S'(A) + S'(A)$	$2/5$
Within subjects			
3 B'	$b-1$	$P'(C'(B')'S'(A)) + C'(B')'S'(A) + C'(B')*A + C'(B') + B'*S'(A) + B'$	$3/(5 + 6 - 8)^b$
4 B'*A	$(b-1)(a-1)$	$P'(C'(B')'S'(A)) + C'(B')'S'(A) + C'(B')*A + B'*S'(A) + B'*A$	$4/(5 + 7 - 8)^b$
5 B'*S'(A)	$(b-1)(n-1)a$	$P'(C'(B')'S'(A)) + C'(B')'S'(A) + B'*S'(A)$	$5/8$
6 C'(B')	$(c-1)b$	$P'(C'(B')'S'(A)) + C'(B')'S'(A) + C'(B')$	$6/8^c$
7 C'(B')*A	$(c-1)b(a-1)$	$P'(C'(B')'S'(A)) + C'(B')'S'(A) + C'(B')*A$	$7/8$
8 C'(B')*S'(A)	$(c-1)b(n-1)a$	$P'(C'(B')'S'(A)) + C'(B')'S'(A)$	**No test**
9 P'(C'(B')'S'(A))	0	$P'(C'(B')'S'(A))$	–
Total variation	$ncba-1$		

[a] There is no exact denominator for this test (see page 40). If B'*A has $P > 0.25$ but S'(A) has $P < 0.25$, however, *post hoc* pooling can be used to eliminate B'*A from the mean square for A, making S'(A) its error mean square. If both S'(A) and B'*A have $P > 0.25$, use the pooled error mean square: $[SS\{S'(A)\} + SS\{B'*A\} + SS\{C'(B')*S'(A)\}]/[(n-1)a + (b-1)(a-1) + (c-1)b(n-1)a]$. See page 38.

[b] There is no exact denominator for this test (see page 40). If higher-order interactions contributing to the mean square have $P > 0.25$, however, they can be removed from the mean square in *post hoc* pooling to derive an exact denominator (applying the same technique as for A above; see page 38).

[c] An unrestricted model tests the MS for C'(B') over the MS for its interaction with A (F-ratio = **6/7**). See page 242.

203

Model 6.4(iii) A', B' and C' are all random factors, S' is a random subject:

Mean square	d.f.	Components of variation estimated in population	F-ratio
Between subjects			
1 A'	$a-1$	P'(C'(B')*S'(A')) + C'(B')*S'(A') + C'(B')*A' + B'*S'(A') + B'*A' + S'(A') + A'	$1/(2+4-5)$[a]
2 S'(A')	$(n-1)a$	P'(C'(B')*S'(A')) + C'(B')*S'(A') + B'*S'(A') + S'(A')	2/5
Within subjects			
3 B'	$b-1$	P'(C'(B')*S'(A')) + C'(B')*S'(A') + C'(B')*A' + C'(B') + B'*S'(A') + B'*A' + B'	$3/(4+6-7)$[b]
4 B'*A'	$(b-1)(a-1)$	P'(C'(B')*S'(A')) + C'(B')*S'(A') + C'(B')*A' + B'*S'(A') + B'*A'	$4/(5+7-8)$[b]
5 B'*S'(A')	$(b-1)(n-1)a$	P'(C'(B')*S'(A')) + C'(B')*S'(A') + B'*S'(A')	5/8
6 C'(B')	$(c-1)b$	P'(C'(B')*S'(A')) + C'(B')*S'(A') + C'(B')*A' + C'(B')	6/7
7 C'(B')*A'	$(c-1)b(a-1)$	P'(C'(B')*S'(A')) + C'(B')*S'(A') + C'(B')*A'	7/8
8 C'(B')*S'(A')	$(c-1)b(n-1)a$	P'(C'(B')*S'(A')) + C'(B')*S'(A')	No test
9 P'(C'(B')*S'(A'))	0	P'(C'(B')*S'(A'))	—
Total variation	$ncba-1$		

[a] There is no exact denominator for this test (see page 40). If B'*A' has $P > 0.25$ but S'(A') has $P < 0.25$, however, *post hoc* pooling can be used to eliminate B'*A' from the mean square for A', making S'(A') its error mean square. If both S'(A') and B'*A' have $P > 0.25$, use the pooled error mean square: $[SS\{S'(A')\} + SS\{B'*A'\} + SS\{C'(B')*S'(A')\}]/[(n-1)a + (b-1)(a-1) + (c-1)b(n-1)a]$. See page 38.

[b] There is no exact denominator for this test (see page 40). If higher-order interactions contributing to the mean square have $P > 0.25$, however, then they can be removed from the mean square in *post hoc* pooling to derive an exact denominator (applying the same technique as for A' above; see page 38).

204

6.5 Three-factor model with repeated measures on two cross factors

Model

$$Y = C|B|S'(A)$$

Test hypothesis

Variation in the response Y is explained by A cross factored with repeated measures on C cross factored with B.

Description

Replicate subjects (S′) are assigned to each level of treatment A, and repeated observations (P′) are taken on each subject, once at each combination of levels of cross factors C and B.

Factors	Levels	Repeated measures on S′
A	a	no
B	b	yes
C	c	yes
S′	n	–

Allocation table

The table shows $n = 2$ replicate subjects S′ nested in each of $a = 2$ levels of factor A, and each subject observed once at each of $c = 2$ levels of factor C in each of $b = 2$ levels of treatment B.

Examples

(1) *Subject-by-trial design*: H_1: Systolic and diastolic blood Pressure (C) of Patients (S′) responds to Ingestion (B with two levels: before and after) of Medicine (A with two levels: drug and placebo).

(2) *Subject-by-trial design*: H_1: Barnacle settlement depends upon background recruitment, elevation up shore, and substrate aspect, tested by measuring barnacle density on cb Patches (P′) of rock at different Elevations (B) and Aspects (C) on n Shores (S′) nested in a background rates of Recruitment (A). For example, east- and west-facing sides of the shore are sampled at low- and mid-shore on four shores at high and four at low background rates of recruitment.

(3) *Subject-by-treatment design*: H_1: Performance of athletes depends on Drink treatment (C with two levels: isotonic glucose electrolyte and water) and Vitamin supplement (B with two levels: vitamin tablet and placebo). Performance is measured by clocking the running times of athletes (S′) over a 10 km course after taking each combination of drink and vitamin supplement. Each athlete receives the four treatments in a particular Order (A with ten levels).

Comparisons

Model 6.5 is an extension of repeated-measures model 6.2 to include a between-subjects factor, and is an extension of repeated-measures model 6.3 to include a second within-subjects factor.

The test for the main effect of A is identical to a fully replicated one-factor ANOVA (model 1.1) on the mean value of the response for each subject pooled across levels of B and C. When $c = 2$, the interaction of C with B|S′(A) is identical to the repeated-measures split-plot model 6.3 on a treatments, tested with b responses per subject each comprising the value of C_2 subtracted from C_1. When both c and $b = 2$, the interaction of C*B with A is identical to a fully replicated one-factor ANOVA on a treatments (model 1.1), tested with one response per subject comprising the value of $[(C_2 - C_1)$ at $B_2] - [(C_2 - C_1)$ at $B_1]$.

Model 6.5 is equivalent to split-plot model 5.7, where subject corresponds with block (S′), except that the cb levels of factors B and C are tested sequentially on each subject rather than being randomly assigned within each block. It is therefore inherently susceptible to practice and carryover effects from the sequential application of treatments in repeated measures.

In testing the combined effect of three crossed factors, model 6.5 has similar objectives to cross-factored models 3.2, 4.3, 5.2, 5.3, 5.4, 5.5, 5.7, 5.9 and 6.7. Crucially, it differs from completely randomised, randomised-block and split-plot models in that the levels of factors B and C are tested sequentially on each subject. Model 6.5 differs from repeated-measures model 6.7 in that it has one between-subjects factor and two within-subjects factors, rather than two between-subjects factors and one within-subjects factor.

Special assumptions (see also general assumptions of repeated measures on page 183)

The model cannot test the interactions of B and C with S′, because the lack of replication means that there is no residual error term (shaded grey in the ANOVA tables below). Interpretation of non-significant terms amongst B, C, C*B and their interactions with A is compromised because the result could mean either no effect, or opposing effects on different subjects. The assumption of no significant treatment-by-subject interactions can be tested if independent, replicate observations (P′) are made for each of the *bc* combinations of factors B and C on each subject. The interpretation of a significant treatment by-subject interaction is nevertheless problematic because the treatment effect may depend upon any of the multiple sources of variation encompassed by the subject factor. Thus, the causal mechanisms underlying a significant treatment-by-subject effect cannot be interpreted without further experimentation.

ANOVA tables for analysis of terms C|B|A + C|B|S(A) – C*B*S(A)

Model 6.5(i) A, B and C are fixed factors, S' is a random subject:

Mean square	d.f.	Components of variation estimated in population	F-ratio
Between subjects			
1 A	$a-1$	$P'(C*B*S'(A)) + S'(A) + A$	1/2
2 S'(A)	$(n-1)a$	$P'(C*B*S'(A)) + S'(A)$	No test[a]
Within subjects			
3 B	$b-1$	$P'(C*B*S'(A)) + B*S'(A) + B$	3/5[c]
4 B*A	$(b-1)(a-1)$	$P'(C*B*S'(A)) + B*S'(A) + B*A$	4/5[c]
5 B*S'(A)	$(b-1)(n-1)a$	$P'(C*B*S'(A)) + B*S'(A)$	No test[b]
6 C	$c-1$	$P'(C*B*S'(A)) + C*S'(A) + C$	6/8[c]
7 C*A	$(c-1)(a-1)$	$P'(C*B*S'(A)) + C*S'(A) + C*A$	7/8[c]
8 C*S'(A)	$(c-1)(n-1)a$	$P'(C*B*S'(A)) + C*S'(A)$	No test[b]
9 C*B	$(c-1)(b-1)$	$P'(C*B*S'(A)) + C*B*S'(A) + C*B$	9/11[c]
10 C*B*A	$(c-1)(b-1)(a-1)$	$P'(C*B*S'(A)) + C*B*S'(A) + C*B*A$	10/11[c]
11 C*B*S'(A)	$(c-1)(b-1)(n-1)a$	$P'(C*B*S'(A)) + C*B*S'(A)$	No test
12 P'(C*B*S'(A))	0	$P'(C*B*S'(A))$	–
Total variation	$ncba - 1$		

[a] An unrestricted model has an inexact F-ratio denominator (see page 242).
[b] An unrestricted model tests the MS for B*S'(A) and for C*S'(A) over the MS for C*B*S'(A). See page 242.
[c] Model-2 analysis for a split plot uses p[5 + 8 + 11] for the denominator MS.

Model 6.5(ii) *A and C are fixed factors, B' is a random factor, S' is a random subject:*

Mean square	d.f.	Components of variation estimated in population	F-ratio
Between subjects			
1 A	$a-1$	$P'(C*B'*S'(A)) + B'*S'(A) + B'*A + S'(A) + A$	$1/(2+4-5)$[a]
2 S'(A)	$(n-1)a$	$P'(C*B'*S'(A)) + B'*S'(A) + S'(A)$	$2/5$[c]
Within subjects			
3 B'	$b-1$	$P'(C*B'*S'(A)) + B'*S'(A) + B'$	$3/5$[c]
4 B'*A	$(b-1)(a-1)$	$P'(C*B'*S'(A)) + B'*S'(A) + B'*A$	$4/5$[c]
5 B'*S'(A)	$(b-1)(n-1)a$	$P'(C*B'*S'(A)) + B'*S'(A)$	No test[d]
6 C	$c-1$	$P'(C*B'*S'(A)) + C*B'*S'(A) + C*B' + C*S'(A) + C$	$6/(8+9-11)$[b]
7 C*A	$(c-1)(a-1)$	$P'(C*B'*S'(A)) + C*B'*S'(A) + C*B'*A + C*S'(A) + C*A$	$7/(8+10-11)$[b]
8 C*S'(A)	$(c-1)(n-1)a$	$P'(C*B'*S'(A)) + C*B'*S'(A) + C*S'(A)$	$8/11$
9 C*B'	$(c-1)(b-1)$	$P'(C*B'*S'(A)) + C*B'*S'(A) + C*B'$	$9/11$[e]
10 C*B'*A	$(c-1)(b-1)(a-1)$	$P'(C*B'*S'(A)) + C*B'*S'(A) + C*B'*A$	$10/11$
11 C*B'*S'(A)	$(c-1)(b-1)(n-1)a$	$P'(C*B'*S'(A)) + C*B'*S'(A)$	No test
12 P'(C*B'*S'(A))	0	$P'(C*B'*S'(A))$	–
Total variation	$ncba - 1$		

[a] There is no exact denominator for this test (see page 40). If S'(A) and/or B'*A have $P > 0.25$, however, then *post hoc* pooling can be used to derive an exact denominator for A. If S'(A) has $P > 0.25$ (but B'*A has $P < 0.25$), then eliminate S'(A) from the mean square for A, making B'*A its error mean square. If B'*A has $P > 0.25$ (but S'(A) has $P < 0.25$), eliminate B'*A from the mean square for A, making S'(A) its error mean square. If both S'(A) and B'*A have $P > 0.25$, use the pooled error mean square: $[SS\{S'(A)\} + SS\{B'*A\} + SS\{B'*S'(A)\}]/[(n-1)a + (b-1)(a-1) + (b-1)(n-1)a]$. See page 38.

[b] There is no exact denominator for this test (see page 40). If higher-order interactions contributing to the mean square have $P > 0.25$, however, then they can be removed from the mean square in *post hoc* pooling to derive an exact denominator (applying the same technique as for A above; see page 38).

[c] An unrestricted model has an inexact F-ratio denominator (see page 242).

[d] An unrestricted model tests the MS for B'*S'(A) over the MS for C*B'*S'(A) (F-ratio = **5/11**). See page 242.

[e] An unrestricted model tests the MS for C*B' over the MS for its interaction with A (F-ratio = **9/10**). See page 242.

Model 6.5(iii) *A is a fixed factor, B' and C' are random factors, S' is a random subject:*

Mean square	d.f.	Components of variation estimated in population	F-ratio
Between subjects			
1 A	$a-1$	P'(C'*B'*S'(A)) + C'*B'*S'(A) + C'*B'*A + C'*S'(A) + C'*A + B'*S'(A) + B'*A + S'(A) + A	1/(2+4−5+7−8−10+11)[a]
2 S'(A)	$(n-1)a$	P'(C'*B'*S'(A)) + C'*B'*S'(A) + C'*S'(A) + B'*S'(A) + S'(A)	2/(5+8−11)[a]
Within subjects			
3 B'	$b-1$	P'(C'*B'*S'(A)) + C'*B'*S'(A) + C'*B' + B'*S'(A) + B'	3/(5+9−11)[b]
4 B'*A	$(b-1)(a-1)$	P'(C'*B'*S'(A)) + C'*B'*S'(A) + C'*B'*A + B'*S'(A) + B'*A	4/(5+10−11)[b]
5 B'*S'(A)	$(b-1)(n-1)a$	P'(C'*B'*S'(A)) + C'*B'*S'(A) + B'*S'(A)	5/11
6 C'	$c-1$	P'(C'*B'*S'(A)) + C'*B'*S'(A) + C'*B' + C'*S'(A) + C'	6/(8+9−11)[b]
7 C'*A	$(c-1)(a-1)$	P'(C'*B'*S'(A)) + C'*B'*S'(A) + C'*B'*A + C'*S'(A) + C'*A	7/(8+10−11)[b]
8 C'*S'(A)	$(c-1)(n-1)a$	P'(C'*B'*S'(A)) + C'*B'*S'(A) + C'*S'(A)	8/11
9 C'*B'	$(c-1)(b-1)$	P'(C'*B'*S'(A)) + C'*B'*S'(A) + C'*B'	9/11[c]
10 C'*B'*A	$(c-1)(b-1)(a-1)$	P'(C'*B'*S'(A)) + C'*B'*S'(A) + C'*B'*A	10/11
11 C'*B'*S'(A)	$(c-1)(b-1)(n-1)a$	P'(C'*B'*S'(A)) + C'*B'*S'(A)	No test
12 P'(C'*B'*S'(A))	0	P'(C'*B'*S'(A))	–
Total variation	$ncba-1$		

[a] There is no exact denominator for this test (see page 40). If B'*S'(A) and/or C'*S'(A) have $P > 0.25$, however, then *post hoc* pooling can be used to derive an exact denominator for S'(A). If B'*S'(A) has $P > 0.25$ (but C'*S'(A) has $P < 0.25$), then eliminate B'*S'(A) from the mean square for S'(A), making C'*S'(A) its error mean square. If C'*S'(A) has $P > 0.25$ (but B'*S'(A) has $P < 0.25$), eliminate C'*S'(A) from the mean square for S'(A), making B'*S'(A) its error mean square. If both B'*S'(A) and C'*S'(A) have $P > 0.25$, use the pooled error mean square: $[\text{SS}\{\text{B'*S'(A)}\} + \text{SS}\{\text{C'*S'(A)}\} + \text{SS}\{\text{C'*B'*S'(A)}\}]/[(b-1)(n-1)a + (c-1)(n-1)a + (c-1)(b-1)(n-1)a]$. See page 38.

[b] There is no exact denominator for this test (see page 40). If higher-order interactions contributing to the mean square have $P > 0.25$, however, then they can be removed from the mean square in *post hoc* pooling to derive an exact denominator (applying the same technique as for S'(A) above; see page 38).

[c] An unrestricted model tests the MS for C'*B' over the MS for its interaction with A (F-ratio = **9/10**). See page 242.

Model 6.5(iv) *A' is a random factor, B and C are fixed factors, S' is a random subject:*

Mean square	d.f.	Components of variation estimated in population	F-ratio
Between subjects			
1 A'	$a-1$	$P'(C*B*S'(A')) + S'(A') + A'$	1/2[a]
2 S'(A')	$(n-1)a$	$P'(C*B*S'(A')) + S'(A')$	No test[a]
Within subjects			
3 B	$b-1$	$P'(C*B*S'(A')) + B*S'(A') + B*A' + B$	3/4
4 B*A'	$(b-1)(a-1)$	$P'(C*B*S'(A')) + B*S'(A') + B*A'$	4/5[a]
5 B*S'(A')	$(b-1)(n-1)a$	$P'(C*B*S'(A')) + B*S'(A')$	No test[b]
6 C	$c-1$	$P'(C*B*S'(A')) + C*S'(A') + C*A' + C$	6/7
7 C*A'	$(c-1)(a-1)$	$P'(C*B*S'(A')) + C*S'(A') + C*A'$	7/8[a]
8 C*S'(A')	$(c-1)(n-1)a$	$P'(C*B*S'(A')) + C*S'(A')$	No test[b]
9 C*B	$(c-1)(b-1)$	$P'(C*B*S'(A')) + C*B*S'(A') + C*B*A' + C*B$	9/10
10 C*B*A'	$(c-1)(b-1)(a-1)$	$P'(C*B*S'(A')) + C*B*S'(A') + C*B*A'$	10/11
11 C*B*S'(A')	$(c-1)(b-1)(n-1)a$	$P'(C*B*S'(A'))$	No test
12 P'(C*B*S'(A'))	0	$P'(C*B*S'(A'))$	–
Total variation	$ncba-1$		

[a] An unrestricted model has an inexact F-ratio denominator (see page 242).
[b] An unrestricted model tests the MS for B*S'(A') and for C*S'(A') over the MS for C*B*S'(A'). See page 242.

211

Model 6.5(v) A' and B' are random factors, C is a fixed factor, S' is a random subject:

Mean square	d.f.	Components of variation estimated in population	F-ratio
Between subjects			
1 A'	$a-1$	$P'(C*B'*S'(A')) + B'*S'(A') + B'*A' + S'(A') + A'$	$1/(2+4-5)^{ac}$
2 S'(A')	$(n-1)a$	$P'(C*B'*S'(A')) + B'*S'(A') + S'(A')$	$2/5^c$
Within subjects			
3 B'	$b-1$	$P'(C*B'*S'(A')) + B'*S'(A') + B'*A' + B'$	$3/4^c$
4 B'*A'	$(b-1)(a-1)$	$P'(C*B'*S'(A')) + B'*S'(A') + B'*A'$	$4/5^c$
5 B'*S'(A')	$(b-1)(n-1)a$	$P'(C*B'*S'(A')) + B'*S'(A')$	No test^d
6 C	$c-1$	$P'(C*B'*S'(A')) + C*B'*S'(A') + C*B'*A' + C*B' + C*S'(A') + C*A' + C$	$6/(7+9-10)^{bc}$
7 C*A'	$(c-1)(a-1)$	$P'(C*B'*S'(A')) + C*B'*S'(A') + C*B'*A' + C*S'(A') + C*A'$	$7/(8+10-11)^{bc}$
8 C*S'(A')	$(c-1)(n-1)a$	$P'(C*B'*S'(A')) + C*B'*S'(A') + C*S'(A')$	$8/11$
9 C*B'	$(c-1)(b-1)$	$P'(C*B'*S'(A')) + C*B'*S'(A') + C*B'*A' + C*B'$	$9/10$
10 C*B'*A'	$(c-1)(b-1)(a-1)$	$P'(C*B'*S'(A')) + C*B'*S'(A') + C*B'*A'$	$10/11$
11 C*B'*S'(A')	$(c-1)(b-1)(n-1)a$	$P'(C*B'*S'(A')) + C*B'*S'(A')$	No test
12 P'(C*B'*S'(A'))	0	$P'(C*B'*S'(A'))$	–
Total variation	$ncba-1$		

[a] There is no exact denominator for this test (see page 40). If S'(A') and/or B'*A' have $P > 0.25$, however, then *post hoc* pooling can be used to derive an exact denominator for A'. If S'(A') has $P > 0.25$ (but B'*A' has $P < 0.25$), eliminate S'(A') from the mean square for A', making B'*A' its error mean square. If B'*A' has $P > 0.25$ (but S'(A') has $P < 0.25$), then eliminate B'*A' from the mean square for A', making S'(A') its error mean square. If both S'(A') and B'*A' have $P > 0.25$, use the pooled error mean square: [SS{S'(A')} + SS{B'*A'} + SS{B'*S'(A')}]/[$(n-1)a+(b-1)(a-1)+(b-1)(n-1)a$]. See page 38.

[b] There is no exact denominator for this test (see page 40). If higher-order interactions contributing to the mean square have $P > 0.25$, however, then they can be removed from the mean square in *post hoc* pooling to derive an exact denominator (applying the same technique as for A' above; see page 38).

[c] An unrestricted model has an inexact F-ratio denominator (see page 242).

[d] An unrestricted model tests the MS for B'*S'(A') over the MS for C*B'*S'(A') (F-ratio = **5/11**). See page 242.

Model 6.5(*vi*) A', B' and C' *are random factors, S' is a random subject:*

Mean square	d.f.	Components of variation estimated in population	F-ratio
Between subjects			
1 A'	$a-1$	P(C'*B'*S'(A')) + C'*B'*S'(A') + C'*B'*A' + C'*S'(A') + C'*A' + B'*S'(A') + B'*A' + S'(A') + A'	1/(2 + 4 − 5 + 7 − 8 − 10 + 11)
2 S'(A')	$(n-1)a$	P(C'*B'*S'(A')) + C'*B'*S'(A') + C'*S'(A') + B'*S'(A') + S'(A')	2/(5 + 8 − 11)[a]
Within subjects			
3 B'	$b-1$	P(C'*B'*S'(A')) + C'*B'*S'(A') + C'*B'*A' + C'*B' + B'*S'(A') + B'*A' + B'	3/(4 + 9 − 10)[b]
4 B'*A'	$(b-1)(a-1)$	P(C'*B'*S'(A')) + C'*B'*S'(A') + C'*B'*A' + B'*S'(A') + B'*A'	4/(5 + 10 − 11)[b]
5 B'*S'(A')	$(b-1)(n-1)a$	P(C'*B'*S'(A')) + C'*B'*S'(A') + B'*S'(A')	5/11
6 C'	$c-1$	P(C'*B'*S'(A')) + C'*B'*S'(A') + C'*B'*A' + C'*B' + C'*S'(A') + C'*A' + C'	6/(7 + 9 − 10)[b]
7 C'*A'	$(c-1)(a-1)$	P(C'*B'*S'(A')) + C'*B'*S'(A') + C'*B'*A' + C'*S'(A') + C'*A'	7/(8 + 10 − 11)[b]
8 C'*S'(A')	$(c-1)(n-1)a$	P(C'*B'*S'(A')) + C'*B'*S'(A') + C'*S'(A')	8/11
9 C'*B'	$(c-1)(b-1)$	P(C'*B'*S'(A')) + C'*B'*S'(A') + C'*B'*A' + C'*B'	9/10[c]
10 C'*B'*A'	$(c-1)(b-1)(a-1)$	P(C'*B'*S'(A')) + C'*B'*S'(A') + C'*B'*A'	10/11
11 C'*B'*S'(A')	$(c-1)(b-1)(n-1)a$	P(C'*B'*S'(A')) + C'*B'*S'(A')	No test
12 P(C'*B'*S'(A'))	0	P(C'*B'*S'(A'))	–
Total variation	$ncba-1$		

[a] There is no exact denominator for this test (see page 40). If B'*S'(A') and/or C'*S'(A') have $P > 0.25$, however, then *post hoc* pooling can be used to derive an exact denominator for S'(A'). If B'*S'(A') has $P > 0.25$ (but C'*S'(A') has $P < 0.25$), then eliminate B'*S'(A') from the *mean square* for S'(A'), making C'*S'(A') its error mean square. If C'*S'(A') has $P > 0.25$ (but B'*S'(A') has $P < 0.25$), eliminate C'*S'(A') from the mean square for S'(A'), making B'*S'(A') its error mean square. If both B'*S'(A') and C'*S'(A') have $P > 0.25$, use the pooled error mean square: [SS{B'*S'(A')} + SS{C'*S'(A')} + SS{C'*B'*S'(A')}]/[(b−1)(n−1)a + (c−1)(n−1)a + (c−1)(b−1)(n−1)a]. See page 38.

[b] There is no exact denominator for this test (see page 40). If higher-order interactions contributing to the mean square have exact $P > 0.25$, however, then they can be removed from the mean square in *post hoc* pooling to derive an exact denominator (applying the same technique as for S'(A') above; see page 38).

[c] Planned *post hoc* pooling is permissible for C'*B' if C'*B'*A' has $P > 0.25$. Use the pooled error mean square: [SS{C'*B'*A'} + SS{C'*B'*S'(A')}]/[(c−1)(b−1)(a−1) + (c−1)(b−1)(n−1)a]. See page 38.

213

6.6 Nested model with repeated measures on a cross factor

Model

$$Y = C|S'(B(A))$$

Test hypothesis

Variation in the response Y is explained by repeated-measures treatment C combined with treatment A and with grouping factor B nested in A.

Description

Replicate subjects (S') are nested in groups (B') which are themselves nested in levels of treatment A, and repeated observations (P') are taken on each subject, once at each level of factor C.

Factors	Levels	Repeated measures on S'
A	a	no
B(A)	b	no
C	c	yes
S'	n	–

Allocation table

The table shows $n = 2$ replicate subjects S' nested in each of $b = 2$ groups B' nested in each of $a = 2$ levels of treatment A, and each subject observed once at each of $c = 4$ levels of treatment C.

Examples

(1) *Subject-by-trial design*: H_1: Blood pressure of Patients (S′) responds to drug treatment over Time (C with two levels: before and after) according to Doctor (B′) nested in Medicine (A with two levels: drug and placebo). This analysis assumes that doctors are allocated randomly to patients and that medicines are assigned randomly to doctors.

(2) *Subject-by-treatment design*: H_1: Social interactions in Groups of captive lemurs (S′) depend on public Viewing (C with two levels: open and closed to view) according to Zoo (B′) nested in Management regime (A with two levels: single-species cages and mixed-species cages). n groups of lemurs are studied in each of b zoos in each of a management regimes. The order in which each group of lemurs is opened and closed to view is randomised. This analysis assumes that the effect of management is not confounded by other factors, such as number of individuals per cage.

Comparisons

Model 6.6 is an extension of model 2.1, in which each subject (S′) is tested sequentially in every level of an extra cross factor (C). If $c = 2$, tests for interactions with C are numerically equivalent to nested model 2.1 using a response of $C_2 - C_1$.

Model 6.6 is equivalent to split-plot model 5.8, where subject corresponds with block (S′), except that the c levels of factor C are tested sequentially on each subject rather than being randomly assigned within each block. It is therefore inherently susceptible to practice and carryover effects from the sequential application of treatments in repeated measures.

Special assumptions (see also general assumptions of repeated measures on page 183)

The model cannot test the C*S′ interaction, because the lack of replication means that there is no residual error term (shaded grey in the ANOVA tables below). Interpretation of non-significant C or C*A is compromised because the result could mean either no effect, or opposing effects on different subjects. The assumption of no significant C*S′ interaction can be tested if independent, replicate observations (P′) are made for each of the c levels of factor C in each subject. The interpretation of a significant treatment-by-subject interaction is nevertheless problematic because the treatment effect may depend upon any of the multiple sources of variation encompassed by the subject factor. Thus, the causal mechanisms underlying a significant treatment-by-subject effect cannot be interpreted without further experimentation.

ANOVA tables for analysis of terms C|A + C|B(A) + S(B A)

Model 6.6(i) A and C are fixed factors, B' is a random factor, S' is a random subject:

Mean square	d.f.	Components of variation estimated in population	F-ratio
Between subjects			
1 A	$a-1$	P'(C*S'(B'(A))) + S'(B'(A)) + B'(A) + A	1/2[a]
2 B'(A)	$(b-1)a$	P'(C*S'(B'(A))) + S'(B'(A)) + B'(A)	2/3[b]
3 S'(B'(A))	$(n-1)ba$	P'(C*S'(B'(A))) + S'(B'(A))	No test[c]
Within subjects			
4 C	$c-1$	P'(C*S'(B'(A))) + C*S'(B'(A)) + C*B'(A) + C	4/6[d]
5 C*A	$(c-1)(a-1)$	P'(C*S'(B'(A))) + C*S'(B'(A)) + C*B'(A) + C*A	5/6[e]
6 C*B'(A)	$(c-1)(b-1)a$	P'(C*S'(B'(A))) + C*S'(B'(A)) + C*B'(A)	6/7
7 C*S'(B'(A))	$(c-1)(n-1)ba$	P'(C*S'(B'(A))) + C*S'(B'(A))	No test
8 P'(C*S'(B'(A)))	0	P'(C*S'(B'(A)))	–
Total variation	$ncba-1$		

[a] Planned *post hoc* pooling is permissible for A if B'(A) has $P>0.25$. Use the pooled error mean square: [SS{B'(A)} + SS{S'(B'(A))}]/[$(b-1)a+(n-1)ba$]. See page 38.

[b] An unrestricted model has an inexact F-ratio denominator (see page 242).

[c] An unrestricted model tests the MS for S'(B'(A)) over the MS for its interaction with C (F-ratio = **3/7**). See page 242.

[d] Planned *post hoc* pooling is permissible for C if C*B'(A) has $P>0.25$. Use the pooled error mean square: [SS{C*B'(A)} + SS{C*S'(B'(A))}]/[$(c-1)(b-1)a+(c-1)(n-1)ba$]. See page 38.

[e] Planned *post hoc* pooling is permissible for C*A if C*B'(A) has $P>0.25$. Use the pooled error mean square: [SS{C*B'(A)} + SS{C*S'(B'(A))}]/[$(c-1)(b-1)a+(c-1)(n-1)ba$]. See page 38.

Model 6.6(ii) *A is a fixed factor, B′ and C′ are random factor, S′ is a random subject:*

Mean square	d.f.	Components of variation estimated in population	F-ratio
Between subjects			
1 A	$a-1$	$P'(C'*S'(B'(A))) + C'*B'(A) + C'*A + S'(B'(A)) + B'(A) + A$	$1/(2+5-6)^a$
2 B′(A)	$(b-1)a$	$P'(C'*S'(B'(A))) + C'*S'(B'(A)) + C'*B'(A) + S'(B'(A)) + B'(A)$	$2/(3+6-7)^b$
3 S′(B′(A))	$(n-1)ba$	$P'(C'*S'(B'(A))) + C'*S'(B'(A)) + S'(B'(A))$	3/7
Within subjects			
4 C′	$c-1$	$P'(C'*S'(B'(A))) + C'*S'(B'(A)) + C'*B'(A) + C'$	$4/6^{ce}$
5 C′*A	$(c-1)(a-1)$	$P'(C'*S'(B'(A))) + C'*S'(B'(A)) + C'*B'(A) + C'*A$	$5/6^d$
6 C′*B′(A)	$(c-1)(b-1)a$	$P'(C'*S'(B'(A))) + C'*S'(B'(A)) + C'*B'(A)$	6/7
7 C′*S′(B′(A))	$(c-1)(n-1)ba$	$P'(C'*S'(B'(A))) + C'*S'(B'(A))$	No test
8 P′(C′*S′(B′(A)))	0	$P'(C'*S'(B'(A)))$	—
Total variation	$ncba-1$		

[a] There is no exact denominator for this test (see page 40). If C′*A has $P > 0.25$, eliminate C′*A from the mean square for A, making B′(A) its error mean square. Further pooling can be done if C′*B′(A) has $P > 0.25$. See page 38.

[b] There is no exact denominator for this test (see page 40). If S′(B′(A)) and/or C′*B′(A) have $P > 0.25$, however, then *post hoc* pooling can be used to derive an exact denominator for B′(A). If S′(B′(A)) has $P > 0.25$ (but C′*B′(A) has $P < 0.25$), then eliminate S′(B′(A)) from the mean square for B′(A), making C′*B′(A) its error mean square. If C′*B′(A) has $P > 0.25$ (but S′(B′(A)) has $P < 0.25$), eliminate C′*B′(A) from the mean square for B′(A), making S′(B′(A)) its error mean square. If both S′(B′(A)) and C′*B′(A) have $P > 0.25$, use the pooled error mean square: $[SS\{S'(B'(A))\} + SS\{C'*B'(A)\} + SS\{C'*S'(B'(A))\}]/[(n-1)ba + (c-1)(b-1)a + (c-1)(n-1)ba]$. See page 38.

[c] Planned *post hoc* pooling is permissible for C′ if C′*B′(A) has $P > 0.25$. Use the pooled error mean square: $[SS\{C'*B'(A)\} + SS\{C'*S'(B'(A))\}]/[(c-1)(b-1)a + (c-1)(n-1)ba]$. See page 38.

[d] Planned *post hoc* pooling is permissible for C′*A if C′*B′(A) has $P > 0.25$. Use the pooled error mean square: $[SS\{C'*B'(A)\} + SS\{C'*S'(B'(A))\}]/[(c-1)(b-1)a + (c-1)(n-1)ba]$. See page 38.

[e] An unrestricted model tests the MS for C′ over the MS for its interaction with A (F-ratio = **4/5**). See page 242.

Model 6.6(iii) A' and B' are random factors, C is a fixed factor, S' is a random subject:

Mean square	d.f.	Components of variation estimated in population	F-ratio
Between subjects			
1 A'	$a-1$	$P'(C*S'(B'(A'))) + S'(B'(A')) + B'(A') + A'$	$1/2$[ab]
2 $B'(A')$	$(b-1)a$	$P'(C*S'(B'(A'))) + S'(B'(A')) + B'(A')$	$2/3$[b]
3 $S'(B'(A'))$	$(n-1)ba$	$P'(C*S'(B'(A'))) + S'(B'(A'))$	No test[c]
Within subjects			
4 C	$c-1$	$P'(C*S'(B'(A'))) + C*S'(B'(A')) + C*B'(A') + C*A' + C$	$4/5$[d]
5 $C*A'$	$(c-1)(a-1)$	$P'(C*S'(B'(A'))) + C*S'(B'(A')) + C*B'(A') + C*A'$	$5/6$[e]
6 $C*B'(A')$	$(c-1)(b-1)a$	$P'(C*S'(B'(A'))) + C*S'(B'(A')) + C*B'(A')$	$6/7$
7 $C*S'(B'(A'))$	$(c-1)(n-1)ba$	$P'(C*S'(B'(A'))) + C*S'(B'(A'))$	No test
8 $P'(C*S'(B'(A')))$	0	$P'(C*S'(B'(A')))$	–
Total variation	$ncba-1$		

[a] Planned *post hoc* pooling is permissible for A' if $B'(A')$ has $P > 0.25$. Use the pooled error mean square: $[SS\{B'(A')\} + SS\{S'(B'(A'))\}]$ $/[(b-1)a + (n-1)ba]$. See page 38.

[b] An unrestricted model has an inexact F-ratio denominator (see page 242).

[c] An unrestricted model tests the MS for $S'(B'(A))$ over the MS for its interaction with C (F-ratio $= 3/7$). See page 242.

[d] Planned *post hoc* pooling is permissible for C if $C*A'$ has $P > 0.25$. Use the pooled error mean square: $[SS\{C*A'\} + SS\{C*B'(A')\}]/[(c-1)$ $(a-1) + (c-1)(b-1)a]$. Further pooling is permissible if $C*B'(A')$ has $P > 0.25$. See page 38.

[e] Planned *post hoc* pooling is permissible for $C*A'$ if $C*B'(A')$ has $P > 0.25$. Use the pooled error mean square: $[SS\{C*B'(A')\} + SS\{C*S'(B'$ $(A'))\}]/[(c-1)(b-1)a + (c-1)(n-1)ba]$. See page 38.

218

Model 6.6(iv) A', B' and C' are random factors, S' is a random subject:

Mean square	d.f.	Components of variation estimated in population	F-ratio
Between subjects			
1 A'	$a-1$	$P(C'*S'(B'(A'))) + C'*S'(B'(A')) + C'*B'(A') + C'*A' + S'(B'(A')) + B'(A') + A'$	$1/(2+5-6)^a$
2 B'(A')	$(b-1)a$	$P(C'*S'(B'(A'))) + C'*S'(B'(A')) + C'*B'(A') + S'(B'(A')) + B'(A')$	$2/(3+6-7)^b$
3 S'(B'(A'))	$(n-1)ba$	$P(C'*S'(B'(A'))) + C'*S'(B'(A')) + S'(B'(A'))$	$3/7$
Within subjects			
4 C'	$c-1$	$P(C'*S'(B'(A'))) + C'*S'(B'(A')) + C'*B'(A') + C'*A' + C'$	$4/5^c$
5 C'*A'	$(c-1)(a-1)$	$P(C'*S'(B'(A'))) + C'*S'(B'(A')) + C'*B'(A') + C'*A'$	$5/6^d$
6 C'*B'(A')	$(c-1)(b-1)a$	$P(C'*S'(B'(A'))) + C'*S'(B'(A')) + C'*B'(A')$	$6/7$
7 C'*S'(B'(A'))	$(c-1)(n-1)ba$	$P(C'*S'(B'(A'))) + C'*S'(B'(A'))$	No test
8 P(C'*S'(B'(A')))	0	$P(C'*S'(B'(A')))$	–
Total variation	$ncba-1$		

[a] There is no exact denominator for this test (see page 40). If C'*A' has $P > 0.25$, eliminate C'*A' from the mean square for A', making B'(A') its error mean square. Further pooling can be done if C'*B'(A') has $P > 0.25$. See page 38.

[b] There is no exact denominator for this test (see page 40). If S'(B'(A')) and/or C'*B'(A') have $P > 0.25$, however, then post hoc pooling can be used to derive an exact denominator for B'(A'). If S'(B'(A')) has $P > 0.25$ (but C'*B'(A') has $P < 0.25$), then eliminate S'(B'(A')) from the mean square for B'(A'), making C'*B'(A') its error mean square. If C'*B'(A') has $P > 0.25$ (but S'(B'(A')) has $P < 0.25$), eliminate C'*B'(A') from the mean square for B'(A'), making S'(B'(A')) its error mean square. If both S'(B'(A')) and C'*B'(A') have $P > 0.25$, use the pooled error mean square: [SS{S'(B'(A'))} + SS{C'*S'(B'(A'))}]/[(n-1)ba + (c-1)(n-1)ba]. See page 38.

[c] Planned post hoc pooling is permissible for C' if C'*A' has $P > 0.25$. Use the pooled error mean square: [SS{C'*A'} + SS{C'*B'(A')}] /[[(c-1)(a-1) + (c-1)(b-1)a]. Further pooling is permissible if C'*B'(A') has $P > 0.25$. See page 38.

[d] Planned post hoc pooling is permissible for C'*A' if C'*B'(A') has $P > 0.25$. Use the pooled error mean square: [SS{C'*B'(A')} + SS{C'*S' (B'(A'))}]/[[(c-1)(b-1)a + (c-1)(n-1)ba]. See page 38.

6.7 Three-factor model with repeated measures on one factor

Model

$$Y = C|S'(B|A)$$

Test hypothesis

Variation in the response Y is explained by the interaction of repeated-measures treatment C with factors A and B combined.

Description

Each of ba combinations of levels of treatments B and A is randomly allocated n subjects (S'), and repeated observations (P') are taken on each subject, once at each level of factor C.

Allocation table

Factors	Levels	Repeated measures on S'
A	a	no
B	b	no
C	c	yes
S'	n	–

The table shows $n = 2$ replicate subjects S' nested in each of $ba = 4$ combinations of levels of cross factors B and A, and each subject observed once at each of $c = 4$ levels of treatment C.

P'(C|S'(B|A))	A_1				A_2			
	B_1		B_2		B_1		B_2	
	S_1	S_2	S_3	S_4	S_5	S_6	S_7	S_8
C_1	P_1	P_n	...	P_{nb}	...	...	...	P_{nba}
C_2	...	...	...	...	...	...	...	...
C_3	...	...	...	...	...	...	...	...
C_4	...	...	...	...	...	...	...	P_{ncba}

Examples

(1) *Subject-by-trial design*: H_1: Species diversity of lichens on Trees (S')
depends on Aspect (C with two levels: north and south side), tree
Species (B with two levels: oak and beech) and Ivy (A, with two levels:
present or absent).

(2) *Subject-by-trial design*: H_1: Blood pressure of Patients (S') responds
over Time (C with two levels: before and after) to ingestion of
Medicine (A with two levels: drug and placebo) depending upon
Gender (B with two levels: male and female).

(3) *Subject-by-treatment design*: H_1: Performance of Athletes (S') depends
on Drink treatment (C with two levels: isotonic glucose electrolyte and
water) and Gender (B). Performance is measured by clocking the
running times of Athletes (S') over a 10 km course after drinking either
isotonic glucose electrolyte or water, and clocking them again after
swapping their treatments. Each athlete receives the two treatments in
a particular Order (A with two levels: electrolyte first and water first).

(4) *Subject-by-treatment design*: H_1: Social interactions in Groups of
captive lemurs (S') depend on public Viewing (C with two levels:
open and closed to view), Zoo (B') and Management regime (A with
two levels: single-species cages and mixed-species cages). n groups of
lemurs in single-species cages and n groups of lemurs in mixed-species
cages are studied in each of b zoos. The order in which each group of
lemurs is opened and closed to view is randomised. This analysis
assumes that the effect of management is not confounded by other
factors, such as number of individuals per cage.

Comparisons

Model 6.7 is an extension of model 3.1 in which each subject is tested
sequentially in every level of a third crossed factor C. It is also an extension
of repeated-measures model 6.3 to include an additional between-subjects
factor. If $c = 2$, tests for interactions with C are numerically equivalent to
fully replicated two-factor model 3.1 using a response of $C_2 - C_1$.

Model 6.7 is equivalent to split-plot model 5.9, where subject corresponds with block (S'), except that the c levels of factor C are tested
sequentially on each subject rather than being randomly assigned within
each block. It is therefore inherently susceptible to practice and carryover effects from the sequential application of treatments in repeated
measures.

In testing the combined effect of three crossed factors, model 6.7 has similar objectives to cross-factored models 3.2, 4.3, 5.2, 5.3, 5.4, 5.5, 5.7, 5.9 and 6.5. Crucially, it differs from completely randomised, randomised-block and split-plot models in that the c levels of factor C are tested sequentially on each subject. Model 6.7 differs from repeated-measures model 6.5 in that it has two between-subjects factors and one within-subjects factor, rather than one between-subjects factor and two within-subjects factors.

Special assumptions (see also general assumptions of repeated measures on page 183)

The model cannot test the C*S′ interaction, because the lack of replication means that there is no residual error term (shaded grey in the ANOVA tables below). Interpretation of non-significant terms amongst C and its interactions with A and B is compromised because the result could mean either no effect, or opposing effects on different subjects. The assumption of no significant C*S′ interaction can be tested if independent, replicate observations (P′) are made for each of the c levels of factor C on each subject. The interpretation of a significant C*S′ is nevertheless problematic because the treatment effect may depend upon any of the multiple sources of variation encompassed by the subject factor.

ANOVA tables for analysis of terms C|B|A + S(B A)

Model 6.7(i) A, B and C are fixed factors, S' is a random subject:

Mean square	d.f.	Components of variation estimated in population	F-ratio
Between subjects			
1 A	$a-1$	P'(C*S'(B*A))+S'(B*A)+A	1/4
2 B	$b-1$	P'(C*S'(B*A))+S'(B*A)+B	2/4
3 B*A	$(b-1)(a-1)$	P'(C*S'(B*A))+S'(B*A)+B*A	3/4
4 S'(B*A)	$(n-1)ba$	P'(C*S'(B*A))+S'(B*A)	No test[a]
Within subjects			
5 C	$c-1$	P'(C*S'(B*A))+C*S'(B*A)+C	5/9
6 C*A	$(c-1)(a-1)$	P'(C*S'(B*A))+C*S'(B*A)+C*A	6/9
7 C*B	$(c-1)(b-1)$	P'(C*S'(B*A))+C*S'(B*A)+C*B	7/9
8 C*B*A	$(c-1)(b-1)(a-1)$	P'(C*S'(B*A))+C*S'(B*A)+C*B*A	8/9
9 C*S'(B*A)	$(c-1)(n-1)ba$	P'(C*S'(B*A))+C*S'(B*A)	No test
10 P'(C*S'(B*A))	0	P'(C*S'(B*A))	–
Total variation	$ncba-1$		

[a] An unrestricted model tests the MS for S'(B*A) over the MS for its interaction with C (F-ratio = **4/9**). See page 242.

223

Model 6.7(ii) A and B are fixed factors, C is a random factor, S' is a random subject:

Mean square	d.f.	Components of variation estimated in population	F-ratio
Between subjects			
1 A	$a-1$	$P'(C*S'(B*A)) + C*S'(B*A) + S'(B*A) + C*A + A$	$1/(4+6-9)$[a]
2 B	$b-1$	$P'(C*S'(B*A)) + C*S'(B*A) + S'(B*A) + C*B + B$	$2/(4+7-9)$[a]
3 B*A	$(b-1)(a-1)$	$P'(C*S'(B*A)) + C*S'(B*A) + S'(B*A) + C*B*A + B*A$	$3/(4+8-9)$[a]
4 S'(B*A)	$(n-1)ba$	$P'(C*S'(B*A)) + C*S'(B*A) + S'(B*A)$	$4/9$
Within subjects			
5 C'	$c-1$	$P'(C*S'(B*A)) + C*S'(B*A) + C'$	$5/9$[b]
6 C*A	$(c-1)(a-1)$	$P'(C*S'(B*A)) + C*S'(B*A) + C*A$	$6/9$[c]
7 C*B	$(c-1)(b-1)$	$P'(C*S'(B*A)) + C*S'(B*A) + C*B$	$7/9$[c]
8 C*B*A	$(c-1)(b-1)(a-1)$	$P'(C*S'(B*A)) + C*S'(B*A) + C*B*A$	$8/9$
9 C*S'(B*A)	$(c-1)(n-1)ba$	$P'(C*S'(B*A)) + C*S'(B*A)$	No test
10 P'(C*S'(B*A))	0	$P'(C*S'(B*A))$	–
Total variation	$ncba-1$		

[a] There is no exact denominator for this test (see page 40). If higher-order interactions contributing to the mean square have exact $P > 0.25$, however, then they can be removed from the mean square in *post hoc* pooling to derive an exact denominator (see page 38).
[b] An unrestricted model has an inexact F-ratio denominator (see page 242).
[c] An unrestricted model tests the MS for C*A and for C*B over the MS for the interaction term C*B*A. See page 242.

Model 6.7(iii) A and C are fixed factors, B' is a random factor, S' is a random subject:

Mean square	d.f.	Components of variation estimated in population	F-ratio
Between subjects			
1 A	$a-1$	$P'(C*S'(B'*A)) + S'(B'*A) + B'*A + A$	1/3[a]
2 B'	$b-1$	$P'(C*S'(B'*A)) + S'(B'*A) + B'$	2/4[b]
3 B'*A	$(b-1)(a-1)$	$P'(C*S'(B'*A)) + S'(B'*A) + B'*A$	3/4[b]
4 S'(B'*A)	$(n-1)ba$	$P'(C*S'(B'*A)) + S'(B'*A)$	No test[c]
Within subjects			
5 C	$c-1$	$P'(C*S'(B'*A)) + C*S'(B'*A) + C*B' + C$	5/7[e]
6 C*A	$(c-1)(a-1)$	$P'(C*S'(B'*A)) + C*S'(B'*A) + C*B'*A + C*A$	6/8[f]
7 C*B'	$(c-1)(b-1)$	$P'(C*S'(B'*A)) + C*S'(B'*A) + C*B'$	7/9[d]
8 C*B'*A	$(c-1)(b-1)(a-1)$	$P'(C*S'(B'*A)) + C*S'(B'*A) + C*B'*A$	8/9
9 C*S'(B'*A)	$(c-1)(n-1)ba$	$P'(C*S'(B'*A)) + C*S'(B'*A)$	No test
10 P'(C*S'(B'*A))	0	$P'(C*S'(B'*A))$	—
Total variation	$ncba-1$		

[a] Planned *post hoc* pooling is permissible for A if B'*A has $P > 0.25$. Use the pooled error mean square: $[SS\{B'*A\} + SS\{S'(B'*A)\}]/[(b-1)(a-1) + (n-1)ba]$. See page 38.

[b] An unrestricted model has an inexact F-ratio denominator (see page 242).

[c] An unrestricted model tests the MS for S'(B'*A) over the MS for its interaction with C (*F*-ratio = **4/9**). See page 242.

[d] An unrestricted model tests the MS for C*B' over the MS for its interaction with A (*F*-ratio = **7/8**). See page 242.

[e] Planned *post hoc* pooling is permissible for C if C*B' has $P > 0.25$. Use the pooled error mean square: $[SS\{C*B'\} + SS\{C*S'(B'*A)\}]/[(c-1)(b-1) + (c-1)(n-1)ba]$. See page 38.

[f] Planned *post hoc* pooling is permissible for C*A if C*B'*A has $P > 0.25$. Use the pooled error mean square: $[SS\{C*B'*A\} + SS\{C*S'(B'*A)\}]/[(c-1)(b-1)(a-1) + (c-1)(n-1)ba]$. See page 38.

Model 6.7(iv) A is a fixed factor, B' and C' are random factors, S' is a random subject:

Mean square	d.f.	Components of variation estimated in population	F-ratio
Between subjects			
1 A	$a-1$	P'(C'*S'(B'*A)) + C'*S'(B'*A) + S'(B'*A) + C'*B'*A + C'*A + B'*A + A	**1/(3 + 6 − 8)**[a]
2 B'	$b-1$	P'(C'*S'(B'*A)) + C'*S'(B'*A) + S'(B'*A) + C'*B' + B'	**2/(4 + 7 − 9)**[a]
3 B'*A	$(b-1)(a-1)$	P'(C'*S'(B'*A)) + C'*S'(B'*A) + S'(B'*A) + C'*B'*A + B'*A	**3/(4 + 8 − 9)**[a]
4 S'(B'*A)	$(n-1)ba$	P'(C'*S'(B'*A)) + C'*S'(B'*A) + S'(B'*A)	**4/9**
Within subjects			
5 C'	$c-1$	P'(C'*S'(B'*A)) + C'*S'(B'*A) + C'*B' + C'	**5/7**[db]
6 C'*A	$(c-1)(a-1)$	P'(C'*S'(B'*A)) + C'*S'(B'*A) + C'*B'*A + C'*A	**6/8**[e]
7 C'*B'	$(c-1)(b-1)$	P'(C'*S'(B'*A)) + C'*S'(B'*A) + C'*B'	**7/9**[c]
8 C'*B'*A	$(c-1)(b-1)(a-1)$	P'(C'*S'(B'*A)) + C'*S'(B'*A) + C'*B'*A	**8/9**
9 C'*S'(B'*A)	$(c-1)(n-1)ba$	P'(C'*S'(B'*A)) + C'*S'(B'*A)	**No test**
10 P'(C'*S'(B'*A))	0	P'(C'*S'(B'*A))	–
Total variation	$ncba-1$		

[a] There is no exact denominator for this test (see page 40). If higher-order interactions contributing to the mean square have exact $P > 0.25$, however, then they can be removed from the mean square in *post hoc* pooling to derive an exact denominator (see page 38).

[b] An unrestricted model has an inexact F-ratio denominator (see page 242).

[c] An unrestricted model tests the MS for C'*B' over the MS for its interaction with A (*F*-ratio = **7/8**). See page 242.

[d] Planned *post hoc* pooling is permissible for C' if C'*B' has $P > 0.25$. Use the pooled error mean square: [SS{C'*B'} + SS{C'*S'(B'*A)}]/ [$(c-1)(b-1) + (c-1)(n-1)ba$]. See page 38.

[e] Planned *post hoc* pooling is permissible for C'*A if C'*B'*A has $P > 0.25$. Use the pooled error mean square: [SS{C'*B'*A} + SS{C'*S' (B'*A)}]/[$(c-1)(b-1)(a-1) + (c-1)(n-1)ba$]. See page 38.

Model 6.7(v) A' and B' are random factors, C is a fixed factor, S' is a random subject:

Mean square	d.f.	Components of variation estimated in population	F-ratio
Between subjects			
1 A'	$a-1$	$P'(C*S'(B'*A')) + S'(B'*A') + B'*A' + A'$	$1/3^{a,b}$
2 B'	$b-1$	$P'(C*S'(B'*A')) + S'(B'*A') + B'*A' + B'$	$2/3^{a,b}$
3 B'*A'	$(b-1)(a-1)$	$P'(C*S'(B'*A')) + S'(B'*A') + B'*A'$	$3/4^{b}$
4 S'(B'*A')	$(n-1)ba$	$P'(C*S'(B'*A')) + S'(B'*A')$	No test[c]
Within subjects			
5 C	$c-1$	$P'(C*S'(B'*A')) + C*S'(B'*A') + C*B'*A' + C*B' + C*A' + C$	$5/(6+7-8)^{d}$
6 C*A'	$(c-1)(a-1)$	$P'(C*S'(B'*A')) + C*S'(B'*A') + C*B'*A' + C*A'$	$6/8^{e}$
7 C*B'	$(c-1)(b-1)$	$P'(C*S'(B'*A')) + C*S'(B'*A') + C*B'*A' + C*B'$	$7/8^{e}$
8 C*B'*A'	$(c-1)(b-1)(a-1)$	$P'(C*S'(B'*A')) + C*S'(B'*A') + C*B'*A'$	$8/9$
9 C*S'(B'*A')	$(c-1)(n-1)ba$	$P'(C*S'(B'*A')) + C*S'(B'*A')$	No test
10 P'(C*S'(B'*A'))	0	$P'(C*S'(B'*A'))$	–
Total variation	$ncba-1$		

[a] Planned *post hoc* pooling is permissible for A' and B' if B'*A' has $P > 0.25$. Use the pooled error mean square: $[SS\{B'*A'\} + SS\{S'(B'*A')\}]/[(b-1)(a-1) + (n-1)ba]$. See page 38.

[b] An unrestricted model has an inexact F-ratio denominator (see page 242).

[c] An unrestricted model tests the MS for S'(B'(A)) over the MS for its interaction with C (F-ratio = **4/9**). See page 242.

[d] There is no exact denominator for this test (see page 40). If higher-order interactions contributing to the mean square have exact $P > 0.25$, however, then they can be removed from the mean square in *post hoc* pooling to derive an exact denominator (see page 38).

[e] Planned *post hoc* pooling is permissible for C*A' and C*B' if C*B'*A' has $P > 0.25$. Use the pooled error mean square: $[SS\{C*B'*A'\} + SS\{C*S'(B'*A')\}]/[(c-1)(b-1)(a-1) + (c-1)(n-1)ba]$. See page 38.

Model 6.7(*vi*) A', B' and C' are random factors, S' is a random subject:

Mean square	d.f.	Components of variation estimated in population	F-ratio
Between subjects			
1 A'	$a-1$	P'(C'*S'(B'*A')) + C'*S'(B'*A') + S'(B'*A') + C'*B'*A' + C'*A' + B'*A' + A'	$1/(3+6-8)$[a]
2 B'	$b-1$	P'(C'*S'(B'*A')) + C'*S'(B'*A') + S'(B'*A') + C'*B'*A' + C'*B' + B'*A' + B'	$2/(3+7-8)$[a]
3 B'*A'	$(b-1)(a-1)$	P'(C'*S'(B'*A')) + C'*S'(B'*A') + S'(B'*A') + C'*B'*A' + B'*A'	$3/(4+8-9)$[a]
4 S'(B'*A')	$(n-1)ba$	P'(C'*S'(B'*A')) + C'*S'(B'*A') + S'(B'*A')	4/9
Within subjects			
5 C'	$c-1$	P'(C'*S'(B'*A')) + C'*S'(B'*A') + C'*B'*A' + C'*B' + C'*A' + C'	$5/(6+7-8)$
6 C'*A'	$(c-1)(a-1)$	P'(C'*S'(B'*A')) + C'*S'(B'*A') + C'*B'*A' + C'*A'	$6/8$[b]
7 C'*B'	$(c-1)(b-1)$	P'(C'*S'(B'*A')) + C'*S'(B'*A') + C'*B'*A' + C'*B'	$7/8$[b]
8 C'*B'*A'	$(c-1)(b-1)(a-1)$	P'(C'*S'(B'*A')) + C'*S'(B'*A') + C'*B'*A'	8/9
9 C'*S'(B'*A')	$(c-1)(n-1)ba$	P'(C'*S'(B'*A')) + C'*S'(B'*A')	No test
10 P'(C'*S'(B'*A'))	0	P'(C'*S'(B'*A'))	–
Total variation	$ncba - 1$		

[a] There is no exact denominator for this test (see page 40). If higher-order interactions contributing to the mean square have exact $P > 0.25$, however, then they can be removed from the mean square in *post hoc* pooling to derive an exact denominator (see page 38).

[b] Planned *post hoc* pooling is permissible for C'*A' and C'*B' if C'*B'*A' has $P > 0.25$. Use the pooled error mean square: [SS {C'*B'*A'} + SS{C'*S'(B'*A')}]/[(c − 1)(b − 1)(a − 1) + (c − 1)(n − 1)ba]. See page 38.

228

7

Unreplicated designs

Every model in Chapters 2 and 3 has one or more equivalents without full replication. For model 2.1 it is 1.1, for 2.2 it is 2.1, for 3.1 it is 4.1 or 6.1, for 3.2 it is 4.2 or 6.2, for 3.3 it is 5.6 or 6.3, and for 3.4 it is 3.1. Here we give two further versions of factorial models 3.1 and 3.2 without full replication. The lack of replicated sampling units means that at least one of the factors must be random, as demonstrated by model 7.1(*i*) below in comparison to (*ii*) and (*iii*). Factorial designs that lack full replication must further assume that there are no significant higher-order interactions between factors, which cannot be tested by the model since there is no measure of the residual error among replicate observations (subjects). This is problematic because lower-order effects can only be interpreted fully with respect to their higher-order interactions (chapter 3). Falsely assuming an absence of higher-order interactions will cause tests of lower-order effects to overestimate the Type I error (rejection of a true null hypothesis) and to underestimate the Type II error (acceptance of a false null hypothesis). Without testing for interactions, causality cannot be attributed to significant main effects, and no conclusion can be drawn about non-significant main effects. For some analyses, the existence of a significant main effect when levels of an orthogonal random block are pooled together may hold interest regardless of whether or not the effect also varies with block; the main effect indicates an overall trend averaged across levels of the random factor.

The sampling unit for a given treatment level or combination in unreplicated designs is the plot, neither nested in a sample (as in Chapters 1 to 3) nor in a block (as in Chapters 4 to 6):

7.1 Two-factor cross-factored unreplicated model

Model

$$Y = B|A$$

Test hypothesis

Variation in the response Y is explained by additive effects of factors A and B.

Description

Each combination of levels of cross factors B and A are randomly assigned to a different subject or plot (S′). Each subject (or plot) is measured once.

Factors	Levels	Repeated measures on S′
A	*a*	no
B	*b*	no

Allocation table

The table illustrates $ba = 16$ combinations of levels of cross factors B and A assigned randomly amongst ba subjects or plots. For plots, note that the table does not indicate the spatial distribution of treatment combinations, which must be randomised.

S′(B|A)	A_1	A_2	A_3	A_4
B_1	S_1	...	...	S_a
B_2	...	...	...	...
B_3	...	...	...	...
B_4	...	...	...	S_{ba}

Example

(1) H_1: Crop yield depends upon sowing Density (A), with one of a sowing density treatments and one of b levels of a Watering regime (B′) randomly assigned to each of ba Plots (S′).

Comparisons

This design is an unreplicated version of a two-factor ANOVA (model 3.1). It assumes no two-way interaction, and it is logically testable only if at least one of the two factors is random. It differs from a one-factor randomised-block design (model 4.1) in that the levels of the random factor are randomly assigned to sampling units S′, rather than being blocked in space. Were it not for the lack of full replication, such a factor could otherwise be treated as fixed (see discussion of fixed and random factors on page 16).

Example 1 is suitable for analysis (*ii*) below if the replicate plots for each level of watering are not blocked together. Such a design might be used to test for an effect of sowing density over the natural range of rainfall likely to be experienced across years. If watering level is grouped in space, for example by a natural gradient in moisture, use randomised-block model 4.1. The design is fully interpretable only if A and B have additive effects, since there is no within-plot replication with which to test the interaction. If the response to the sowing density may depend on soil moisture, then use the fully replicated two-factor model 3.1.

ANOVA tables for analysis of terms A + B

Model 7.1(*i*) *A and B are both fixed factors:*

Mean square	d.f.	Components of variation estimated in population	F-ratio
1 A	$a-1$	S′(B*A) + A	**No test**[a]
2 B	$b-1$	S′(B*A) + B	**No test**[a]
3 B*A	$(b-1)(a-1)$	S′(B*A) + B*A	**No test**[a]
4 S′(B*A)	0	S′(B*A)	–
Total variation	$ba-1$		

[a] A, B and B*A are all untestable because the residual error cannot be estimated. Use the fully replicated two-factor model 3.1(*i*).

Model 7.1(*ii*) *A is a fixed factor, B' is a random factor:*

Mean square	d.f.	Components of variation estimated in population	*F*-ratio
1 A	$a-1$	$S'(B'*A)+B'*A+A$	**1/3**
2 B'	$b-1$	$S'(B'*A)+B'$	**No test**[a]
3 B'*A	$(b-1)(a-1)$	$S'(B'*A)+B'*A$	**No test**
4 S'(B'*A)	0	$S'(B'*A)$	–
Total variation	$ba-1$		

[a] An unrestricted model tests the MS for B' over the MS for its interaction with A (*F*-ratio = **2/3**). See page 242.

Model 7.1(*iii*) *A' and B' are both random factors:*

Mean square	d.f.	Components of variation estimated in population	*F*-ratio
1 A'	$a-1$	$S'(B'*A')+B'*A'+A'$	**1/3**
2 B'	$b-1$	$S'(B'*A')+B'*A'+B'$	**2/3**
3 B'*A'	$(b-1)(a-1)$	$S'(B'*A')+B'*A'$	**No test**
4 S'(B'*A')	0	$S'(B'*A')$	–
Total variation	$ba-1$		

7.2 Three-factor cross-factored unreplicated model

Model

$$Y = C|B|A$$

Test hypothesis

Response Y depends on factors A, B, C and their two-factor interactions.

Description

Each combination of levels of cross factors C, B and A are randomly assigned to a different subject or plot (S'). Each subject (or plot) is measured once.

Factors	Levels	Repeated measures on S'
A	a	no
B	b	no
C	c	no

Allocation table

The table illustrates $cba = 16$ combinations of levels of cross factors C, B and A assigned randomly amongst cba subjects or plots. For plots, note that the table does not indicate the spatial distribution of treatment combinations, which must be randomised.

S'(C|B|A)	A_1		A_2	
	B_1	B_2	B_1	B_2
C_1	S_1	S_b	...	S_{ba}
C_2	...	...	...	...
C_3	...	...	...	...
C_4	...	...	...	S_{cba}

Example

(1) H_1: Crop yield depends upon Fertiliser (A) and Shading (C), with one of ca combinations of Fertiliser and Shading treatments and one of b levels of a Watering regime (B′) randomly assigned to each of cba Plots (S′).

Comparisons

The design is an unreplicated version of a three-factor ANOVA (model 3.2). It assumes no three-way interaction and is logically testable only if at least one of the three factors is random. It differs from a two-factor randomised-block design (model 4.2) in that it does not assume homogeneous covariances for randomised blocks.

Example 1 is suitable for analysis (*ii*) below, provided that the replicate plots at each of the levels of moisture and shading are fully independent, and not grouped together spatially. Alternative field designs for blocking a natural gradient in soil moisture (or shading) are described by model 4.2 and model 5.1. If plots are grouped both for moisture and shading, the treatment effect may be tested more efficiently with a Latin square design (page 125).

ANOVA tables for analysis of terms C|B|A – C*B*A

Model 7.2(i) A, B and C are all fixed factors:

Mean square	d.f.	Components of variation estimated in population	F-ratio
1 A	$a-1$	$S'(C*B*A)+A$	**No test**[a]
2 B	$b-1$	$S'(C*B*A)+B$	**No test**[a]
3 B*A	$(b-1)(a-1)$	$S'(C*B*A)+B*A$	**No test**[a]
4 C	$c-1$	$S'(C*B*A)+C$	**No test**[a]
5 C*A	$(c-1)(a-1)$	$S'(C*B*A)+C*A$	**No test**[a]
6 C*B	$(c-1)(b-1)$	$S'(C*B*A)+C*B$	**No test**[a]
7 C*B*A	$(c-1)(b-1)(a-1)$	$S'(C*B*A)+C*B*A$	**No test**[a]
8 S'(C*B*A)	0	$S'(C*B*A)$	–
Total variation	$cba-1$		

[a] A, B, C and their interactions are all untestable because the residual error cannot be estimated. Use the fully replicated three-factor model 3.2(i).

Model 7.2(ii) A and C are fixed factors, B' is a random factor:

Mean square	d.f.	Components of variation estimated in population	F-ratio
1 A	$a-1$	$S'(C*B'*A)+B'*A+A$	**1/3**
2 B'	$b-1$	$S'(C*B'*A)+B'$	**No test**[a]
3 B'*A	$(b-1)(a-1)$	$S'(C*B'*A)+B'*A$	**No test**[b]
4 C	$c-1$	$S'(C*B'*A)+C*B'+C$	**4/6**
5 C*A	$(c-1)(a-1)$	$S'(C*B'*A)+C*B'*A+C*A$	**5/7**
6 C*B'	$(c-1)(b-1)$	$S'(C*B'*A)+C*B'$	**No test**[b]
7 C*B'*A	$(c-1)(b-1)(a-1)$	$S'(C*B'*A)+C*B'*A$	**No test**
8 S'(C*B'*A)	0	$S'(C*B'*A)$	–
Total variation	$cba-1$		

[a] An unrestricted model has an inexact *F*-ratio denominator (see page 242).
[b] An unrestricted model tests the MS for B'*A and for C*B' over the MS for the interaction term C*B'*A. See page 242.

Model 7.2(iii) *A is a fixed factor, B' and C' are random factors:*

Mean square	d.f.	Components of variation estimated in population	F-ratio
1 A	$a-1$	$S'(C'*B'*A)+C'*B'*A+C'*A+B'*A+A$	1/(3+5−7)[a]
2 B'	$b-1$	$S'(C'*B'*A)+C'*B'+B'$	2/6[b]
3 B'*A	$(b-1)(a-1)$	$S'(C'*B'*A)+C'*B'*A+B'*A$	3/7
4 C'	$c-1$	$S'(C'*B'*A)+C'*B'+C'$	4/6[b]
5 C'*A	$(c-1)(a-1)$	$S'(C'*B'*A)+C'*B'*A+C'*A$	5/7
6 C'*B'	$(c-1)(b-1)$	$S'(C'*B'*A)+C'*B'$	No test[c]
7 C'*B'*A	$(c-1)(b-1)(a-1)$	$S'(C'*B'*A)+C'*B'*A$	No test
8 S'(C'*B'*A)	0	$S'(C'*B'*A)$	–
Total variation	$cba-1$		

[a] There is no exact denominator for this test (see page 40). If B'*A and/or C'*A have $P>0.25$, however, then *post hoc* pooling can be used to derive an exact denominator for A. If B'*A has $P>0.25$ (but C'*A has $P<0.25$), eliminate B'*A from the mean square for A, making C'*A its error mean square. If C'*A has $P>0.25$ (but B'*A has $P<0.25$), then eliminate C'*A from the mean square for A, making B'*A its error mean square. If both B'*A and C'*A have $P>0.25$, use the pooled error mean square: $[SS\{B'*A\}+SS \{C'*A\}+SS\{C'*B'*A\}]/[(b-1)(a-1)+(c-1)(a-1)+(c-1)(b-1)(a-1)]$. Further pooling can be done if C'*B'*A has $P>0.25$. See page 38.

[b] An unrestricted model has an inexact F-ratio denominator (see page 242).

[c] An unrestricted model tests the MS for C'*B' over the MS for its interaction with A (*F*-ratio = **6/7**). See page 242.

235

Model 7.2(*iv*) A', B' and C' are all random factors:

Mean square	d.f.	Components of variation estimated in population	F-ratio
1 A'	$a-1$	S'(C'*B'*A') + C'*B'*A' + C'*A' + B'*A' + A'	$1/(3+5-7)$[a]
2 B'	$b-1$	S'(C'*B'*A') + C'*B'*A' + C'*B' + B'*A' + B'	$2/(3+6-7)$[a]
3 B'*A'	$(b-1)(a-1)$	S'(C'*B'*A') + C'*B'*A' + B'*A'	$3/7$
4 C'	$c-1$	S'(C'*B'*A') + C'*B'*A' + C'*B' + C'*A' + C'	$4/(5+6-7)$[a]
5 C'*A'	$(c-1)(a-1)$	S'(C'*B'*A') + C'*B'*A' + C'*A'	$5/7$
6 C'*B'	$(c-1)(b-1)$	S'(C'*B'*A') + C'*B'*A' + C'*B'	$6/7$
7 C'*B'*A'	$(c-1)(b-1)(a-1)$	S'(C'*B'*A') + C'*B'*A'	**No test**
8 S'(C'*B'*A')	0	S'(C'*B'*A')	–
Total variation	$cba-1$		

[a] There is no exact denominator for this test (see page 40). If higher-order interactions contributing to the mean square have $P > 0.25$, however, then they can be removed from the mean square in *post hoc* pooling to derive an exact denominator (applying the same technique as for A in model (*iii*). above; see page 38).

Further topics

Balanced and unbalanced designs

Balanced designs have the same number of replicate observations in each sample. Thus a one-factor model $Y = A + \varepsilon$ will be balanced if sample sizes all take the same value n at each of the a levels of factor A. Balanced designs are generally straightforward to analyse because factors are completely independent of each other and the total sum of squares (SS) can be partitioned completely among the various terms in the model. The SS explained by each term is simply the improvement in the residual SS as that term is added to the model. These are often termed 'sequential SS' or 'Type I SS'.

Designs become unbalanced when some sampling units are lost, destroyed or cannot be measured, or when practicalities mean that it is easier to sample some populations than others. For nested models, imbalance may result from unequal nesting as well as unequal sample sizes. Thus a nested model $Y = B'(A) + \varepsilon$ will be balanced only if each of the a levels of factor A has b levels of factor B', and each of the ba level of B' has n replicate observations. For factorial models, an imbalance means that some combinations of treatments have more observations than others. An extreme case of unbalanced data arises in factorial designs where there are no observations for one or more combinations of treatments, resulting in missing samples and a substantially more complicated analysis. Missing data are particularly problematic for unreplicated designs, such as randomised-block, split-plot or repeated-measures models, where each data point represents a unique combination of factor levels. Where this is a risk, avoid such designs in favour of fully replicated models.

Unbalanced one-factor ANOVA presents few problems other than increased sensitivity to the assumptions, particularly of homogeneity of variances. Unbalanced designs with more than one factor are likewise less robust to violations of the assumptions (including homogeneity of covariances for randomised-block, split-plot and repeated-measures designs, pages 118, 143 and 183).

Imbalance in nested designs causes no difficulties for computing SS and MS, but results in inexact F-tests for all but the last term in the model (Underwood 1997). Under certain conditions, Satterthwaite's approximation will provide adjusted F-ratios that follow a true F distribution (Sokal and Rohlf 1995). Alternatively, randomly sub-sampling an equal number of replicates per level can reinstate balance, with the consequent reduction in replication being offset by a likely gain in homogeneity of sample variances.

Loss of balance in factorial models can cause the factors to become correlated with each other, and therefore non-orthogonal (i.e., non-independent), with the result that the sequential SS cannot partition the total SS straightforwardly amongst the various terms in the model. This loss of orthogonality applies to categorical factors just as to covariates, and it can be an inherent feature even of certain balanced designs (e.g., balanced incomplete blocks and Youden squares on pages 124 and 127). It will always arise among covariates that take observed values as opposed to values set by experimental manipulation, unless the two covariates have a correlation coefficient equal to zero. To determine the independent effect of a term, its SS must be adjusted to factor out the correlated effects of other terms in the model (see box on page 240). The analysis of variance is then done on these 'adjusted SS'. Be aware that if two factors are highly correlated as a result of severe imbalance, it may be impossible to determine the independent effect of each predictor using adjusted SS. Neither factor may add additional predictive power after controlling for the effect of the other, even though the model as a whole is significant. In such cases consider testing just one of the correlated variables in a simpler model, or use a technique such as principal components analysis to reduce the number of variables in the analysis to strictly orthogonal components which can then be tested with factorial ANOVA.

Although an unequal distribution of sample sizes can be planned to avoid loss of orthogonality (Grafen and Hails 2002), the usual outcome of measuring some combinations of factor levels less than others is that the factors lose their independence and adjusted SS differ from sequential SS. The adjustment may raise or lower the SS of a particular term, depending on whether the factor is made more or less informative by accounting for the other sources of variation. If the explanatory power of a factor A is increased in the presence of another factor B, then any correlation between them raises the adjusted SS above the sequential SS for A when B is included in the model. In contrast, if factor A shares information on the response with factor B, then any correlation between them reduces the adjusted SS below the sequential SS for A.

This difference is illustrated by considering the example of rate of increase in the size of a population of breeding insects. A population of size N_t in year t, has a per capita rate of increase measured from births minus deaths that approximates to $r = -\ln(N_t) + \ln(N_{t+1})$. If the population is free to grow without density limitation, growth rate r will be independent of N_t and the covariate $\ln(N_t)$ will therefore have little or no power to explain variation in r with a statistical model of the form $Y = A + \varepsilon$. However, the two covariates $\ln(N_t)$ and $\ln(N_{t+1})$ in combination will explain all or virtually all variation in r with a model of the form $Y = A + B + \varepsilon$. In this two-factor model, the first-entered predictor $\ln(N_t)$ will have sequential SS close to zero, but a large adjusted SS reflecting its high explanatory power when $\ln(N_{t+1})$ is already included in the model (Figure 11a). In contrast, if the population is density limited, growth rate r will decrease as population size increases and the covariate $\ln(N_t)$ will therefore have high explanatory power when tested with a statistical model of the form $Y = A + \varepsilon$. However,

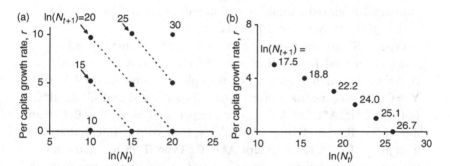

Figure 11 Contrasting datasets of population growth rate r on the y-axis as a function of population size $\ln(N_t)$ on the x-axis. Each point has an associated value of $\ln(N_{t+1})$ and broken lines join points with equal $\ln(N_{t+1})$. Both graphs are analysed with the same statistical covariate model $r = \ln(N_t) + \ln(N_{t+1}) + \varepsilon$. (a) With density independent population growth, the first entered term $\ln(N_t)$ has sequential SS close to zero because it has almost no explanatory power in the absence of the second term. Analysis with adjusted SS is more informative, showing both terms to be highly significant as an additive combination. (b) With density-dependent population growth, both main effects are non-significant when analysed with adjusted SS, because of a strong correlation between $\ln(N_t)$ and $\ln(N_{t+1})$. Analysis with sequential SS is more informative in this case, indicating a highly significant linear trend with $\ln(N_t)$, as suggested by the graph, and little additional explanatory power provided by $\ln(N_{t+1})$.

its SS will now be adjusted downwards on adding a second covariate $\ln(N_{t+1})$ because of a strong positive correlation between $\ln(N_t)$ and $\ln(N_{t+1})$. The adjusted SS may become so small as to render a clear trend apparently insignificant (Figure 11b).

Sums of squares in non-orthogonal factorial models

Two factors A and B are orthogonal if the distribution of levels of B is independent of the distribution of levels of A (i.e., they are uncorrelated with each other). Orthogonal designs are analysed with sequential (Type I) SS that are not influenced by their order of entry into the model. Non-orthogonal designs have sequential SS with values that depend on their order of entry into the model. These models can be analysed with adjusted SS that are computed by one of two methods, termed Type II and Type III. The merits of these alternative types of adjustment have received much attention and are a subject of ongoing debate (Shaw and Mitchell-Olds 1993; Grafen and Hails 2002; Quinn and Keough 2002). Type II and III SS are computed from sequential SS by comparing the residual SS of full and appropriately reduced models.

Type II SS are the reduction in residual SS obtained by adding a term to a model consisting of all the other terms that do not contain the term in question. For example, in a three-factor ANOVA: $Y = C|B|A + \varepsilon$, the main effect A is adjusted for B and C and B*C, but not A*B, A*C or A*B*C, by comparing $Y = B + C + B*C$ with model $Y = B + C + B*C + A$. Similarly, the two-way interaction A*B is adjusted for all terms except A*B*C. Type II SS use marginal means weighted by the sample sizes and so test hypotheses that are complex functions of the sample sizes. Type II SS are suitable for models with fixed cross factors but unsuitable for models with random cross factors (Searle *et al.* 1992).

Type III SS are the reduction in residual SS obtained by adding a term to a model that contains all other terms. This is equivalent to the SS explained by a term when it is the last to enter the model. Continuing the three-factor ANOVA example, the SS explained by A is found by comparing $Y = B + C + A*B + A*C + B*C + A*B*C$ with $Y = B + C + A*B + A*C + B*C + A*B*C + A$. Type III SS are based on unweighted marginal means, and so tests of hypotheses are unaffected by the imbalance in the data. Type III SS are suitable for models with random cross factors, but unsuitable for models with only fixed cross factors.

The problem with using Type III SS in fixed-factor models is that terms are illogically adjusted for their own higher-order interactions (Grafen and Hails 2002). As a result, Type III SS violate the principle of marginality, that terms be tested in hierarchical order (see how F-ratios are constructed on page 35). The hierarchical ordering is logical, because the test of an interaction includes tests of its constituent main effects. A significant interaction means by definition that the main effects of which it is composed must also be important, since the effect of each on the response is deemed to depend on the other (regardless of the significance of each as an individual main effect – detailed on page 77). Because an interaction contains a main effect, it makes no sense to include it when testing the explanatory power of the main effect, yet the interaction does get included with a Type III SS that is being adjusted for the influence of all other variables in the model.

The adjustment of SS by comparison of full and reduced models is automated in many statistics packages, and you should check which methods your statistics package offers and which is used as the default. If your SS have been adjusted for higher-order interactions (a Type III adjustment), this will be evident in non-identical sequential and adjusted SS for the last entered main effect in the model. Some packages only do Type III SS, and therefore cannot avoid adjusting for higher-order interactions in fixed effects, which thereby violates the principle of marginality (see box above). You can nevertheless obtain Type II SS by requesting sequential SS and running the GLM as many times as there are main effects, each time changing their order of entry into the model and keeping the sequential SS (and its MS and F) only for the last-entered main effect and its interactions. In that way you ensure that the retained SS will have been correctly adjusted for all terms other than those containing the term in question.

The process of comparing full and reduced models is also used to simplify complex unbalanced models. The highest-order interaction is tested first, followed by lower-order interactions and main effects, pooling non-significant terms into the residual term en route (Crawley 2002). Whilst this is a valid method of *model simplification* to find the most parsimonious of unbalanced models and useful for deriving predictive models, the indiscriminate and uncritical use of pooling means that it is not the best approach to hypothesis testing (see the section on *post hoc* pooling on page 38, in particular the problems associated with pooling up). Formal significance testing of specific terms should be achieved using the ANOVA table and *F*-tests that follow from the design of the experiment, as set out in the tables in this book.

The analysis of unbalanced designs with missing whole samples poses substantial difficulties. In factorial designs, the imbalance may prevent testing of some main effects and interactions. Certain hypotheses may still be tested, however, either by running a one-factor ANOVA to compare all the sample means and then partitioning the variation using planned contrasts (page 245), or by analysing balanced subsets of the full dataset (e.g., worked examples in Quinn and Keough 2002). For unreplicated models, including randomised-block and repeated-measures designs, omitting any blocks or subjects that have missing values is the easiest solution but may result in a considerably reduced dataset for analysis. Balance can also be reinstated by estimating missing values from the marginal means and adjusting the residual d.f. accordingly (Sokal and Rohlf 1995; Underwood 1997). This technique has the advantage of not losing any data but relies on the assumption that there are no interactions between treatment and block or subject. A third option is to compute the SS for each term by comparing appropriate full and reduced models (detailed in Quinn and Keough 2002).

Restricted and unrestricted mixed models

A mixed model is one with both random and fixed factors. It is termed 'restricted' or 'unrestricted' according to the method of constructing error mean squares of its random factors (see box).

The choice of model does not change the mean squares or their associated degrees of freedom but it does affect the estimated variance components, the expected mean squares and, most critically, some error terms used to calculate *F*-ratios. For example: in model 3.3(i) (page 101), the random factor $B'(A)$ estimates the following independent components of variation:

- *Restricted model*: $S'(C*B'(A)) + B'(A)$, with error estimated by the MS for $S'(C*B'(A))$;
- *Unrestricted model*: $S'(C*B'(A)) + C*B'(A) + B'(A)$, with error estimated by the MS for $C*B'(A)$.

In the restricted model, C*B′(A) does not contribute to the independent components of variation estimated by B′(A) because it sums to zero over the *a* levels of fixed factor A.

What are restricted and unrestricted models?

To distinguish the two types, it is necessary to define an important characteristic of fixed factors. All fixed factors and their interactions with each other have a zero sum for the deviation of their sample means from the grand mean $\bar{y}$ (e.g., Winer *et al.* 1991). Worked example 3 on page 51 illustrates the principle. Let us use the coding of model 3.3(*i*) to denote the mean value for the 18 measures at high Recruitment as $\bar{y}_{A1}$, and for the 12 measures at Treatment level '2' as $\bar{y}_{C1}$, and for the six measures at Treatment level '2' and high Recruitment as $\bar{y}_{C1A1}$. Then:

across columns: $\sum_{i=1}^{a} (\bar{y}_{Ai} - \bar{y}) = 0$,

and across rows: $\sum_{k=1}^{c} (\bar{y}_{Ck} - \bar{y}) = 0$, and also $\sum_{k=1}^{c} \sum_{i=1}^{a} (\bar{y}_{CkAi} - \bar{y}) = 0$

Consider now all random factors and their interactions with other factors, whether random or fixed. These are each assumed to contribute a random component of variation with a normal distribution around a mean of zero. In the worked example, the deviations from $\bar{y}$ by each mean of the nine measures per Site: $\bar{y}_{B'(A)j}$ sum to zero across the four levels of Site; likewise, the 12 deviations $(\bar{y}_{CkB'(A)j} - \bar{y})$ sum to zero. A restricted mixed model requires in addition that the random components with crossed, mixed factors (C*B′(A) in the worked example) sum to zero over the levels of each fixed factor. An 'unrestricted' mixed model does not require this constraint, and in consequence all its random components are considered to be independent of each other.

The reasons for choosing one form over the other have not been clearly defined in the statistical literature (Quinn and Keough 2002). Most textbooks adhere to the restricted model and this is the one we use because it is consistent with the method of generating error terms from the principles described on page 35. The unrestricted model is appropriate for unbalanced data (Searle 1971), and is the default option for many statistics packages, though some will allow optional use of the restricted form for balanced designs. If your statistics package does not provide this option

and you wish to use the restricted model, then manually recalculate the
F-ratios using the correct error terms provided by the tables in this book.

Magnitude of effect

Analysis of variance provides information on the magnitude of an effect in
addition to testing its significance as a source of variation. Although this
book focuses on the hypothesis-testing applications of ANOVA, its more
exploratory uses often concern predictions about effect sizes. The size of an
effect cannot be gauged from its significance alone, since significance
depends also on the amount of background variation and the sample size.
An effect of small magnitude can be strongly significant if it is sampled
with little residual variation from many replicates. Conversely, an apparently large effect may have no significance if it is sampled with large
residual variation or from few replicates. Here we summarise briefly the
issues involved in measuring the magnitude of a significant effect. For
more detailed analysis, we recommend Searle *et al.* (1992), Graham and
Edwards (2001) and Quinn and Keough (2002).

The magnitude of an effect is measured in different ways depending on
the type of effect. The size of a fixed categorical effect is estimated in
terms of deviations of sample means from the grand mean, which are zero
in the case of no effect. The impact of a covariate is estimated by the
steepness of the regression slope, which is horizontal in the case of no
covariation. The size of a random effect is estimated by the magnitude of
between-sample variance, which is zero in the case of no effect.

Effect sizes for fixed factors should be measured for the highest-order
significant fixed effects in the model hierarchy. Thus, in the event of a
significant interaction B*A, measure deviations from the global mean of
the *ba* sample means, rather than the deviations of the *a* means of main
effect A and the *b* means of B. Effect sizes may be illustrated most
succinctly with an interaction plot, or main-effects plots if there is no
interaction. In the event of a significant interaction with a random factor,
B'*A, the size of a significant A effect can be measured from the deviations of the *a* means of main effect A, because the significance of A is
estimated over and above that of the interaction with the random factor.

Regression slopes for covariates should be measured and graphed only
for significant effects. The slope is the increment or decrement in the
response Y with each unit of increment in the covariate X. In the event of
a significant interaction of a covariate with a categorical fixed factor:
X*A, the magnitude of the interaction is given by the amount of variation

between the *a* slopes. The coefficient of determination, r^2, is an alternative measure of effect size for a covariate, since its estimate of the proportion of explained variation is informative about how tightly the data are grouped around the regression line.

Variance components for random factors are measured for nested random effects, which are deemed significant if they have non-zero variance between their sample means. A variance component for a random effect is given by the increase in the effect MS over its error MS, divided by its pooled sample size. For example, model 2.2: $Y = C'(B'(A)) + \varepsilon$, has a variance component for subjects S' (nested in C' nested in B' nested in A) given directly by the residual MS. At the next step up in the hierarchy, the variance component for C' is $(MS[C'] - MS[\varepsilon])/n$. Finally, the variance component for B' is $(MS[B'] - MS[C'])/nc$. All variance components should be positive or zero, reflecting the increasing number of components of variation estimated in the population at each step up in the model hierarchy. A negative value has no meaning, and is conventionally returned as zero. The relative contribution of each step in the hierarchy is given by the variance component as a percentage of the sum of all variance components. This information can be useful for improving the efficiency of a design. For example, the power to test a treatment factor A in the above model may be enhanced by focussing replication at the scale with the largest variance component. Any imbalance in the nested design poses problems for estimating variance components and GLIM methods are then preferred, such as restricted maximum likelihood estimation (REML), discussed in detail in Searle *et al.* (1992).

A priori planned contrasts and *post hoc* unplanned comparisons

A significant categorical factor allows us to reject the null hypothesis that group means are equal, but for fixed effects with more than two levels it does not indicate how they are unequal. Additional tests are available to find out which groups differ from which others, either as an integral part of the analysis or as a supplementary analysis. The two approaches are a priori planned contrasts and *post hoc* unplanned comparisons.

A priori *planned contrasts* are pre-meditated tests of specific subsidiary hypotheses concerning group means within fixed effects. They can be made on a factor of interest even if it returns a non-significant effect in the ANOVA. Planned contrasts compare the mean of the response among groups or combinations of groups. For instance, one could compare the mean of group 1 to the mean of group 2, or compare the mean of group 1 to the weighted average of groups 2 and 3. Each contrast has d.f. $= k - 1$, where k is the number of groups, or combinations of groups, being compared. Contrasts are tested for significance using an F-ratio test with the same denominator MS as that used for the original test of overall significance.

A set of planned contrasts is orthogonal if each contrast is independent of all other contrasts – i.e., if the outcome of each contrast does not influence the outcome of any other contrast. A treatment factor with $a > 2$ levels has explained SS that can be partitioned completely into $a - 1$ planned orthogonal contrasts. There is often more than one way to construct a set of orthogonal contrasts for a particular treatment factor and the choice will depend upon the hypotheses to be tested. Provided they are orthogonal, planned contrasts use the same pre-determined significance level (e.g., $\alpha = 0.05$) for rejecting the null hypothesis as the original test of overall significance.

Planned orthogonal contrasts are particularly useful for analysing factors that are incompletely crossed by design. For example, the one-factor ANOVA model 1.1 on page 62 might be used to test the influence of a commercial egg Harvest (A) on breeding success of gull pairs (S′). An experiment could have $a = 3$ levels of impact: undisturbed control, disturbed by collectors, harvested by collectors. If it were possible to remove eggs without disturbance, then disturbance and harvest could have been treated as independent and fully crossed factors using model 3.1 (page 78). Since harvesting inevitably involves disturbance, however, we cannot sample a harvested–undisturbed combination. Instead, planned contrasts can firstly test for a general effect of disturbance by comparing the mean of the undisturbed control with the weighted mean of the disturbed-by-collectors and the harvested-by-collectors treatments. The contrasts can independently test for an effect of harvesting by comparing the mean breeding success of gulls that are disturbed and harvested with those that are disturbed only. In general for contrasts within a factor A, a contrast B between a control (B_1) and the average of two or more experimental treatments (B_2) has one d.f., and a contrast $C(B_2)$ between the c treatments nested in B_2 has $a - 2$ d.f., with $SS(B + C(B_2)) = SS(A)$. These particular contrasts can be done in a GLM model that requests analysis of terms: $B + C(B)$, where $C(B)$ tests variation amongst experiments around the overall experimental mean, and the error term $\varepsilon = MS[S'(A)]$ as in the one-way test.

A set of planned contrasts is non-orthogonal if the outcome of each contrast influences the outcome of any other contrast. Performing simultaneously a number of non-independent contrasts inflates the family-wise error rate (the probability of making at least one Type I error in a set of tests) by an unknown amount. A variety of procedures are available to limit this error rate by adjusting α, the threshold for significance of each individual test (Day and Quinn 1989; Quinn and Keough 2002). For example, Dunnett's test specifically contrasts a control group against all other groups, while the sequential Bonferroni method or the Dunn–Sidák procedure can be useful for other sets of non-orthogonal contrasts (but see cautions in Moran 2003).

Post hoc *unplanned comparisons* explore a significant main effect by comparing all possible pairs of group means. Unplanned comparisons, as the name suggests, should be used when the researcher has no premeditated subsidiary hypotheses to test and desires simply to identify which groups differ from which others. Unplanned comparisons are invariably non-orthogonal and, just as with planned contrasts, simultaneously performing multiple non-independent tests inflates the family-wise error rate. Again, a variety of procedures have been developed to control the excessive rate of Type I error that otherwise accrues in multiple exploratory comparisons (Day and Quinn 1989; Quinn and Keough 2002). For example, Ryan's test provides the most powerful pairwise comparisons, and Tukey's honestly significant difference test is practical for hand-calculation of unplanned comparisons.

In multi-factor models with significant nested or crossed effects, *post hoc* unplanned comparisons should be used to explore only the significant source(s) of variation at the highest level in the hierarchy of sources. For example, if the model $Y = B|A + \varepsilon$ produces a significant interaction B*A, then a *post hoc* test should be used to compare all combinations of levels of B with A. If only the main effects have a significant influence on the response, then levels of main effect A can be compared with each other (pooling levels of B), and levels of main effect B can be compared with each other (pooling levels of A).

Choosing experimental designs

Empirical research invariably requires making informed choices about the design of data collection. Although the number and identity of experimental treatments is determined by the question(s) being addressed, the investigator must decide at what spatial and temporal scales to apply them and whether to include additional fixed or random factors to extend the generality of the study. The investigator can make efficient use of resources by balancing the cost of running the experiment against the power of the experiment to detect a biologically significant effect. In practice this means either minimising the resources required to achieve a desired level of statistical power or maximising the statistical power that can be attained using the finite resources available. An optimum design can be achieved only by careful planning before data collection, particularly in the selection of an appropriate model and allocation of sampling effort at appropriate spatial and temporal scales.

Inadequate statistical power continues to plague biological research (Jennions and Møller 2003; Ioannidis 2005), despite repeated calls to incorporate it into planning (Peterman 1990; Greenwood 1993; Thomas and Juanes 1996). Yet efficient experimentation has never been more in demand. Journal editors and grant review panels are increasingly scrutinizing the statistical power of studies submitted for publication or funding (McClelland 1997). At the same time, increased competition for funding imposes financial constraints on replication, and animal welfare guidelines require researchers to minimise the number of animals used in their experiments.

Statistical power

To provide a robust test of the hypotheses of interest, an experiment should have a reasonable chance of detecting a biologically important effect if it truly occurs. In statistical terms this means having a low Type II error rate – the probability β of accepting a false null hypothesis. The probability that a test *will* reject a false null hypothesis $(1 - \beta)$ is therefore a measure of the sensitivity of the experiment, and is known as statistical power.

The power of an experiment can be calculated retrospectively to demonstrate that a study producing a non-significant result had sufficient power to detect a real effect. Such calculations commonly work on the sampled effect and error mean squares, however, in which case the retrospective power contains no other information than that provided by the *P*-value (Hoenig and Heisey 2001). A non-significant effect from a powerful test can be more persuasively demonstrated simply by graphing fitted values with their confidence intervals (Colegrave and Ruxton 2003).

Power analysis is far more useful if used prospectively to ensure that a proposed experiment will have adequate power to detect a given difference between population means, known as the effect size. Prospective, or a priori, power analysis can be employed to optimise the design of a study in two ways: either it can determine the minimum amount of resources (i.e., replication) required to detect a specified effect size, or it can determine the minimum detectable effect size for a fixed total quantity of resources. These calculations require an estimate of the error variance, specification of the desired power and significance threshold, and a knowledge of either the total quantity of resources available or the minimum effect size that we wish to detect.

The statistical power $(1 - \beta)$ to detect a given effect size (θ) increases with the significance threshold (α) and the number of replicates (n), and decreases with increasing error variance (σ^2). The error variance (σ^2) may be estimated from a pilot experiment, previously published data or from personal experience. Whatever source is used, it is important that the conditions under which the variance is estimated match as closely as possible the conditions of the future experiment (Lenth 2001; Carey and Keough 2002).

Since a smaller significance threshold (α) has the effect of reducing power $(1 - \beta)$, it is rarely possible in practice to achieve the ideal of α close to zero and $1 - \beta$ close to unity. The trade-off is usually resolved by a compromise, many investigators arbitrarily setting α at 0.05 and power at 0.80, respectively – the so-called 'five-eighty convention' (Di Stefano 2003), which sets the probability of Type I and Type II errors at 5 % and 20 %, respectively. Adopting this convention implies an acceptance that the cost of making a Type I error is four times more important than the cost of making a Type II error (Cohen 1988; Di Stefano 2003). However, Type II errors may be more critical than Type I errors, for example when assessing environmental impacts, testing the toxicity of chemicals, or managing natural resources (Mapstone 1995; Dayton 1998; Field *et al.* 2004). The relative costs of making Type I and Type II errors should therefore be taken into account when deciding on an acceptable level of statistical power. More flexible methods that evaluate these relative costs are described by Mapstone (1995) and Keough and Mapstone (1997).

The effect size (θ) measures absolute change in the response variable, usually relative to a control group. The specified effect size should be the minimum change in the response that is biologically meaningful. This is often difficult to decide in practice, especially for complex and poorly understood systems (Lenth 2001). It can be tempting to use arbitrary effect sizes. For example, Cohen (1988) took the standardised difference between group means ($[\bar{y}_2 - \bar{y}_1]/\sigma$) as a measure of the effect size, in order to quantify 'large', 'medium' and 'small' effects as 0.8, 0.5 and 0.2, respectively. This 'off-the-shelf' approach suffers two main drawbacks: the effects may or may not be biologically important, and it takes no account of measurement precision (Lenth 2001). Given the difficulty of specifying a single meaningful effect size, an alternative approach is to plot the attainable power or required sample size for a range of effect sizes to get an idea of the sensitivity of the experiment (Lenth 2001; Quinn and Keough 2002).

Armed with this information, power analysis can be used to compare alternative models and determine the optimal allocation of resources within a given design.

Evaluating alternative designs

Power analysis is a useful tool for evaluating the relative efficiency of different experimental designs. Investigators can achieve considerable gains in efficiency by choosing between alternatives on the basis of their statistical power at a given level of replication, or their cost in replication required to detect a specified effect size (Allison *et al.* 1997).

The exact formulae to be used depend upon the model being evaluated. Detailed descriptions of power-analysis calculations are beyond the scope of this book; interested readers should consult more specialist texts, and use power-analysis software freely available on the web. Each hypothesis requires a separate calculation, and it may be necessary to prioritise them to ensure that the experiment has adequate power to detect the key hypotheses.

The main limitation of power analysis is that it requires reliable estimates of the error variation. Whilst this can be fairly straightforward for simple designs, more complex designs may require comprehensive pilot studies. For example, to calculate the power of a test for A in the fully replicated model A|B′, one needs to know the expected variance of the A*B′ interaction (which forms the denominator of the F-ratio), which may be difficult to estimate without conducting a large-scale pilot study.

If the error variation cannot be estimated from earlier studies and there are insufficient resources to conduct a pilot study, sensible design decisions can still be made without a formal power analysis, by adhering to the following general rules.

(1) Prioritise your hypotheses and focus on those of most interest. Since more complex designs usually require more resources than simple designs, trying to answer too many questions at once may mean that resources are insufficient to answer any of them adequately.

(2) Ensure that a valid F-ratio is available to test key hypotheses. For example, the unreplicated two-factor design B|A (model 7.1(i)) has no residual variation with which to test any of its terms – although your statistics package may go ahead and test them anyway.

(3) Be aware of the problems of interpreting unreplicated, repeated-measures and split-plot designs; interpretation of results will be clearer and easier to justify to your audience if you can use a completely randomised and fully replicated design.

(4) An unreplicated randomised complete block will be more powerful than an equivalent unblocked design only if it has a reduction in the residual MS that more than compensates for the reduction in residual d.f. from lack of replication. In the absence of good pilot data, a decision to block without replication must be made on the likely magnitude of variation between blocks relative to that within blocks. In the event that blocks (or repeated measures) are used, and the block effect turns out to be non-significant, avoid the temptation to simplify the model *post hoc* by removing block (or subject) from the main effects declared in the model. Failure to detect a significant effect in samples does not necessarily mean that there is no effect in the population. Removing the effect from the model biases the error MS and consequently the validity of the treatment F-ratios.

(5) Avoid subjecting a null hypothesis to more than one test. Incorporate multiple factors into a single ANOVA rather than doing several

one-factor ANOVAs, which ignore nesting or interactions and accrue excessive Type I errors as a result of not partitioning the total variation into distinct sources. Likewise, use one-factor ANOVA rather than multiple t tests. As an example of just how excessive the Type I errors can be in multiple tests of the same null hypothesis, consider a response that has been measured across ten samples of a factor. The sensible analysis is one-factor ANOVA, but suppose instead that you wish to probe the data with an unplanned search for any significant differences amongst the 45 sample pairs. You might be tempted to do 45 t tests all of the same null hypothesis H_0: no difference between any pair of means. The approach is disastrous, however, because it leads to a 90 % chance of falsely rejecting H_0 on at least one test. This 'family-wise' Type I error rate is calculated from one minus the probability of not making a Type I error in any of the 45 individual tests: $1 - (1 - 0.05)^{45} = 0.90$ (e.g., Moran 2003). Setting $\alpha = 0.05$ means that we are willing to falsely reject the null hypothesis on up to 5 % of occasions. In 45 tests, we may thus expect to falsely reject the null hypothesis on as many as 2–3 occasions with this α. ANOVA avoids the problem of multiple tests by partitioning the variance in the data into distinct sources and testing one unique null hypothesis per partition. It is possible to do unplanned *post hoc* tests after an ANOVA, in order to seek where differences lie amongst sample means, but these are designed specifically to control the family-wise error rate (see page 245).

(6) There is little point in doing a very weak test with only one or a few error degrees of freedom, because a significant difference would be obviously different anyway and no conclusions could be drawn from a non-significant difference. Conversely, there may be little extra power to be gained from having hundreds rather than tens of error d.f., and usually little opportunity of obtaining large numbers of truly independent replicates. For example, the critical value of F at $\alpha = 0.05$ for a test with one and six degrees of freedom is $F_{1,6 [0.05]} = 5.99$. This means that an effect will register as significant only if the measure of explained variance given by the test mean square is at least six times greater than the unexplained (error) variance. This threshold increases in incrementally bigger steps with fewer error d.f., until $F_{1,1[0.05]} = 161$, and it tails off going the other way, until $F = 1.00$. For a given test and workload of total observations, the

critical F depends on the distribution of data points between levels of sampling units and treatments. Figure 12 illustrates the rapid increase in threshold as the error d.f. drop below six, and the rapidly diminishing returns in power as the error d.f. increase in the other direction. For a given total of N data points, the critical F will tend to be smaller in designs that partition N between more samples, as opposed to more replicates per sample (illustrated by circles in Figure 12). This is particularly true for mixed models, where the number of levels of the random factor determine the error degrees of freedom.

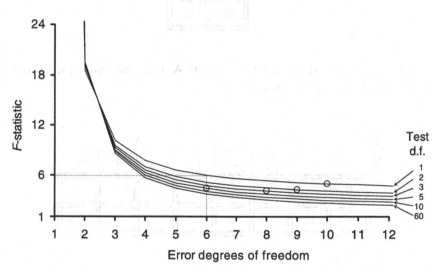

Figure 12 Upper 5% points of the F distribution for given test degrees of freedom. Dotted lines show the threshold ratio of test to error MS for one and six d.f.; circles show thresholds for one-factor analyses of two, three, four and six samples (right to left), all with the same total number of observations ($N=12$).

When comparing alternative designs it can be informative to consider how many subjects in total are required to obtain a given number of error d.f. for the main hypotheses of interest. For example, the following models all test a two-level fixed factor A with six error d.f. but require collection of vastly different quantities of data:

1.1. One-factor model $Y = A + \varepsilon$ tests A with one and six d.f. from error $MS[S'(A)]$ on $N = 8$ subjects:

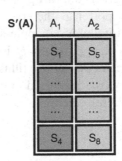

2.1(*i*) Nested model $Y = B'(A) + \varepsilon$ tests A with one and six d.f. from error $MS[B'(A)]$ on $N \geq 16$ subjects:

S'(B'(A))	A₁				A₂			
	B₁	B₂	B₃	B₄	B₅	B₆	B₇	B₈
	S₁	...	...	...	...	...	...	S₁₅
	S₂	...	...	...	...	...	...	S₁₆

3.1. Cross factored models ...

    (*i*) $Y = B|A + \varepsilon$ tests A with one and six d.f. from error $MS[S'(B*A)]$ on $N = 12$ subjects:

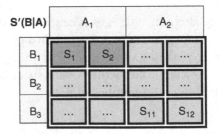

(*ii*) $Y = B'|A + \varepsilon$ tests A with one and six d.f. from error MS[B'*A] on $N \geq 28$ subjects:

S'(B'|A)	A_1		A_2	
B_1	S_1	S_2	...	...
B_2	...	...	...	...
B_3	...	...	...	...
B_4	...	...	...	...
B_5	...	...	...	...
B_6	...	...	...	...
B_7	...	...	S_{27}	S_{28}

4.1(*i*) or 6.1(*i*) Randomised-block or repeated-measures model $Y = S'|A$ tests A with one and six d.f. from error MS[S'*A] on $N = 7$ blocks or subjects:

P'(S'|A)	S_1	S_2	S_3	S_4	S_5	S_6	S_7
A_1	P_1	...	...	...	...	...	...
A_2	...	...	...	...	...	...	P_{14}

5.6(*i*) or 6.3(*i*). Split-plot or repeated-measures model $Y = B|S'(A)$ tests A with one and six d.f. from error MS[S'(A)] on $N = 8$ blocks or subjects:

P'(B|S'(A))	A_1				A_2			
	S_1	S_2	S_3	S_4	S_5	S_6	S_7	S_8
B_1	P_1	...	...	...	...	...	...	...
B_2	...	...	...	...	...	...	...	P_{16}

We end this chapter with a caution that some types of scientific endeavour will always be more susceptible than others to false claims, regardless of the design of data collection. Although a more powerful design will increase the chance of forming true conclusions from a test, a claimed finding may yet have low probability of being true. This is because its chance of being true depends on the prevalence of the effect in the population, in addition to the Type I and II error rates for the test. This should not pose a problem for tests of an effect with putative 100 % prevalence. For example, we may suppose that crop yield either does or does not depend on watering regime, always and everywhere within the defined environment of interest. If it does not, then we can expect a false positive result on 5 % of trials given an $\alpha = 0.05$; if it does, then we can expect a false negative on 20 % of trials given a $\beta = 0.20$. Problems arise, however, when statistics are used to claim a finding of some rare attribute or event. Rare findings attract high profile attention and thus tend to be claimed with vigour, but the statistical evidence must be interpreted with great caution to avoid later embarrassment in the face of contradictory results.

The frequency of false positive results can be extremely high in studies that trawl many thousands of suspects for a few rare dependencies (Ioannidis 2005). For example, if a heritable disease is likely to be associated with around ten gene polymorphisms out of 100 000 available for testing, then a claim to have identified one of these polymorphisms with $P < 0.01$ will have no more than 1 % chance of being true even with the most powerful test (i.e., with $\beta \sim 0$). This is because an analysis with $\alpha = 0.01$ must sanction 1000 false positive results in the total 100 000 tests that would embrace the $\sim$10 true polymorphisms, yielding $\sim$10/1010 chance of a given positive result being true. If the test has only 60 % power ($\beta = 0.4$), then about four of the $\sim$10 true results are likely to be misdiagnosed, resulting in $\sim$0.6 % chance that the positive result is a true find. With such a high likelihood of error, it can be only a matter of time before the claim is contradicted by other independent studies of the same polymorphism. Indeed, claims and counter-claims are a recurrent feature of scientific endeavour of this sort (Ioannidis 2005). The positive result nevertheless serves a valuable purpose, even in the face of counter-claims, inasmuch as it reveals $\sim$60-fold increase in probability for that polymorphism, relative to the pre-test probability. Similar issues arise with diagnostic screening for rare diseases (see example on page 268). These kinds of studies should draw probabilistic conclusions with respect to the known rarity of relationships, rather than claiming to reveal a truth.

In general, a statistically significant result is more likely true than false only if the expected ratio of wrongly to correctly rejected null hypotheses $(\alpha/(1 - \beta))$ is less than the actual ratio of false to true null hypotheses in the field of research. In fact, in order to have as little as a 1 % chance of a false positive result from a test with $\alpha = 0.01$ would require the putative effect to have at least 99 % prevalence in the population (and more if $\beta > 0$). If such an effect is known to be so prevalent, however, there is nothing to be gained by testing for it. This is an example of the unavoidable trade-off between certainty and utility that can seem to reduce statistical analysis to a dispenser of either useless truths or false claims. It emphasises the importance of identifying a correct statistical approach with respect to the objectives of the study. The method of falsification, which is the great strength of hypothesis-testing statistics, is severely undermined in applications that involve screening for a sought-after result. These endeavours are much better suited to the more subjective approach of Bayesian inference, which concerns the impact of new information on a previous likelihood. The method of testing a falsifiable null hypothesis for which statistics such as ANOVA were developed is best suited to studies that can obtain persuasive evidence from a single test.

How to request models
in a statistics package

You will need to declare any random factors and covariates as such. For balanced designs you may have an option to use the restricted form of the model (see page 242).

For a fully replicated design, most packages will give you all main effects and their interactions if you request the model in its abbreviated form. For example, the design $Y = C|B|A + \varepsilon$ (model 3.2) can be requested as: 'C|B|A'. Where a model has nested factors, you may need to request it with expansion of the nesting. For example the design $Y = C|B'(A) + \varepsilon$ (model 3.3) is requested with 'C|A + C|B(A)'.

Repeated-measures and unreplicated designs have no true residual variation. The package may require residual variation nevertheless, in which case declare all the terms except the highest-order term (always the last row with non-zero d.f. in the ANOVA tables in this book). For example, for the design $Y = B|S'(A)$ (model 6.3) request: 'B|A + B|S(A) − B*S(A)', and the package will take the residual from the subtracted term. Likewise, for the design $Y = S'|A$ (model 4.1) request: 'S|A − S*A', and the package will take the residual from the subtracted term; or equally, request 'A + S', and the package will take the residual from the one remaining undeclared term: S*A.

Where models contain nesting of the form B(A), factor B may need to have its levels coded as 1, 2, ..., b repeated within each level of A. Where a model has nesting into more than one factor simultaneously, you may need to simplify the description of the model. For example, the designs $Y = C'(B'(A)) + \varepsilon$ and $Y = C'(B|A) + \varepsilon$, of models 2.2 and 3.4 respectively, both need factor C to be written as 'C(B A)'. The first is analysed by requesting: 'A + B(A) + C(B A)', and the second by requesting: 'B|A + C(B A)'. The same structure of the input is required for both these requests, and also for $Y = C|B|A + \varepsilon$ and $Y = C|B'(A) + \varepsilon$ (models 3.2 and 3.3).

For example, a response Y measured on two subjects at each of two levels of factors C, B and A is input in the following form regardless of nesting or cross factoring:

A	B	C	Y
1	1	1	9.2
1	1	1	9.4
1	1	2	8.5
1	1	2	9.7
1	2	1	8.3
1	2	1	9.1
1	2	2	9.2
1	2	2	7.9
2	1	1	8.2
2	1	1	9.6
2	1	2	9.2
2	1	2	9.5
2	2	1	7.8
2	2	1	9.1
2	2	2	8.9
2	2	2	9.4

Because your data will be correctly analysed by only one model, it is obviously vital that you request the correct one. Find the appropriate model in the book with the help of the guide to model construction on page 58, and the diagrams on p. 288. Remember that a factor is nested in another if each of its levels belongs to only one level of the other (e.g., subject nested in gender, plot nested in treatment). It is cross factored if each of its levels are represented in each level of the other. All repeated measures on replicate subjects or blocks are cross factored with the replicate.

Best practice in presentation of the design

How to report your designs and analyses

The objective of a Methods section to a report is to allow anyone to repeat all of your procedures. You therefore need to explain what you did and report all decisions relevant to the design of data collection and its analysis.

In the Methods, write out the statistical model either fully or in its contracted form (e.g., $Y = B|A + \varepsilon$). The residual variation should be indicated by ε in a fully replicated model, to distinguish it from unreplicated or repeated-measures designs that do not have true residual variation. Clearly identify your sampling or observational unit, from which you draw each data point. Explain which factors are fixed and which random. Explain the function served by any random factors, and detail how these influence the construction of F-ratios. Where an analysis will not be testing for some interactions, explain why not. The reason is likely to have to do with intrinsic design features, for example of some split-plot and other non-orthogonal designs, or because of insufficient replication. That an interaction may be deemed biologically uninteresting is not a good reason for dropping it from the analysis, because to do so pools up the interaction with the error term and changes the estimates of the main effects.

Also in the Methods, justify the assumptions of random and independent observations, and report results of tests or checks for homogeneity of variances and normality of residuals (after any necessary transformations). If *post hoc* pooling is an option, show that this has been planned into the data-collection design.

The objective of the Results section to a report is to interpret the outcomes of your analyses (according to protocols described in the

Methods), showing sufficient detail of the analysis to allow your audience to evaluate the interpretation. So remember to fulfil the formal requirements of showing degrees of freedom or sample sizes, in addition to emphasising the result that you consider most important.

In the Results, try to summarise principal differences and trends graphically. If possible, show one graph per analysis of variance. An 'interaction plot' may suit a cross-factored analysis with significant interactions, showing sample means without associated variation and linking means of the same factor. Otherwise, always attach a measure of variation to any mean, clearly identifying which measure it is (standard deviation, standard error, or confidence intervals, etc.). If the analysis required transformed data, then show back-transformed means and confidence intervals on the graph and in the text. More than two factors may require panels of graphs, or a table to summarise sample means and confidence intervals. In graphs, use the minimum necessary axis marks, labelled to sensible decimal places. In tables, give all non-integer values to whatever numbers of decimal places are appropriate to the scale and accuracy of measurement. If space permits, show statistics for all sources, regardless of significance, because non-significant results have the same biological validity as significant ones. For each source of variation, report the value of F, the two values of d.f., and P. For analyses with more than two factors, this may be achieved most succinctly in a table listing each source, its d.f., MS, F and P. Always interpret such a table from the bottom up, because interactions take precedence over main effects. In complex analyses consider how to get more from the global test by comparing magnitudes of effect (page 244) or using *post hoc* comparisons of sample means (page 245).

A one-factor ANOVA can be completely described by a single sentence, such as: 'Body weights differed by sex (mean ± s.e. of males = 23.6 ± 3.3 g, females = 18.2 ± 3.4 g; $F_{1,8} = 6.48$, $P < 0.05$).' There is no need to talk about a 'significant difference' because that only opens the door to nonsensical permutations such as 'males were heavier than females but the difference was not significant' when an analysis has not yielded a desired result. The statistic provides the evidence that the factor levels either did differ at a probability α of rejecting a true null hypothesis, or did not differ at a probability β of accepting a false null hypothesis. Be informative about what is revealed by each result. To state that 'the results were significant' is uninformative, and that 'the results are presented in Table 1' is lazy. Obviously, avoid annoying your audience with statements of the type: 'The data were significant'.

Where factors vary on a continuous scale, show regression lines only for significant trends. For each source of variation, report the value of F, the two values of d.f., P, and the r^2 which represents the proportion of variation explained by the model. A linear regression is completely described in one sentence, such as: 'The per capita birth rate day^{-1} declined with population density m^{-2} ($y = 3.4 - 0.2x$, $F_{1,12} = 8.32$, $P < 0.01$, $r^2 = 0.41$).'

How to understand the designs and analyses reported by others

Authors often omit to make any explicit mention of design in their Methods, either because it is simple and self-evident, or because it is complicated and they have let a statistics package sort out that bit for them. If you suspect the latter, then treat the analyses and their inferences with suspicion. Statistical analyses should not be judged correct simply by virtue of having been published, but by virtue of well-justified explanations of the logic underpinning design choices.

Graphs or tables of principal results will usually provide clues to the appropriate design, if not to the actual design used by the authors. If error bars are attached to means, then the data probably suit an ANOVA or related analysis. If means have no error bars, then again think of ANOVA remembering that, except for interaction plots, means should always be given with their errors. A graph with two or more types of data point or bar is likely to need factorial ANOVA; equally a graph with two or more regression lines is likely to need a factorial ANCOVA. Analysis of residuals is not an acceptable substitute for ANCOVA (see page 32).

Authors use different measures of variation around sample means to represent their data, and they don't always clearly identify what the measure is. Standard errors are always smaller than s.d. and confidence limits, but all of these measures can show up any non-homogeneity of variances (unless the graph shows only the pooled standard deviation from the error MS).

If the report shows an ANOVA table, then use the relevant tables in this book to check that effects have been tested with the appropriate error MS. This is particularly important in mixed models and nested designs where omitting to identify random factors as random can lead to grossly inflated levels of significance (e.g., compare F-ratios for factor A in models 3.1(i) and (ii)). Where tables are not shown, the values of error d.f. will generally reveal which source of variation was used for the error

MS. If no error d.f. are shown, then treat the results as highly suspect because of the failure to report the amount of replication underpinning the inferences. If error d.f. are very large, then question whether they refer to genuinely independent replicates. For example, do they correspond to the number of subjects or plots? If not, has subject or plot been factored into the analysis in a repeated-measures design?

Troubleshooting problems during analysis

Correctly identifying the appropriate model to use (see page 57) is the principal hurdle in any analysis, but running the chosen model in your favourite statistics package also presents a number of potential pitfalls. If you encounter problems when using a statistics package, do refer to its help routines and tutorials in order to understand the input requirements and output formats, and to help you interpret error messages. If that fails then look to see if you have encountered one of these common problems.

Problems with sampling design

If I just want to identify any differences amongst a suite of samples, can I do t *tests on all sample pairs?* No, the null hypothesis of no difference requires a single test yielding a single P-value. Multiple P-values are problematic in any unplanned probing of the data with more than one test of the same null hypothesis, because the repeated testing inflates the Type I error rate (illustrated by an example on page 252). If an ANOVA reveals a general difference between samples, explore where the significance lies using *post hoc* tests designed to account for the larger family-wise error (page 245).

How can I get rid of unwanted variation? In experimental designs, a treatment applied to a group of sampling units should be compared to a control group which is the same in all respects other than the test manipulation. Full control is often not logistically feasible, particularly in field experiments, and mensurative studies typically have no controls. It is then important to declare all the components of random variation in the model, so that the analysis can test the factors of interest independently of other sources of variation. This needs thinking about at the design stage, because the different sources of random variation will influence the amount of replication for testing effects of interest. See sections on nesting, blocking and covariates (pages 21, 25, 29).

I have applied a treatment factor to whole sampling units but have taken replicate measurements from within each sampling unit. Use a nested model to account for the nesting of replicate measurements within sampling units (see the introduction to nesting on page 21, worked example 1 on page 47 and the models in Chapter 2).

Allocation of treatment levels cannot be fully randomised, because of natural gradients in the landscape. Use stratified random sampling in a randomised-block design (see the introduction to blocking on page 25 and the models in Chapter 4).

Cross-factored treatments are applied to sampling units at different spatial scales. If one factor has treatment levels assigned to blocks, while another factor has treatment levels assigned to plots nested in blocks, then use a split-plot design (see the introduction to blocking on page 25, and the models in Chapter 5).

Some combinations of factor levels cannot be measured in principle. Redefine the existing combinations as levels of a single factor and analyse with orthogonal contrasts (page 245).

Do the levels of a random blocking factor need to be independent of each other? The mean responses per block need to vary independently of each other around the overall mean response for the block factor. Check for an absence of correlation between the responses per block.

Do the values of a covariate need to be independent or evenly spaced? It is only the response residuals that need to provide independent information in ANOVA and ANCOVA. There is no special requirement for covariate values to be evenly spaced, though a skewed distribution can cause the few values in the long tail to have a high leverage – i.e., to exert an undue influence on the regression slope. A covariate cross factor should be measured at the same or similar level for each level of the other factor, if possible, and adjusted SS used to adjust for any discrepancies (see the discussion of unbalanced designs on page 237).

Can I use the same test many times over to screen a population for a rare phenomenon? Hypothesis testing is not well suited to finding a few rare dependencies amongst a large number of suspects. For example, a positive result with $P < 0.05$ is more likely false than true if the effect occurs in less than 5% of the population available for testing, regardless of the power of the analysis (page 256).

Problems with model specification

I just want to do a one-way ANOVA on three samples, but the statistics package demands information on a 'response' and 'factors'. All analyses of variance use statistical models, and the package is simply asking for the elements of your model, in this case a response variable containing all the measured data and an explanatory variable which describes the factor level or covariate value applied to each observation. Most statistics packages require the response and each factor or covariate to be arranged in columns of equal length (as described in the worked examples, pages 48, 51, 54). Make sure that the model you request will contain all the testable sources of variation present in your design, even those that account only for nuisance variation.

How do I get rid of nuisance variables? If your design has not controlled for unwanted variation, then any nuisance variables will need to be factored into the model. Failure to declare all sources of variation as factors will result in their contributions to variation becoming pooled into the residual variation. Although this raises the residual MS, it also increases the residual d.f. which can greatly inflate the Type I error for the test.

If I am only interested in main effects from a multi-factor analysis, is it wrong to not request the interactions? Interactions can provide valuable additional information about the significance of main effects (see page 77) and it is generally advisable to include them in hypothesis-testing designs. In more exploratory analyses, you can consider dropping non-significant interactions as part of model simplification (page 40). In designs without full replication (Chapters 4 to 7), some or all interactions cannot be tested and are assumed to be zero, though they still need to be entered into the model as (untestable) sources of variation. Such models cannot be fully interpreted without testing the assumption of no interaction, which would require full replication (using models in Chapters 1 to 3).

A factor of interest varies on a continuous scale, but has been measured in discrete increments; should it be declared as a categorical factor or as a covariate? Either is feasible, and which you choose depends on the nature of the response and the desired hypothesis. Plot a graph of the response against the continuous factor to find out whether the relationship is linear or whether the response and/or the factor can be transformed to make the relationship linear. If so, modelling it as a covariate may give a more parsimonious model and allow you to interpolate between the measured values of the covariate. It can also increase the residual d.f. which increases the power to detect some or all declared effects in the model (though not always those of most interest – see worked example 3 on page 51).

If a categorical factor of interest has levels arranged on an ordinal scale, can it be analysed as a covariate? It may be reasonable to designate a set of ordered categories as a covariate for the purpose of testing a null hypothesis of no systematic increase or decrease in response. The ANCOVA cannot be used to predict the value of the response, however, unless a covariate is measured on an interval scale, such that the interval between values of one and two has the same value as that between two and three, etc. This may not necessarily be the case with ordered categories that measure qualitative degrees, for example of the health of a subject, or the shadiness of a plot.

I am trying to do an analysis of variance on a categorical factor, but my statistics package insists on treating the factor as a covariate. Some statistics packages automatically treat a factor with numerical values as a covariate unless you identify it as a categorical factor. This problem will not arise if levels of a factor are coded using words or letters rather than numbers.

The statistics package won't give me the interaction term in a two-factor ANOVA. Make sure that you have asked it to by requesting 'B|A', or 'A + B + B*A' instead of just 'A + B'. The two-factor ANOVA can only estimate an interaction if the design is fully replicated, with more than one measure at each combination of levels of A and B.

I have many possible explanatory factors – should I include them all in the model? If your goal is to explore a dataset to identify which of many competing factors most influence a response, then ANOVA can be used as a tool to select the most parsimonious model. If your goal is to test specific hypotheses rather than to develop a predictive model, then you would be wise to keep things simple. Each additional cross factor added to an ANOVA design adds an extra dimension to the analysis, multiplies up the number of potential sources of variance and creates extra complexity that can be difficult to interpret. In addition, it can reduce the power of the analysis to detect a significant effect, unless an appropriate increase is planned in the number of measures to be taken on the response. A good design is therefore one that samples the minimum number of factors necessary to answer the question of interest, and measures sufficient replicates to estimate all potential sources of variance amongst those chosen few factors.

Not all samples contain the same number of replicate observations (or more generally, the nesting is not symmetrical). This is not a problem for one-factor analyses, though it increases sensitivity to the assumptions of the analysis. For designs with more than one factor, use adjusted sums of squares in a general linear model (see page 237). If the GLM package cannot avoid adjusting for higher-order interactions between fixed factors, request only sequential SS and run the GLM as many times as there are main effects, each time changing their order of entry into the model and keeping results only for the last-entered main effect and its interactions. Alternatively, resample from the data to reinstate symmetry, whereupon sequential and adjusted SS will be equal.

The data are not normally distributed. It is the residuals that are assumed by ANOVA to be normally distributed, not the raw data (see page 14). The residuals are the squared distance of each data point from its sample mean (or from the regression line in ANCOVA), from which is calculated the unexplained (residual) variation on the assumption that this is adequately represented for all samples by the same normal distribution. Most statistical packages will calculate and store residuals for you, which you can then test for normality using a normal probability plot. If you suspect there is a significant departure from normality, then consider applying a transformation to the response (see assumptions of ANOVA on page 14 and of ANCOVA on page 32).

Sample variances differ, or residuals are not normally distributed around sample means. Consider applying a transformation to the response (see assumptions of ANOVA on page 14 and of ANCOVA on page 32).

Problems with results

A diagnostic test for a disease has a Type I error rate of 1 %; if it returns a positive result ($P < 0.01$) on a patient's sample, does the patient have $> 99 \%$ chance of carrying the disease? No, the error rate indicates a 1 % chance of the analysis returning a false positive, but the probability of this particular diagnosis being true depends also on the prevalence of the disease and the Type II error rate of the test. For a disease carried by 1 in 5000 of the population, a test with $\alpha = 0.01$ will return 100 false positives on average for every couple of true positives. If the test has $\beta = 0.5$, then one of these true positives will be missed on average, and the patient returning a positive result will have a 1 in 101 chance of carrying the disease – in other words $> 99 \%$ chance of *not* having it! The test has nevertheless served a purpose, by reporting a 50-fold increase in the patient's probability of being a carrier relative to the pre-test probability of 1 in 5000 (see also page 256).

The statistics package returns an ANOVA table with only one set of d.f. assigned to each term. Should I report the treatment effect as '$F_2 = 9.78$' *etc?* No, always report two sets of d.f. for an ANOVA result. The first set is the test d.f., which provides information about the number of levels of the effect. The second set is the error d.f., which provides information on the amount of replication available for testing the effect. For an ANOVA without random factors, this will be the residual d.f. in the last line of the table before the total d.f. For any other type of ANOVA, use the tables in this book to determine the correct error d.f. for each term. Then check that the package has used the correct error terms by dividing the effect MS by the error MS to get the same F-value as that returned by the package.

Can I transform the data in order to improve their fit to the model? The data represent your best estimate of reality and so cannot be fitted to a model. The purpose of statistics is to compare the fit of alternative models to the data (see page 2). The validity of any model inevitably depends on its underlying assumptions. Although many types of biological data violate the assumptions of ANOVA, it is often possible to apply some form of transformation to correct the problem (see pages 14 and 32). The sole purpose of transformations is therefore to allow valid tests of model hypotheses.

The data contain numerous zeros. If these contribute to violating the assumptions of ANOVA, this will present a problem that cannot be resolved by transformation. Consider redefining the hypothesis to exclude zeros from consideration. Regression analyses can be severely biased by a heavy weighting of zeros in the response and/or covariate even without violating underlying assumptions. For example, consider a test of 'camera traps' deployed to photograph jaguars patrolling forest trails, which pairs a camera with a new type of heat-sensitive trigger against one with a standard infra-red trigger of known efficiency. The frequency of captures by the new type might bear no relation to that by the standard type, but it will appear as strongly correlated if the analysis includes the many trap points where neither camera was triggered by a jaguar. These locations may simply contain no jaguars, and they can be excluded from the analysis on this assumption.

Adjusted sums of squares differ from sequential sums of squares. The explanatory factors are not orthogonal, requiring care in the interpretation of main effects (page 237). If two continuous variables are strongly correlated with each other, they may both show as non-significant even when each has a clear linear relationship to the response. This is because the effect of each is measured after adjusting for the other. SS should not be adjusted for higher-order interactions between their fixed effects.

The statistics package returns an F-*test denominator of zero, or zero error d.f.* Erase from the input model the last-entered (and highest-order) term, which then becomes the residual error term (see pages 57 and 258).

The statistics package returns an inexact F-*test.* The design permits only a quasi *F*-ratio, although *post hoc* pooling may present a viable alternative (see page 40 and footnotes to tables of the model structures).

The statistics package calculates the F-*ratio for some random factors using a different denominator to that prescribed in this book.* It may be using an unrestricted mixed model (see page 242 and footnotes to tables of the model structures).

In a design with many crossed factors, is there a problem with getting multiple P-*values in the ANOVA table of results?* Multiple *P*-values are not a problem when they are generated by an ANOVA that has partitioned sources of variation in the response, because each tests a different null hypothesis. This is true also of a priori contrasts, but unplanned *post hoc* tests must account for an inflated Type I error that results from multiple tests of the same null hypothesis (page 245).

My ANOVA on three samples is not significant, but when I do a t *test on each pair of samples, one of them does give a significant result.* All that the multiple tests have given you is an excessive Type I error rate. See the section on evaluating alternative designs (page 250, and particularly point 5 on page 252). Consider use of *post hoc* tests designed to account for the inflated error (page 245).

There are few error degrees of freedom for one or more F-*ratios.* Investigate options for *post hoc* pooling (see page 38 and footnotes to tables of the model structures). If pooling is not possible then reflect on the need to plan the analysis before collecting the data (see the example on page 51).

Glossary

Adjusted sums of squares   Adjustment to the sum of squares used in general linear models (GLM) to account for designs without orthogonality. A Type II adjustment to the SS of a term involves adjusting for all other terms in the model that do not contain the term in question. A Type III adjustment involves adjusting for all other terms in the model, including those containing the term in question. Only Type II SS are suitable for models with fixed cross factors, and only Type III SS are suitable for models with random cross factors.

Analysis of covariance (ANCOVA)   Analysis of variance on a model containing one or more covariates, usually in addition to one or more categorical factors. Each covariate X is tested for a linear trend with the continuous response Y.

Analysis of variance (ANOVA)   An analysis of the relative contributions of explained and unexplained sources of variance in a continuous response variable. In this book, we use the term 'ANOVA' in its broad sense to include explanatory factors that vary on continuous as well as categorical scales, with a focus on balanced designs. Parametric ANOVA and GLM partition the total variance in the response by measuring sums of squared deviations from modelled values. Significant effects are tested with the F statistic, which assumes a normal distribution of the residual error, homogeneous variances and random sampling of independent replicates.

A priori tests   Tests that are integral to the original hypothesis.

Assumptions   These are the necessary preconditions for fitting a given type of model to data. No form of generalisation from particular data is possible without assumptions. They provide the context for, and the means of evaluating, scientific statements purporting to truly explain reality. As with any statistical test, ANOVA assumes unbiased sampling from the population of interest. Its other assumptions concern the error variation against which effects are tested by the ANOVA model. Underlying assumptions should be tested where possible, and otherwise acknowledged as not testable for a given reason of design or data deficiency.

271

Balance   A balanced design has the same number of replicate observations in each sample. Balance is a desirable attribute particularly of cross-factored models, where loss of balance generally (though not inevitably) leads to loss of orthogonality. The consequent complications to the partitioning of sources of variance in the response are accommodated by general linear models.

Block   A level of a random factor designated to sample unmeasured variation in the environment.

Blocking factor   A random factor designated to sample unmeasured variation in the environment.

Categorical factor   A factor with levels that are classified by categories (e.g., factor Sex with levels male and female). A factor may vary on a continuous scale (e.g., distance in km, or time in hours) but still be treated as categorical if it is measured at fixed intervals (e.g., before and after a place or event).

Control   A treatment level used to factor out extraneous variation by mimicking the test procedure in all respects other than the manipulation of interest. For example, a liquid fertiliser applied to a crop needs to be tested against a control of an equal quantity of liquid without the fertiliser ingredients. Failure to do so can result in a false positive induced by the carrier medium alone.

Correlation   Any co-variation of continuous factors with each other or with a continuous response. Correlation between explanatory factors is a form of non-orthogonality.

Covariate   A factor X that varies at least on an ordinal scale, and usually on a continuous scale (such as time, distance, etc.) and is therefore a covariate of the response Y. Analysis of covariance assumes that the response has a linear relation to the covariate, and transformations of response or covariate may be necessary to achieve this prior to analysis.

Crossed factor   One factor is crossed with another when each of its levels is tested in each level of the other factor. For example, watering regime is crossed with sowing density if the response to the wet regime is tested at both high and low sowing density, and so is the response to the dry regime (assuming both factors have just two levels).

Data   The measurements of the response at given levels of factors of interest.

Degrees of freedom (d.f.)   The number of independent pieces of information required to measure the component of variation, subtracted from the total number of pieces contributing to that variation. Analysis of variance always has two sets of d.f.: the first informs on the number of test samples and the second informs on the amount of replication available for testing the effect. For example, a result $F_{2,12} = 3.98$, $P < 0.05$ indicates a significant effect with three levels allocated between 15 sampling units.

Effect   A term in the statistical model accounting for one of several independent sources of variance in the response. For example the cross-factored model $Y = B|A + \varepsilon$ has two main effects (A and B) and one interaction effect (B*A).

Effect size   The magnitude of an effect, measured in terms of deviations of sample means from the grand mean (fixed factor), or the steepness of the regression slope from horizontal (covariate), or the magnitude of between-sample variance (random factor). The significance of an effect depends upon a combination of its size, the amount of background variation and the sample size. An effect of small magnitude can thus be strongly significant if it is sampled with little residual variation from many replicates. Conversely, an apparently large effect may have no significance if it is sampled with large residual variation or from few replicates.

Error variance   The random variation in the response against which an effect is tested, containing all of the same components of variation estimated in the population except for the test effect. The validity of ANOVA depends on three assumptions about the error variance: (i) that the random variation around fitted values is the same for all sample means of a factor, or across the range of a covariate; (ii) that the residuals contributing to this variation are free to vary independently of each other; (iii) that the residual variation approximates to a normal distribution.

Experiment   A manipulative study involving the application of one or more treatments under controlled conditions. Where possible, treatment levels are randomly assigned to sampling units, and effects compared against a control.

Factor   A source of variance in the response. A categorical factor is measured in categorical levels, whereas a covariate factor is measured on a scale of continuous (or sometimes ordinal) variation. A model might be constructed to test the influence of a factor as the sole explanation ($Y = A + \varepsilon$) or as one of many factors variously crossed with each other or nested within each other.

Factorial model   A model containing crossed factors in which every level of each factor is tested in combination with every level of the other factors. Fully replicated factorial designs test whether the effect of one factor is moderated by interaction with another.

False negative   The result of making a Type II error by accepting a false null hypothesis. This type of error can incur severe consequences for sampling units, such as patients being screened for a disease or rivers being screened for a pollutant. The Type II error rate β can be minimised by using a design with sufficient replication to ensure high power for distinguishing true effects.

False positive   The result of making a Type I error by rejecting a true null hypothesis. Tests that are deemed significant if $P < 0.05$ must sanction a false positive arising once in every 20 runs on average. This causes problems particularly in studies that apply the same test to a large number of datasets to screen for a phenomenon with low incidence in the population. A positive identification is more likely false than true if incidence $< \alpha$, the Type I error rate.

Fitted values   The values of the response predicted by the model for each data point. Fitted values are the sample means for categorical factors, or points on a regression line for a covariate.

Fixed factor   A factor with levels that are fixed by the design and could be repeated without error in another investigation. The factor has a significant effect if sample means differ by considerably more than the background variation, or for a covariate, if the variation of the regression line from horizontal greatly exceeds the variation of data points from the line.

F statistic   The test statistic used in ANOVA and GLM, named in honour of R. A. Fisher, who first described the distribution and developed the method of analysis of variance in the 1920s. The continuous *F* distribution for a given set of test and error d.f. is used to determine the probability of obtaining at least as large a value of the observed ratio of explained to unexplained variation, given a true null hypothesis. The associated *P*-value reports the significance of the test effect on the response.

Fully replicated design   A design with replicate sampling units at each factor level, or for designs with more than one factor, each combination of factor levels. Such designs have residual variation given by these nested random sampling units, which permits the ANOVA to test all sources of variance in the response. A design without full replication has the random sampling unit cross-factored with other terms, contributing to the variance in the response having one or more untestable sources.

General linear model (GLM)   Generic term for parametric analyses of variance that can accommodate combinations of factors and covariates, and unbalanced and non-orthogonal designs. GLMs generally use an unrestricted model for analysing combinations of fixed and random factors.

Generalised linear model (GLIM)   Generic term for analyses of variance that can accommodate combinations of factors and covariates, and can permit the residuals to follow any distribution from the exponential family, which includes Gaussian, Poisson, binomial and gamma distributions. Components of variation are partitioned using maximum likelihood rather than sums of squares.

Hypothesis test   An analysis of data to test for pattern against the null hypothesis H_0: no pattern. Analysis of variance subjects a dataset to one or more test hypotheses, described by a model. For example, a test of the model $Y = B|A + \varepsilon$ may reject or accept the null hypothesis of no effect of A on the response. Likewise, it rejects or accepts the null hypotheses of no B effect and of no interaction effect. A decision to reject H_0 is taken with some predefined probability α of making a Type I error by rejecting a true null hypothesis. A decision to accept H_0 is taken with a probability β of making a Type II error by accepting a false null hypothesis.

Independent replicates   The power of any statistical test to detect an effect depends on the accumulation of independent pieces of information. ANOVA assumes that replicate data points are independent of each other in the sense that the value of one data point at a given factor level has no influence on the value of another sampled at the same level. The assumption is often violated by the presence of confounding factors. For instance, a sample of ten subjects will not provide ten independent pieces of information about a response if it comprises five pairs of siblings. Independence can be restored by declaring a factor Sibling, or by measuring just one individual at random of each pair. Likewise, a response of leaf area to soil type is tested with replicates given by the number of independent plants not, by the number of leaves.

Interaction   An interaction tests whether the effect of one factor on a response depends on the level of another factor. For example, students may respond to different tutorial systems according to their age, indicated by a significant interaction effect Age*System on the response. If one factor is a covariate, the interaction is illustrated by different regression slopes at each level of the categorical factor. Two covariates show a significant interaction in a curved plane for their combined effect on the response. An interaction effect must always be interpreted before its constituent main effects, because its impact influences interpretation of the main effect.

Linear model   A model with linear (additive) combinations of parameter constants describing effect sizes. Linear models can describe non-linear trends in covariates, for example by transformation of the data or fitting a polynomial model. All the models in this book are linear.

Main effect   A main effect tests whether the effect of one factor on a response occurs irrespective of the level of another factor. For example, students may respond to different tutorial systems regardless of their age. Main effects must always be interpreted after interpreting any interactions.

Marginality   The fundamental principle of ANOVA that terms be tested in hierarchical order. This becomes an issue in non-orthogonal designs, where the variance due to an interaction must be estimated after factoring out the variance due to the terms contained within it.

Mean   The arithmetic average value of the responses in a sample. The sample means provide the fitted values from which effect size is measured in analyses of categorical factors. In covariate analysis, the linear regression pivots on the coordinate for the sample means of response and covariate: $(\bar{x}, \bar{y})$.

Mean square (MS)   The variance measured as variation per degree of freedom. The F-ratio is the ratio of explained to unexplained MS, where the numerator is the MS explained by the model and the denominator is the error MS left unexplained by the model.

Mensurative study   A study that tests the effect of one or more factors on a response without controlled manipulation.

Mixed model   A model with random and fixed factors.

Model   The hypothesised effect(s) on a response, which can be tested with ANOVA for evidence of pattern in the data. An ANOVA model contains one or more terms, each having an effect on the response that is tested against unmeasured error or residual variation. A model with a single factor (whether categorical or covariate) is written: $Y = A + \varepsilon$, and the ANOVA tests the term A against the residual ε. Models with multiple factors require care with declaring all terms in a statistical package. For example, the cross-factored with nesting model: $Y = C|B'(A) + \varepsilon$ is analysed by declaring the terms: $C|A + C|B(A)$. The two-factor randomised-block model: $Y + S'|B|A$ is analysed by declaring the terms: $S|B|A - S*B*A$ for a Model 1 analysis, or the terms: $S + B|A$ for a Model 2 analysis.

Model 1   In designs without full replication, an ANOVA model that assumes the presence of block-by-treatment interactions, even though the design has not allowed for their estimation. Randomised-block designs may be analysed by Model 1 or Model 2. Repeated-measures designs are generally analysed by Model 1.

Model 2   In designs without full replication, an ANOVA model that assumes the absence of block-by-treatment interactions, even though the design has not allowed for any direct test of this assumption. Randomised-block designs may be analysed by Model 1 or 2. Split-plot designs are generally analysed by Model 2.

Multiple tests   Multiple tests of the same hypothesis cause inflation of the Type I error rate. The problem arises in data probing, involving an unplanned search for any significant differences amongst a set of samples. For example, if replicate measures are taken from two levels of a factor A and from three levels of a factor B, then a search for any differences between the five samples might involve a total of ten independent t tests (A_1 versus A_2, A_1 versus B_1, ... etc.). If each has a Type I error rate of 0.05, then the ensemble of ten tests has a probability of $1 - 0.95^{10} = 0.40$ of mistakenly rejecting the null hypothesis of no single difference between any sample means. This unacceptably high rate is avoided only by using a statistical model that respects a planned design of data collection. A cross-factored ANOVA would partition the total variance in the response into three testable sources: A, B, and B*A, each with their own P-value testing a specific null hypothesis.

Nested factor   One factor is nested within another when each of its levels are tested in (or belong to) only one level of the other. For example a response measured per leaf for a treatment factor applied across replicate trees must declare the trees as a random factor nested in the treatment levels. The sampling unit of Leaf is then correctly nested in Tree nested in Treatment.

Nuisance variable   Factors or covariates holding no interest in their own right, but requiring inclusion in the model in order to factor out their contributions to variation in the data.

Null hypothesis (H_0)   The statistically testable hypothesis of no pattern in the data. The null hypothesis is the proposal that nothing interesting is happening, against which to test a model hypothesis of trend in a sample or differences between samples. If the test upholds the null hypothesis, then we conclude that the ANOVA model takes the form $Y = \varepsilon$; otherwise we infer a significant effect of a factor of interest on the response. A null hypothesis must be open to falsification. For example, a null hypothesis of zero difference between samples is capable of falsification. A suitable ANOVA will evaluate the evidence for a difference and accept or reject the null hypothesis accordingly. In contrast, a null hypothesis of a difference between samples is not capable of falsification, because absence of evidence (for a difference) is not evidence of absence.

Ordinary least squares (OLS)   A method of estimating the values of parameters in linear models by minimising the sum of squared deviations of each observation of the response from the model estimate. In ANOVA, this sum is known as the residual sum of squares, $SS_{residual}$, and it partitions out the variation left unexplained by the model.

Orthogonality   A cross-factored design is orthogonal if each of its factors are independent of each other. Two categorical cross factors are orthogonal by design if each level of one is measured at every level of the other. Orthogonal designs partition total variation in the response straightforwardly into testable components using sequential sums of squares for each effect in turn.

Although a balanced design generally (but not inevitably) ensures orthogonality, this can be difficult to achieve in practice, especially with covariates. Two covariates are only orthogonal if they have a correlation coefficient of zero. Loss of orthogonality can reduce or enhance the power of a design to detect effects, and usually requires analysis with the aid of adjusted sums of squares calculated in a GLM.

Parsimony   The principle of sampling the minimum number of factors necessary to answer the question of interest with a single model. Each additional cross factor adds an extra dimension to the design and multiplies up the number of potential sources of variation in the response. For example the one-way model $Y = A + \varepsilon$ has one testable source (A); the two-factor model: $Y = B|A + \varepsilon$ has three testable sources $(A + B + B*A)$; the three factor model $Y = C|B|A + \varepsilon$ has seven testable sources, and so on. Parsimony is not improved by ignoring any nuisance factors that contribute to variation in the data. These must be included in the analysis.

Placebo   A treatment used in medicinal trials to control for extraneous variation by mimicking the test procedure in all respects other than the therapeutic benefit of interest. For example, a drug trial for the effectiveness of a medicinal pill requires a treatment with two levels: drug and placebo, where the placebo is a dummy pill of the same shape and colour as the drug pill except that it does not contain the drug. The need for a control is well illustrated by the 'placebo effect' – the psychological boost to health that can be stimulated by an environment of medical care. For this reason, the treatment levels usually need to be allocated in a 'double blind' trial, whereby neither doctor nor patient can distinguish drug from placebo.

Polynomial predictor   A polynomial equation describes a curvilinear relationship with one or more exponents. Polynomials can be tested with linear models by declaring the covariate more than once. For example, the relationship: $y = a + bx + cx^2$ is tested in GLM by requesting the polynomial predictor in the form: X|X and taking sequential SS.

Pooling   The construction of an error term from more than one source of variance in the response. A priori pooling occurs in designs without full replication, where untestable interactions with random factors are pooled into the residual variation. The analysis then proceeds on the assumption that the interactions are either present (Model 1) or absent (Model 2). Planned *post hoc* pooling is applied to mixed models by pooling a non-significant error term with its own error term. The design is thereby influenced by the outcome of the analysis (in terms of whether or not an error term is itself significant). More generally, pooling can describe the process of joining together samples, for example in calculating a main effect MS by pooling across levels of a cross factor.

Population   In a statistical model for analysis of variance, the population is the theoretical complete set of units from which we sample replicate independent and randomly selected measures for the purposes of testing treatment effects. Any random factor requires a clear definition of the population it describes, so that a given sampling regime can be seen to fairly represent it. For example, do the subjects for a treatment come from a particular age, gender or ethnic group?

Post hoc tests   Tests that are supplementary to the original hypothesis.

Power   The capacity of a statistical test to detect an effect if it truly occurs. A test with high power has a low probability of mistakenly accepting a false null hypothesis (i.e., a low Type II error rate). Power increases with more replication, provided it is applied at an appropriate scale. For example a response measured per leaf for a treatment applied across replicate trees includes trees as a random factor nested in the treatment levels. The power of the design depends on the number of replicate trees per treatment level, and not directly on the number of replicate leaves per tree.

Pseudoreplication   The result of replicates in a sample not being truly independent of each other, which inflates the Type I error rate. ANOVA models are particularly prone to pseudoreplication if they omit to declare sources of nuisance variation in addition to the effects of interest.

Random factor   A factor with levels that sample at random from a defined population. A random factor will be assumed to have a normal distribution of sample means, and homogeneous variance of means, if its MS is the error variance for estimating other effects (e.g., in nested designs). The random factor has a significant effect if the variance among its levels is considerably greater than zero.

Random sampling   Replicate measures of a response to a given factor level must be taken at random if they are to represent the population that is being sampled. As with any statistical test, ANOVA assumes random sampling. This assumption is violated for instance if a test for a gender effect of body weight samples heavier males and lighter females.

Randomised-blocks   A design containing a random blocking factor, crossed with other factor(s) that have a randomised order of levels within each block.

Regression   Analysis of a covariate, or multiple covariates in the case of multiple regression. In this book we refer to such analyses as analyses of covariance, regardless of whether or not the model also includes categorical factors.

Repeated-measures   A design containing a random factor (usually Subject) crossed with one or more treatments having levels that are applied in a fixed sequence (usually temporal). For example, the performance of subjects may be tested before and after imbibing a treatment drink with two levels: tonic and control. The repeated-measures factor is Time with two levels: before and after. The design has no degrees of freedom for testing residual variation.

Repeated-measures factor   A factor (usually temporal) with a fixed sequence of levels that are crossed with a random factor (usually Subject).

Replicates   Randomly selected and independent measurements of the response that together make up a sample of the population of interest.

Replication   A model is fully replicated if it has true residual variation, given by a nesting of sampling units in samples. Full replication requires taking more than one independent, randomly selected measurement of the response at each level of each categorical factor, or at each combination of levels of crossed factors. The true residual variation allows estimation of all the explained components of variation.

Residual variation   All ANOVA models have residual variation defined by the variation amongst sampling units within each sample. This is always given by the last mean square in ANOVA tables, and denoted 'ε' (epsilon) in the descriptions of fully replicated models. Models without full replication may have no degrees of freedom for measuring residual variation (e.g., randomised-block, split-plot and repeated-measures models).

Response   The continuous variable on which data are collected to test for sources of variance. The response is the variable Y on the left of the equals sign in the model equation: $Y = A + \varepsilon$, etc.

Restricted model   A mixed model (i.e., with random and fixed factors) is termed restricted if a random factor is not allowed to have fixed cross factors amongst its components of variation estimated in the population. This restriction influences the choice of error MS for random effects. The ANOVA tables in this book are all constructed with the restricted model.

Sample   A group of replicate measures of the response taken at the same level of a categorical factor (or combination of factor levels if several categorical factors are present), or across a range of values of a covariate.

Sampling unit   The basic unit from which is recorded a single measure or observation of the response.

Significance   The strength of evidence for an effect, measured by a P-value associated with the F-ratio from analysis of variance. A significant effect has a small P-value indicating a small chance of making a Type I error. For example, $P < 0.05$ means a less than 5% chance of mistakenly rejecting a true null hypothesis. For many tests this would be considered a reasonable level of safety for rejecting the null hypothesis of no effect, in favour of the model hypothesis of a significant effect on the response. The significance of an effect is not directly informative about the size of the effect. Thus an effect may be statistically highly significant as a result of low residual variation, yet have little biological significance as a result of a small effect size in terms of the amount of variation between sample means or the slope of a regression. A non-significant effect should be interpreted with reference to the Type II error rate, which depends on the power of the test to detect significant effects.

Split-plot   A design with two or more treatment factors, and the levels of one factor applied at a different scale to those of another. For example, whole blocks might be allocated to wet or dry watering regime, and plots within blocks allocated to dense or sparse sowing density.

Sum of squares (SS)   The sum of squared deviations of each independent piece of information from its modelled value. Analysis of variance partitions the total variation in the response into explained and unexplained sums of squares.

Test hypothesis H_1 The hypothesis describing the statistical model to be tested by analysis of variance. The hypothesis H_1 may have several partitions (e.g., A + B + B*A), which describe putative pattern in the data. The evidence for pattern is tested against the null hypothesis H_0 of no pattern.

Transformation   A re-scaling procedure applied systematically to the response and/or covariates with the purpose of meeting the assumptions of the analysis. For example, measurements of volume and length might be log-transformed to linearise the relationship between them.

Treatment   A factor with levels that are applied in a manipulative experiment. More loosely, a factor of interest (as opposed to a nuisance variable).

Type I error   The mistake of rejecting a true null hypothesis. A maximum acceptable Type I error rate should be set a priori; in the biological sciences it is often taken to be $\alpha = 0.05$. An effect is then considered significant if it returns a $P < 0.05$. The Type I error is particularly susceptible to inflation in multiple tests of the same hypothesis. It is an unavoidable cause of false positives in screening programmes for rare phenomena.

Type II error   The mistake of accepting a false null hypothesis. An acceptable Type II error should be set a priori; in the biological sciences it is often taken to be $\beta = 0.20$. The power of a test is greater the smaller is β. Models without full replication are particularly susceptible to Type II error, as a result of not testing higher-order interactions.

Unrestricted model   A mixed model (i.e., with random and fixed factors) is termed unrestricted if a random factor is allowed to have fixed cross factors amongst its components of variation estimated in the population. This freedom influences the choice of error MS for random effects. The unrestricted model is not used in this book to construct ANOVA tables, though differences are noted in footnotes to the tables. It is generally used for unbalanced designs analysed with GLM.

Variance   The variation in the data, measured as the average squared deviation of the data from the mean. Analysis of variance partitions the total variance into explained and unexplained components and estimates these variances as mean squares (MS).

References

Allison, D. B., Allison, R. L., Faith, M. S., Paultre, F. and Pi-Sunyer, F. X. (1997) Power and money: designing statistically powerful studies while minimizing financial costs. *Psychological Methods*, **2**, 20–33.

Beck, M. W. (1997) Inference and generality in ecology: Current problems and an experimental solution. *Oikos*, **78**, 265–73.

Carey, J. M. and Keough, M. J. (2002) The variability of estimates of variance, and its effect on power analysis in monitoring design. *Environmental Monitoring and Assessment*, **74**, 225–41.

Cohen, J. (1988) *Statistical Power Analysis for the Behavioral Sciences, Second Edition*. New Jersey: Lawrence Erlbaum.

Cohen, J. (1992) Quantitative methods in psychology: a power primer. *Psychological Bulletin*, **112**, 155–9.

Colegrave, N. and Ruxton, G. D. (2003) Confidence intervals are a more useful complement to nonsignificant tests than are power calculations. *Behavioral Ecology*, **14**, 446–450.

Crawley, M. J. (2002) *Statistical Computing. An Introduction to Data Analysis using S-Plus*. Chichester: Wiley.

Darlington, R. B. and Smulders, T. V. (2001) Problems with residual analysis. *Animal Behaviour*, **62**, 599–602.

Davey, A. J. H. (2003) *Competitive interactions in stream fish communities*. Ph.D. thesis, University of Southampton, Southampton.

Day, R. W. and Quinn, G. P. (1989) Comparisons of treatments after an analysis of variance in ecology. *Ecological Monographs*, **59**, 433–63.

Dayton, P. K. (1998) Reversal of the burden of proof in fisheries management. *Science*, **279**, 821–2.

Di Stefano, J. (2003) How much power is enough? Against the development of an arbitrary convention for statistical power calculations. *Functional Ecology*, **17**, 707–9.

Dytham, C. (1999, 2003) *Choosing and Using Statistics: A Biologist's Guide*. Oxford: Blackwell.

Field, S. A., Tyre, A. J., Jonzén, N., Rhodes, J. R. and Possingham, H. P. (2004) Minimizing the cost of environmental management decisions by optimizing statistical thresholds. *Ecology Letters*, **7**, 669–75.

Freckleton, R. P. (2002) On the misuse of residuals in ecology: regression of residuals vs. multiple regression. *Journal of Animal Ecology*, **71**, 542–5.

García-Berthou, E. (2001) On the misuse of residuals in ecology: testing regression residuals vs. the analysis of covariance. *Journal of Animal Ecology*, **70**, 708–11.

Grafen, A. and Hails, R. (2002) *Modern Statistics for the Life Sciences*. Oxford: Oxford University Press.

Graham, M. H. and Edwards, M. S. (2001) Statistical significance versus fit: estimating the importance of individual factors in ecological analysis of variance. *Oikos*, **93**, 505–13.

Greenwood, J. J. D. (1993) Statistical power. *Animal Behaviour*, **46**, 1011.

Hines, W. G. S. (1996) Pragmatics of pooling in ANOVA tables. *The American Statistician*, **50**, 127–39.

Hoenig, J. M. and Heisey, D. M. (2001) The abuse of power: the pervasive fallacy of power calculations for data analysis. *American Statistician*, **55**, 19–24.

Hurlbert, S. H. (1984) Pseudoreplication and the design of ecological field experiments. *Ecological Monographs*, **54**, 187–211.

Ioannidis, J. P. A. (2005) Why most published research findings are false. *Public Library of Science Medicine*, **2**, 696–701.

Janky, D. G. (2000) Sometimes pooling for analysis of variance hypothesis tests: a review and study of a split-plot model. *The American Statistician*, **54**, 269–79.

Jennions, M. D. and Møller, A. P. (2003) A survey of the statistical power of research in behavioral ecology and animal behavior. *Behavioral Ecology*, **14**, 438–45.

Kent, A., Hawkins, S. J. and Doncaster, C. P. (2003) Population consequences of mutual attraction between settling and adult barnacles. *Journal of Animal Ecology*, **72**, 941–52.

Keough, M. J. and Mapstone, B. D. (1997) Designing environmental monitoring for pulp mills in Australia. *Water Science and Technology*, **35**, 397–404.

Keppel, G. and Wickens, T. D. (1973, 1982, 1991, 2004) *Design and Analysis: A Researcher's Handbook*. New Jersey: Prentice-Hall.

Kirk, R. E. (1968, 1982, 1994) *Experimental Design: Procedures for the Behavioural Sciences*. Belmont CA: Wadsworth.

Lenth R. V. (2001) Some practical guidelines for effective sample size determination. *American Statistician*, **55**, 187–93.

Mapstone, B. D. (1995) Scalable decision rules for environmental impact studies: effect size, Type I and Type II errors. *Ecological Applications*, **5**, 401–10.

McClelland, G. H. (1997) Optimal design in psychological research. *Psychological Methods*, **2**, 3–19.

McKillup, S. 2006. *Statistics Explained. An Introductory Guide for Life Scientists*. Cambridge: Cambridge University Press.

Moran, M. D. (2003) Arguments for rejecting the sequential Bonferroni in ecological studies *Oikos*, **100**, 403–5.

Motulsky, H. and Christopoulos, A. (2004) *Fitting Models to Biological Data Using Linear and Nonlinear Regression*. Oxford: Oxford University Press.

Newman, J.A., Bergelson, J. and Grafen, A. (1997) Blocking factors and hypothesis tests in ecology: is your statistics text wrong? *Ecology*, **78**, 1312–20.

Peterman, R.M. (1990) Statistical power analysis can improve fisheries research and management. *Canadian Journal of Fisheries and Aquatic Sciences*, **47**, 2–15.

Quinn, G.P. and Keough, M.J. (2002) *Experimental Design and Data Analysis for Biologists*. Cambridge: Cambridge University Press, UK.

Ratkowski, D.A., Evans, M.A. and Alldredge, J.R. (1993) *Cross-over Experiments. Design, Analysis and Application*. Statistics Textbooks and Monographs. New York: Marcel Dekker.

Resetarits, W.J., Jr. and Bernardo, J. (eds.) (1998) *Experimental Ecology: Issues and Perspectives*. Oxford: Oxford University Press.

Ruxton, G.D. and Colegrave, N. (2003) *Experimental Design for the Life Sciences*. Oxford: Oxford University Press.

Schultz, E.F. (1955) Rules of thumb for determining expectations of mean squares in analysis of variance. *Biometrics*, **11**, 123–35.

Searle, S.R. (1971, 1997) *Linear Models*. New York: John Wiley.

Searle, S.R., Casella G. and McCulloch, C.E. (1992) *Variance Components*. New York: John Wiley & Sons.

Shaw, R.G. and Mitchell-Olds, T. (1993) ANOVA for unbalanced data: an overview. *Ecology*, **74**, 1638–45.

Sokal, R.R. and Rohlf, F.J. (1969, 1981, 1995) *Biometry*. New York: Freeman and Co.

Tagg, N., Innes, D.J. and Doncaster, C.P (2005). Outcomes of reciprocal invasions between genetically diverse and genetically uniform populations of Daphnia obtusa (Kurz). *Oecologia*, **143**, 527–36.

Thomas, L. and Juanes, F. (1996) The importance of statistical power analysis: an example from animal behaviour. *Animal Behaviour*, **52**, 856–9.

Underwood, A.J. (1994) On beyond BACI: sampling designs that might reliably detect environmental disturbance. *Ecological Applications*, **4**, 3–15.

Underwood, A.J. (1997) *Experiments in Ecology: Their Logical Design and Interpretation Using Analysis of Variance*. Cambridge: Cambridge University Press.

Winer, B.J., Brown, D.R. and Michels, K.M. (1962, 1971, 1991) *Statistical Principles in Experimental Design*. New York: McGraw-Hill.

Zar, J.H. (1974, 1984, 1996, 1998) *Biostatistical Analysis*. New Jersey: Prentice Hall.

Index of all ANOVA models with up to three factors

The 29 designs listed below cover all models with up to three treatment factors. Those detailed in Chapters 1 to 3 of the book are all fully replicated designs.

Chapter	Page	Model	Treatments applied to — Sub-sub-plots (R')	Sub-plots (Q')	Plots (P')	Blocks or subjects (S')	Equivalences
Chapter 1: One-factor designs							
1.1	62	$Y = A + \varepsilon$				A	If $a = 2$, a Student's t test
Chapter 2: Nested designs							
2.1	68	$Y = B(A) + \varepsilon$				B(A)	1.1 with sub-sampling
2.2	72	$Y = C(B(A)) + \varepsilon$				C(B(A))	2.1 with sub-sampling
Chapter 3: Fully replicated factorial designs							
3.1	78	$Y = B \mid A + \varepsilon$				B|A	
3.2	86	$Y = C \mid B \mid A + \varepsilon$				C|B|A	
3.3	98	$Y = C \mid B(A) + \varepsilon$				C|B(A)	
3.4	109	$Y = C(B \mid A) + \varepsilon$				C(B|A)	3.1 with sub-sampling
Chapter 4: Randomised-block designs							
4.1	121	$Y = S' \mid A$			A	—	6.1
4.2	128	$Y = S' \mid B \mid A$			B|A	—	6.2
4.3	134	$Y = S' \mid C \mid B \mid A$			C|B|A	—	
Chapter 5: Split-plot designs							
5.1	146	$Y = B \mid P'(S' \mid A)$		B	A	—	
5.2	150	$Y = C \mid P'(S' \mid B \mid A)$		C	B|A	—	
5.3	154	$Y = C \mid B \mid P'(S' \mid A)$		C|B	A	—	
5.4	158	$Y = C \mid Q'(B \mid P'(S' \mid A))$	C	B	A	—	
5.5	163	$Y = C \mid P'(B \mid S'(A))$		C	B	A	
5.6	167	$Y = B \mid S'(A)$			B	A	6.3; 1.1 if $b = 2$, with $Y = B_2 - B_1$
5.7	170	$Y = C \mid B \mid S'(A)$			C|B	A	6.5; 5.6 if $c = 2$, with $Y = C_2 - C_1$
5.8	173	$Y = C \mid S'(B(A))$			C	B(A)	6.6; 2.1 if $c = 2$, with $Y = C_2 - C_1$
5.9	176	$Y = C \mid S'(B \mid A)$			C	B|A	6.7; 3.1 if $c = 2$, with $Y = C_2 - C_1$

Chapter 6: Repeated-measures designs

6.1	$Y = S'|A$	187	A	—	4.1; if $a = 2$, a paired-sample t test
6.2	$Y = S'|B|A$	190	B|A	—	4.2
—	$Y = S'|C|B|A$		C|B|A		4.3
6.3	$Y = B|S'(A)$	195	B	A	5.6; 1.1 if $b = 2$, with $Y = B_2 - B_1$
6.4	$Y = C(B)|S'(A)$	200	C(B)	A	5.7; 6.3 if $c = 2$, with $Y = C_2 - C_1$
6.5	$Y = C|B|S'(A)$	205	C|B	A	5.8; 2.1 if $c = 2$, with $Y = C_2 - C_1$
6.6	$Y = C|S'(B(A))$	214	C	B(A)	5.9; 3.1 if $c = 2$, with $Y = C_2 - C_1$
6.7	$Y = C|S'(B|A)$	220	C	B|A	

Chapter 7: Unreplicated designs

7.1	$Y = B|A$	230	B|A		3.1 without replication
7.2	$Y = C|B|A$	232	C|B|A		3.2 without replication

Index

Categories of model

1. One factor

S'(A)	A₁	A₂	A₃	A_a
	S_1	...	...	...
	...	...	...	...
	...	...	...	...
	S_n	...	...	S_{na}

4. Randomised blocks

P'(S'|B|A)		S_1	S_2	S_3	S_n
A₁	B_1	P_1	...	...	P_n
	B_b	...	...	...	P_{nb}
A_a	B_1	...	...	...	...
	B_b	...	...	...	P_{nba}

2. Fully replicated nested factors

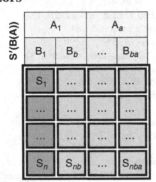

5. Split plot

Q'(B|P'(S'|A))		S_1	S_2	S_3	S_n
A₁	B_1	Q_1	...	...	Q_n
	B_b	...	...	...	Q_{nb}
A_a	B_1	...	...	...	...
	B_b	...	...	...	Q_{nba}

3. Fully replicated crossed factors

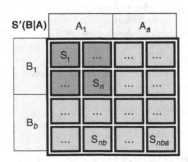

5–6. Split plot + repeated measures

P'(B|S'(A))	A₁		A_a	
	S_1	S_n	...	S_{na}
B_1	P_1	P_n	...	P_{na}
B_2	...	...	...	...
B_3	...	...	...	...
B_b	...	...	...	P_{nba}

Printed in the United States
By Bookmasters